Rate-Controlled Drug Administration and Action

Editor

H. A. J. Struyker-Boudier, Prof.Dr.
Professor of Pharmacology
Department of Pharmacology
University of Limburg, Maastricht
The Netherlands

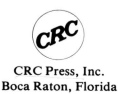

CRC Press, Inc.
Boca Raton, Florida

Library of Congress Cataloging in Publication Data
Main entry under title:

Rate-controlled drug administration and action.

Includes index and bibliography.
1. Drugs--Controlled release.   2. Pharmacokinetics.
3. Drugs--Administration. I. Struyker-Boudier, H. A. J.
RS201.C64R37   1985   615'.191   85-13250
ISBN-0-8493-6151-6

Direct all inquiries to CRC Press, Inc., 2000 Corporate Blvd., N.W., Boca Raton, Florida, 33431.

© 1986 by CRC Press, Inc.

International Standard Book Number 0-8493-6151-6

Library of Congress Card Number 84-13250
Printed in the United States

PREFACE

There is a growing awareness that the design of optimal drug therapy should include the proper design of the dosage form. This has led in the last decade to a wealth of technological innovations in the methodology of controlled drug administration.

The use of some of these systems now allows the specification of drug input as a function of time. No longer is drug input defined as an absolute quantity of the drug, but rather as a rate, i.e., a certain amount per given unit of time. The implications of these new technologies for pharmacology and therapeutics are enormous. An obvious advantage is the better controlled biopharmaceutical behavior of the systems. In the last years, several excellent review books and articles were published on the biopharmaceutical properties of such systems and their impact on the pharmacokinetics of the active drug substance. However, much less attention has been given so far to the implications of rate-controlled drug input for the pharmacodynamic behavior of drugs in man and experimental animals. The ultimate goal of pharmacotherapeutics is to optimize response patterns to drugs rather than kinetic profiles in plasma or other tissues.

This book provides an analysis of the pharmacokinetic theory and pharmacodynamic consequences of rate-controlled drug administration. The idea for this book emerged in the light of an increasing amount of reports in experimental and clinical literature showing that the dynamics of drug action strongly depends on drug input as a function of time. Many discussions with John Urquhart (Palo Alto, California), Jacques van Rossum (Nijmegen) and Jos Smits and Henk Thijssen (Maastricht) contributed to the final realization of this book. I wish to thank them and all other contributors who worked hard to make this book possible. I also wish to express my deepest appreciation to Ms. Els Geurts and Ms. Mia Hogenboom for their excellent secretarial services.

Harry A. J. Struyker-Boudier

INTRODUCTION

When compared to the formidable developments in diagnostic as well as surgical technologies in the last decades, pharmacotherapy until several years ago was based on some rather primitive methods of administering medication. On the diagnostic side of medicine, the strong development of the medical electronics industry after 1950 led to a number of major advances, e.g., automated clinical laboratory facilities, ultrasound diagnostic tools, imaging methods, etc.[1] However, a patient in whom a diagnosis is reached following long and detailed examinations with these advanced technologies is subsequently often exposed to a drug therapy with many uncontrolled factors. With conventional dosage forms, the patient is subjected to widely fluctuating levels of one or more chemicals. These chemicals reach many sites in his body, including those where the underlying disease process is not localized.

During the last 10 to 15 years, the pharmaceutical industry has shifted its attention somewhat from the classical chemical synthesis point of view in drug design towards the design of drug administration systems that provide a better control of drug release as a function of *time*.[2] New technologies now include sustained-release dosage forms, transdermal therapeutic systems, osmotic pressure-driven controlled drug release systems, and matrix diffusion or erosion-controlled drug release systems.[3] Other developments are aimed at a better control of the *site* of delivery of the drug in the body. Such systems include implantable infusion pumps, liposomes, and prodrugs.

Although some of these new technologies still have to prove their clinical utility, they have had already a profound influence on experimental pharmacology. These systems allow the study of the dynamics of drug action on the basis of a given input of drug as a function of time and/or site of delivery.

In experimental pharmacology, this has led to new possibilities to unravel primary sites of action of drugs as well as to analyze the time-dependent responses to different drug input functions. In fact, such studies have led to the important realization that the dynamics of drug action does not always depend on the absolute concentration of the drug in the biophase: a view implicit in classical molecular pharmacology theories of drug action. The use of delivery systems with a control of drug release as a function of time may perhaps contribute to the development of a theory of the dynamics of drug action based truly on time-dependent next to concentration-dependent drug effects.

This book is not aimed at a description of the new systems for rate-controlled drug administration from a technological point of view. Several recent review books and articles have excellently covered this aspect.[3-7] In this book, the major emphasis will be put on the pharmacokinetic theory underlying control of drug administration with respect to time and site of delivery as well as the pharmacodynamic consequences of rate-controlled drug administration. In the first section, Urquhart (Chapter 1) introduces the pertinent history and phenomenology of rate-controlled drug delivery systems. Merkus (Chapter 2) then reviews the major biopharmaceutical properties of these new technologies. The second section is devoted to the pharmacokinetic theory underlying controlled drug administration. Van Rossum and co-workers (Chapter 3) provide a new look at the way the body transfers drug input functions into kinetic drug profiles. Smits and Thijssen (Chapter 4) analyze spatial control of drug action on the basis of pharmacokinetics of target-aimed drug delivery.

The third section of this book reviews some pharmacodynamic consequences of controlling drug input. Fara and Mitchell (Chapter 5) review how the osmotic systems for rate-controlled drug delivery have affected experimental and clinical pharmacological research. The subsequent chapters each deal with a major area of pharmacotherapy. Pickup and Stevenson (Chapter 6) review rate-controlled insulin delivery in physiology and pathophysiology. Struyker-Boudier and co-workers (Chapter 7) give a survey on rate-controlled cardiovascular drug administration and action. Sikic and Carlson (Chapter 8) and Bergeron and LeBel (Chapter 9) review the effects of different schedules of drug administration of cytostatics and antibiotics, respectively. In the final chapter (Chapter 10), Yates and Poston provide a new look at some paradoxical consequences of controlling inputs in the field of the delivery of endocrine agents.

Each chapter itself is a systematic description of one aspect of rate-controlled drug administration and action. Altogether, this book provides, I believe, a comprehensive treatment of the theory and pharmacodynamic consequences of rate-controlled drug administration.

REFERENCES

1. Rushmer, R. F., Alternative futures for biomedical research, *Ann. Biomed. Eng.,* 7, 1, 1979.
2. Struyker-Boudier, H. A. J., Rate-controlled drug delivery: pharmacological, therapeutic and industrial perspectives, *Trends Pharmacol. Sci.,* 3, 162, 1982.
3. Chien, Y. W., *Novel Drug Delivery Systems,* Marcel Dekker, New York, 1982.
4. Roseman, T. J. and Mansdorf, S. Z., Eds., *Controlled Release Delivery Systems,* Marcel Dekker, New York, 1983.
5. Heilmann, K., *Therapeutic Systems, 2nd ed.;* George Thieme Verlag, Stuttgart, 1984.
6. Langer, R. and Wise, D., Eds., *Medical Application of Controlled Release Technology,* CRC Press, Boca Raton, Fla., 1983.
7. Urquhart, J., Rate-controlled drug dosage, *Drugs,* 23, 207, 1982.

THE EDITOR

Harry A. J. Struyker-Boudier, Ph.D., is Professor of Experimental Pharmacology and Chairman of the Department of Pharmacology at the University of Limburg in Maastricht, the Netherlands.

Dr. Struyker-Boudier received his training in pharmacology at the University of Nijmegen in the Netherlands. He did his graduate studies in the Department of Pharmacology of that university (Chairman, Dr. E. J. Ariens) in 1971 and 1972. From 1973 to 1975 he worked on his Ph.D. thesis on catecholamine receptors in nervous tissue under the guidance of Dr. J. M. van Rossum. In 1976 he spent eight months as a postdoctoral research fellow in the Department of Physiology and Biophysics of the University of Mississippi with Dr. A. C. Guyton. During this period he concentrated on the use of quantitative methods of analysis of physiological control systems.

In 1976 Dr. Struyker-Boudier was appointed at the new medical school of the University of Limburg. He was involved in setting up a new curriculum and research program in pharmacology. In 1980 he became professor and chairman of the Department of Pharmacology. His present research interests include cardiovascular pharmacology and physiology, pharmacokinetics, and the quantitative study of the dynamics of drug action. In the latter area he has worked with different systems for controlled drug administration. Dr. Struyker-Boudier is author of eight books and over 100 articles covering his research on catecholamine receptors, cardiovascular pharmacology, blood pressure control, and new systems for drug delivery.

Dr. Struyker-Boudier is a member of the Dutch, German, and American Pharmacological Societies. He serves on the Editorial Board of the Archives Internationales de Pharmacodynamie et de Therapie. He is chairman of the Hypertension Committee of the Dutch Heart Foundation.

CONTRIBUTORS

Michel G. Bergeron
Professor of Microbiology and
  Medicine
Faculte de Medecine and
Chief, Infectious Diseases Service
Le Centre Hospitalier de L'Universite
  Laval
Quebec, Canada

Robert W. Carlson, M.D.
Assistant Professor of Medicine
Department of Medicine
Stanford University
Stanford, California

John W. Fara, Ph.D.
Vice President
New Product Opportunities
ALZA Pharmaceuticals
Palo Alto, California

J. C. S. Kleinjans, Ph.D.
Assistant Professor
Department of Pharmacology
University of Limburg
Maastricht, the Netherlands

Marc LeBel, Pharm.D.
Associate Professor
Ecole de Pharmacie
Universite Laval and
Infectologie, Centre Hospitalier de
  L'Universite Laval
Quebec, Canada

L. M. L. le Noble
Research Fellow
Department of Pharmacology
University of Limburg
Maastricht, the Netherlands

Frans W. H. M. Merkus, Ph.D.
Professor and Chairman
Department of Biopharmaceutics
Faculty of Medicine and Subfaculty of
  Pharmacy
University of Amsterdam
Amsterdam, the Netherlands, and
Department of Clinical Pharmacy
R. C. Hospital
Sittard, the Netherlands

Constance Mitchell
Medical Writer and Managing Editor
Technical Information and Publications
ALZA Corporation
Palo Alto, California

H. M. N. Nievelstein
Research Fellow
Department of Pharmacology
University of Limburg
Maastricht, the Netherlands

J. C. Pickup, B.M., D.Phil.
Senior Lecturer
Honorary Consultant in Chemical
  Pathology
Department of Chemical Pathology
Guys Hospital Medical School
London, England

Timothy Poston
Visiting Associate Professor
Department of Mathematics and
Visiting Associate Researcher
Crump Institute for Medical
  Engineering
University of California, Los Angeles
Los Angeles, California

Branimir Ivan Sikic, M.D.
Associate Professor of Medicine
Divisions of Oncology and Clinical
  Pharmacology
Stanford University
Stanford, California

J. F. M. Smits
Department of Pharmacology
University of Limburg
Maastricht, the Netherlands

H. J. M. Snoeck
Graduate Student
Department of Pharmacology
University of Nijmegen
Nijmegen, the Netherlands

O. M. Steijger
Graduate Student
Department of Pharmacology
University of Nijmegen
Nijmegen, the Netherlands

Ralph W. Stevenson, Ph.D.
Assistant Professor of Physiology
Department of Physiology
Vanderbilt University Medical School
Nashville, Tennessee

H. A. J. Struyker-Boudier, Ph.D.
Professor of Pharmacology
Department of Pharmacology
University of Limburg
Maastricht, the Netherlands

H. W. A. Teeuwen
Postgraduate Student
Department of Pharmacology
University of Nijmegen
Nijmegen, the Netherlands

H. Thijssen
Department of Pharmacology
University of Limburg
Maastricht, the Netherlands

J. T. W. M. Tissen
Graduate Student
Department of Pharmacology
University of Nijmegen
Nijmegen, the Netherlands

John Urquhart
Principal Scientist
Senior Vice President
ALZA Corporation
Palo Alto, California

T. J. F. van Wem
Graduate Student
Department of Pharmacology
University of Nijmegen
Nijmegen, the Netherlands

Jacques M. van Rossum
Professor of Pharmacology
Department of Pharmacology
University of Nijmegen
Nijmegen, the Netherlands

F. Eugene Yates
Director
Crump Institute for Medical
  Engineering
University of California, Los Angeles
Los Angeles, California

TABLE OF CONTENTS

Chapter 1

RATE-CONTROLLED, EXTENDED-DURATION DRUG DELIVERY: PHENOMENOLOGY AND PERTINENT HISTORY

John Urquhart

TABLE OF CONTENTS

I. INTRODUCTION

This chapter has two major themes. The first is that research and development efforts by both firms and universities during the past 2 decades have created something of a critical mass of technical capabilities for controlling the rate of drug administration to humans and animals over extended durations. These advances have involved most of the usual routes of drug administration plus a more or less new one, the transdermal route. Of course, technical wizardry at the bioengineering and pharmaceutical levels does not necessarily lead to therapeutic improvements, so from the practical point of view, one may well ask: so what? Hence, the second theme — the pharmacologic and therapeutic implications of these developments. These have to be considered separately: therapeutic implications follow from what it is possible to do with today's and yesterday's drugs; pharmacologic implications influence what tomorrow's therapeutic agents will be.

One of the aims of this chapter is to show how the advent of rate-controlled, extended-duration (RCED) delivery systems has begun to change some basic pharmacologic ideas and to illustrate how some agents previously thought too impractical for therapeutic use have now become practical. As discussed later, for example, there are already more than a half dozen agents now in therapeutic use that would not be, but for their administration by RCED delivery systems.

To understand the assertion that there is a critical mass of technology for RCED administration of drugs, we have to look not only into the world of pharmacology and pharmaceuticals, but also into the different world of medical devices. We also have to consider a bit of history. In doing so, I shall put special emphasis on the contributions to rate-controlled drug administration that have come from the medical devices field. The reader should note that there has already been a great deal of attention paid to rate-controlled drug delivery in the pharmaceutical context.[1-6] In contrast, the impact of rate-controlled drug delivery via various medical devices has received relatively little attention from pharmacologists and pharmaceutical scientists. My emphasis on developments in the medical device area is an attempt to give some belated balance to the usually overlooked contributions from that side. To keep that emphasis in perspective, however, the reader should recognize that the applications of RCED drug delivery devices (as opposed to pharmaceuticals) are by and large limited to hospitalized patients, often with considerable associated drama. Most RCED pharmaceutical applications, on the other hand, focus on ambulatory patients whose numbers and chronicity of product use far exceed anything that transpires within hospitals.

II. FIRST CLINICAL USE OF RCED DRUG DELIVERY AND ITS IMPACT ON THE FORMAT FOR DESCRIBING DRUG ACTIONS

The first RCED drug delivery systems were the various masks and cones that the 19th century pioneers of ether and chloroform anesthesia invented for administering these dangerous agents, each of which has a very narrow therapeutic index. These first RCED delivery systems solved the problem of converting liquid agent into inhalable gas in a manner that allowed a steady, i.e., rate-controlled, addition of agent to inspired air for extended periods of time, as needed to complete each surgical procedure. Administering these anesthetic agents in the RCED mode revealed their pharmacologic properties in a special way that came to be called "stages" of anesthesia. The stage associated with surgical practicability was further subdivided into "planes". Ether, for example, has four recognizable stages and four recognizable planes within the surgical (third) stage. The concept of stages was already implicit in the writings of John Snow, one of the pioneers of anesthesia in the 1850s, but the concept was codified by Guedel in the early years of this century and extended by Gillespie in the 1940s to include depth-related characteristics of elicited reflexes.

In the teaching of pharmacology, the twin concepts of "depth" and "stages" have been treated as attributes peculiar to the volatile anesthetics. This intellectual construct misses an essential point, however: the concepts of "depth" and "stages" are, in fact, uniquely associated with RCED administration rather than with volatile anesthetics per se.

There are two reasons for this last assertion. First, until recently, the volatile anesthetics were the only class of drugs absolutely requiring RCED administration from the outset of their therapeutic use. Thus, understanding of their pharmacologic actions was unclouded by the special form of confusion created by an initial period of knowing and interpreting a drug's actions only in the nonsteady state of pulse-mode delivery. Second, RCED administration achieved the steady-state drug concentrations and actions that clearly demonstrate the rate- or concentration-dependence of the anesthetics' actions. As we shall see, the concepts of "depth" and "stages" appear to provide a useful format for describing the actions of many nonanesthetic drugs given in the RCED mode.

Continuous, rate-controlled drug administration results in essentially constant concentrations of drug in blood and tissues. Generally, though not always, there is concomitant constancy of drug action. Obviously this persistence makes drug actions easier to recognize and characterize than when they erratically come and go, as is usual with conventional dosing. Recent illustrations of this facilitated recognition include work in animals assessing the estrogenic activities of the 2- and 4-hydroxy metabolites of estradiol.[7,8] In humans, examples are provided by revisions of the pharmacology of scopolamine and pilocarpine, based respectively on their steady-state systemic and topical administration in RCED delivery system forms.[9,10] Figure 1, for example, illustrates how the various actions of scopolamine appear to rank order according to minimum rate needed to elicit each of them.

The definition of concentration- or delivery-rate-dependent "stages" of any drug's actions amounts simply to a rank-ordering of the drug's action by minimum delivery rate (or minimum plasma concentration) required to elicit each action,[11] as illustrated for scopolamine in Figure 1. Certainly not all drugs will fit this simple format: some drug actions manifest tolerance, tachyphylaxis, or subsensitivity development. Those have to be described with a different format, as rate- or concentration-*in*dependent actions; fortunately, such drugs appear to be in the minority.

For most drugs, rank-ordering of actions in relation to minimum effective rate or plasma concentration seems superior to merely listing every action the drug has ever been observed or believed to elicit. Most pharmacology texts and prescribing information is written in this "long list" format. This format may have been satisfactory in an earlier era, but "long lists" have grown increasingly unwieldy as more potent drugs have entered the market and as drug information has proliferated.

For the past few years, new pharmaceuticals have had their side effects rank-ordered by incidence, e.g., occurring in 5 to 10% of patients, 1 to 5%, less than 1%, etc. Generally there is also a statement about the percentage of patients in which the desired therapeutic effect can be obtained. This "incidence-based" format is a useful step forward from strictly qualitative, ever-longer lists of actions and side actions.

A newer format still will probably arise out of the recent pressure by the U.S. Food and Drug Administration for pharmacokinetic screening during premarket clinical trials. The aim is to obtain one or two spot measurements of drug levels in plasma during steady-state dosing in the patient population.[13] This screening has been prompted by growing recognition that within certain populations of patients — especially the elderly — there is often marked interpatient variance in pharmacokinetic

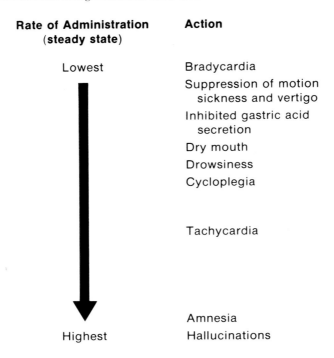

Rate of Administration (steady state) | **Action**

Lowest

Bradycardia

Suppression of motion sickness and vertigo

Inhibited gastric acid secretion

Dry mouth

Drowsiness

Cycloplegia

Tachycardia

Amnesia

Hallucinations

Highest

FIGURE 1.   The evident rank-ordering of the actions of scopolamine by minimum rate of steady-state administration needed to elicit. The basis for this rank-ordering is discussed in References 9 and 11. The inhibition of gastric acid secretion is described in Reference 12.

parameters, such that weight-adjusted dose or rate results in a five- to tenfold plus range of steady-state drug levels in plasma.

If pharmacokinetic screening is done with care and with careful observation of concomitant drug actions, it ought greatly to expand the base of information on concentration-effect relations during steady-state drug administration. Moreover, it ought to support a rank-ordering of drug effects either by minimum concentration needed to elicit or by a probabilistic index, e.g., concentration needed to elicit the effect in N% of the subjects (EC-N). The neoclassical-classical work of Hendeles et al.[14] on the concentration-dependence of the actions of theophylline illustrates the value of a carefully designed study to measure *both* interpatient pharmacokinetic variance *and* concomitant drug actions (Figure 2). Their work defines, in effect, the "stages" or "depth" of the actions of theophylline, although they never used these terms which smell so strongly of ether.

Four conclusions suggest themselves:

1.   Rank ordering (or "staging") of drug actions by minimum concentration needed to elicit or by EC-N will help define the ideal range of plasma levels for achieving maximum selectivity of drug action, as Hendeles and co-workers showed so clearly with theophylline.

2.   Measuring the variance in pharmacokinetic parameters will help specify the various product strengths needed to achieve, in each patient, the defined therapeutic concentration range.

3.   Maintaining plasma concentrations of drug within the defined therapeutic range at all times in the interdose interval will enhance the selectivity of drug action.

4.   Spot checks of drug concentration in plasma to confirm continued accuracy of

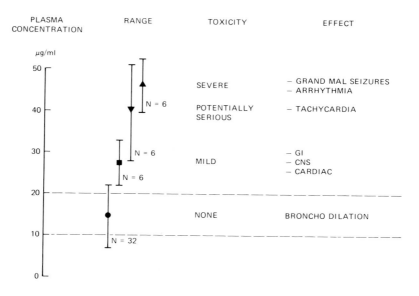

FIGURE 2. Rank-ordering of the actions of theophylline according to minimum plasma concentrations needed to elicit. (Adapted from Hendeles, L. et al., *Drug Intell. Clin. Pharm.* 11, 12, 1977. With permission from *Drug Intelligence and Clinical Pharmacy*, 1241 Broadway, Hamilton, Illinois, 62341.)

dosing are more easily interpreted when concentrations are maintained at near-constancy by RCED administration than when they are allowed to fluctuate widely with conventional pulse-mode dosing.

Recall that the conventional pulse mode of drug administration results in continuously fluctuating concentrations of drug in blood and tissues, generally with concomitant fluctuation of drug actions. Typical interdose fluctuations in drug concentration are such that peak-to-trough concentration ratios range between 5 and 15,[15] with a few examples of 20 or more.[16,17] Continuous fluctuation of both drug concentrations and actions — sometimes out of phase with one another due to pharmacodynamic lags — necessarily complicates or even obscures the perception of concentration- or delivery-rate-dependent "depth" or "stages" of drug action.

III. FURTHER PERSPECTIVES FROM THE HISTORY OF ANESTHESIA

From the beginning of the anesthetic era, proper use of volatile anesthetics has required the constant attention of a skilled professional to regulate the rate of drug administration, so as to maintain the desired depth of anesthesia. The concept of extended duration of anesthetic action is implicit in the option of administering volatile anesthetics continuously for a few minutes or for many hours, as required to complete the surgery. The concept of rate control is implicit in two long-established facts about the maintenance of gaseous anesthesia after induction. (1) There is a narrow range of the agent's partial pressure in arterial blood and brain tissue that gives the surgical stage of anesthesia and even a narrower range within that stage that gives the optimum plane for an adequate mix of anesthesia and muscle relaxation. (2) The patient's ventilation is physiologically self-regulated to meet the metabolic requirement for oxygen while maintaining carbon dioxide balance and is usually essentially constant. Constancy of ventilation calls for a controlled, constant rate of addition of the anesthetic into the stream of inspired air, since ventilation is the sole route by which the volatile anesthetics both enter and leave the body.

Various devices and agents for inhalational anesthesia have come and gone since the 1850s. For the past generation, the dominant inhalational agent has been halothane,[18] and the dominant delivery system for its administration has been the temperature- and flow-compensated vaporizer that was developed jointly in the mid-1950s by Ayerst and ICI as the FLUOTEC® vaporizer. I consider this device to be the first modern, commercially successful RCED drug delivery system. It made halothane a practical agent: without the control provided by the FLUOTEC® vaporizer, the high cost of halothane would have precluded its widespread use by the open-drop technique in which a great deal of agent is lost to ambient air. Also, halothane has an especially narrow therapeutic index which makes it a difficult agent to control by open-drop. In effect, the clinical practicability of halothane depended upon the development of the vaporizer — a RCED delivery system that compensated for two otherwise limiting features of the drug: high cost and very narrow therapeutic index. The clinical superiority of the resulting *therapeutic system* of drug plus delivery system, compared to other types of gaseous anesthesia, has been the basis for the overwhelming dominance of halothane in modern anesthetic practice.

IV. ADVENT OF INFUSION PUMPS AND THEIR THERAPEUTIC IMPACT

A second major line of RCED delivery system developments and another example of the impact of the critical mass phenomenon on drug development started in the early 1970s, when the clinical use of infusion pumps began to be routine. Though infusion pumps had been in laboratory use since the turn of the century, their clinical use had been thwarted by three factors. First, there was little clinically perceived need for the infusion mode of drug administration; the relatively few exceptions relied on the standard i.v. drip set to provide satisfactory rate control. Second, infusion pumps designed primarily for laboratory use were complex to operate, maintain, and calibrate; these difficulties effectively precluded their clinical use. The big impetus to the development of infusion pumps for clinical use was the introduction and rapid growth of total parenteral nutrition, requiring the infusion of about 3 l daily of viscous solutions of amino acids in hypertonic dextrose. Gravity flow systems were too erratic to administer these large volumes of viscous fluid in a dependable way. The advent of the pumps for this application then began to expand their uses into drug infusions.

The concomitant growth in open heart surgery brought the infusion pumps together with two old but hitherto impractical agents, nitroprusside and dopamine. Rate-controlled infusion of these two drugs came into increasing clinical use for acute regulation of the circulation during the first few postoperative days. Both agents combine high potency, short half-life, and a narrow therapeutic index. This combination of attributes mandates administration by rate-controlled infusion with a degree of precision that cannot be had from the conventional i.v. drip set, which is subject to unpredictable, sometimes large fluctuations in drip rate.[19]

Some of the most recently introduced drip sets make claims for much improved reliability of maintaining a given setting. Throughout the 1970s, however, there was a gap between therapeutic need and capability in various intensive care settings that was filled by the infusion pumps or their sister devices, the controllers. (Controllers depend upon gravity as the force for infusate flow but regulate flow electromechanically and permit the user to specify rate. Pumps also control rate, but provide the force for flow, and so they have appropriate safety mechanisms to prevent infusion of air or continued pumping when infiltration is occurring.)

The increasing presence of pumps and controllers in intensive care units has made possible the development of drugs that are uniquely suited to — and, in some cases, even limited to — the infusion mode of administration. Dobutamine,[20] alprostadil,[20] and prostacyclin[20] are recently available drugs for which continuous, rate-controlled i.v. infusion is the only acceptable mode of administration, and it is reasonable to presume that additional infusion-only agents will follow. For example, rapidly adjustable beta blockade may become practical in intensive care if the current clinical trials with continuous infusions of the ultrashort half-life beta blocker, esmolol,[21] are successful. Thus, the use of infusion pumps and controllers has developed to a point of critical mass during the past decade, opening up new avenues of drug development with hitherto impractical agents of exceptionally narrow therapeutic indices and/or exceptionally short pharmacokinetic and pharmacodynamic half-lives. It is also noteworthy that dopamine and the two prostaglandins are substances endogenous to humans; possibly other endogenous substances may find therapeutic uses due to delivery systems.

There is also increasing use of the infusion mode with some older parenteral agents usually given by injection. Heparin for systemic anticoagulation[22] and insulin for treatment of acute diabetic coma[23] are two examples; evidence the superiority of stabilized concentrations of these agents over the fluctuating ones that result from intermittent injections. Bleomycin, as discussed in Chapter 8, is another example: the initial clinical trials and usage were based on the injection mode of administration,[20] but more recent evidence indicates that the infusion mode is superior.[24,25] Thus, the growth of the pumps and controllers has begun to prompt reassessment of whether injections or infusions are preferable for many parenteral agents.

In effect, then, pumps and controllers have created options in parenteral drug regimens: pulse-mode administration, exemplified by injection, vs. continuous, rate-controlled infusion. These two modes of drug administration are kinetic opposites of one another, just as, in a mathematical sense, the impulse is the first time derivative of the step function, and the step function is the time integral of the impulse. There is a growing literature that suggests that there is considerable value in comparative dose-response testing of a given drug with injections vs. infusions. Chapters 5 and 8 consider this important pharmacodynamic point in detail.

While injections and infusions are kinetic opposites, however, sometimes there are occasions to use them together to produce specifically desired temporal patterns of drug concentration in plasma. Also, certain infusion pumps and other RCED delivery systems can be programmed to produce various temporal patterns of drug administration rate. Several RCED pharmaceuticals are already in the market that deliver drug according to a specific time-sequence of rates[20,26] to produce particular time patterns of drug concentration in plasma. This capability poses the question of how to define the optimum regimen for each drug — old as well as new. We shall return to this question.

V. IMPACT OF PUMP MINIATURIZATION

Another trend influencing utilization of RCED drug delivery is the miniaturization of infusion pumps, making pumps of successively smaller size: portable,[27] wearable,[27] and finally, implantable.[27] These developments make intravascular infusions possible in ambulatory patients. Another consequence is to make ultrahigh molar potency a drug attribute of new importance, so that the mass and volume of infused drug and vehicle is not too great to be accommodated within the smallest infusion pumps. This requires total daily doses of drug that are in the range of a few milligrams or less. In effect, then, pump miniaturization is a force for development of drugs of uniquely high molar potencies; drug "miniaturization", in effect. As yet, though, high molar potency drugs have not, per se, been a prominent theme in new drug discovery and development. A notable exception is the Janssen group in Beerse who have made a number of strikingly potent narcotic analgesics, antipsychotics, and other agents. As yet, however, the miniaturized pumps have not had perceptible impact on new drug discovery or development, but they have been widely available for clinical use for only several years.

Even so, the implanted pump has already brought one existing drug, FUDR, into a novel and evidently promising use: chronic infusion into the hepatic artery for the localized treatment of hepatic metastases of bowel neoplasms.[28] Heparin is another agent with which the implantable pump has been used to advantage in patients with chronic tendency to intravascular thrombosis.[29]

It is a curious paradox that the first two uses in humans of implantable pumps have little or no background of pharmacodynamic assessment in animal infusion studies of either drug. A similar paradox is evident in research on anticancer drugs: despite the strikingly positive findings by Sikic and his National Cancer Institute colleagues in their 1978 injection-infusion comparison studies on bleomycin in an animal tumor model[24] and the subsequent clinical confirmation of their findings,[25] there has been no discernible exploration of the infusion mode or of the injection-infusion comparison protocol in other areas of cancer chemotherapy research. Neither has there been any discernible move to extend the technique of regional intra-arterial infusion to evaluations of anticancer drugs in animals, despite the fact that intra-arterial infusion has been a practical possibility in animal studies[30-32] at least since introduction of the osmotic pump implants in 1977. The direction of preclinical testing in the major cancer drug development programs would seem to indicate a lack of appreciation of the significance of the technological developments of the past decade in RCED drug delivery. During 1983, however, the first steps were taken by the National Cancer Institute (NCI) to include infusion studies routinely in the late stages of preclinical evaluation of promising new anticancer drugs. The screening programs, however, appear to be based exclusively on pulse-mode delivery. Given that the NCI screens about a thousand compounds for every one that reaches clinical testing, one might wonder if the injection-infusion comparison protocol might not find good use in earlier stages of the screening program.

VI. RCED DRUG DELIVERY METHODS FOR ANIMAL STUDIES

Animal studies bring an important dimension to the complex matter of defining optimal regimens. Regimen optimization studies are often difficult to carry out in a clinical setting, because the problem of standardizing or pairing the clinical status of individual patients is often overwhelming. Animal studies can therefore play an important role in comparing different modes of drug administration — provided, of course, that such alternative modes are practical in animal models of human disease.

It has always been a theoretical possibility to carry out multiday infusions in rats and mice by arranging a flow path from an external infusion pump to the caged animal. However, either the animal has to be restrained so that it cannot revolve with respect to the flow line, or else the flow line must include a freely rotating, leak-proof swivel joint. Also, the flow line itself must be capable of transmitting sufficient torque without twisting and kinking the line to turn the swivel. Such arrangements require the combined skills of a watchmaker and a plumber, and though described from time to time in the literature,[33,34] they have never attained very wide usage. Portable pumps have been described for larger animals[35] and used in certain studies,[36,37] but have never gained acceptance as a standard method of drug administration in experimental pharmacology.

Only with the development and wide acceptance of polysiloxane[38] and osmotic

Table 1
FULLY DEVELOPED RATE-CONTROLLED PHARMACEUTICAL PRODUCTS

Topical (insert)

Drug	Target tissue/organ	Site of placement	Indication	Duration	Ref.
Pilocarpine	Eye	Conjunctival cul-de-sac	Glaucoma/ocular hypertension	7 days	41
Progesterone	Uterus	Uterine cavity	Contraception	1, 2 years	42, 43

Systemic

Drug	Route	Indication	Duration	Ref.
Theophylline	Oral	Asthma	12 hr	44
Phenylpropanolamine	Oral	Appetite suppression	16 hr	26
Indomethacin	Oral	Arthritis	12—24 hr	45, 46
Scopolamine	Transdermal	Motion sickness, vertigo	3 days	9
Nitroglycerin	Transdermal	Angina pectoris	1 day	47, 48
Clonidine	Transdermal	Hypertension	7 days	49

pump[39] implants has the infusion mode begun to gain wide usage in animal studies. Fara, Willis, and I reviewed the physiological and pharmacological literature on drug delivery systems in drug and hormone research in mid-1983,[40] and found a literature of nearly 1000 publications. Over half, however, have appeared since 1979, even though the polysiloxane capsule implants were first described in 1964. Thus, there appears to be a critical mass phenomenon beginning to operate in basic pharmacologic research since the introduction of miniature osmotic pumps in various sizes, pumping rates, and durations. As noted above, the peculiar hiatus in preclinical testing of anti-cancer drugs illustrates that there are still considerable gaps in exploiting these new developments fully in preclinical drug development.

VII. RCED PHARMACEUTICALS FOR HUMAN USE

On the pharmaceutical side of human therapeutics, a number of rate-controlled pharmaceuticals have been fully developed and either commercialized or are pending registration. These are listed in Table 1.

With only a half-dozen pharmaceuticals that can validly claim inclusion within the RCED delivery classification, no one could claim anything approaching a critical mass in human pharmaceuticals, which include hundreds of drugs and about a thousand products in most countries. Nevertheless, pharmaceutical industry trade papers, such as *Scrip, Labopharma*, and *FD&C Reports*, have reported much industry activity in the pharmaceutical applications of RCED delivery systems. Many product development activities have been announced as underway since about 1980. The first commercial successes have been scored by an oral RCED form of theophylline and the transdermal forms of nitroglycerin. If a reasonable fraction of the announced activities can be translated into marketed products, the critical mass might be approached within the next few years, for they include some very widely used drugs.

One recently introduced RCED oral product, which delivers indomethacin in rate-controlled fashion for 12 hr,[50] has been the subject of controversy about its incidence of indomethacin-related adverse reactions.[51] Its manufacturer has discontinued its marketing. It is not clear what differential, if any, there is in the incidence of these adverse reactions among the various forms and routes of administration of indomethacin, in the various groups of patients with arthritis and concomitant diseases. This episode illustrates, if anyone doubted it *a priori*, that the therapeutic use of any potent drug, however administered, carries with it a certain risk. Moreover, risks more dilute than about 1 in 200 or 300 cannot be detected in premarket clinical trials, which rarely include more than 1000 patients. This episode is also a reminder that RCED drug delivery systems and dosage forms are not a panacea.

Each RCED pharmaceutical thus far introduced has integrated the drug and the delivery capability in such a way that the two cannot be separated after manufacture without destroying the system. These products have not been made by simply placing the new drug into a pre-existing device. Rather, each product has posed a unique mix of problems relating to design, mass transport, formulation, and stability. Recent advances in delivery system technology may provide more "modular" and therefore more easily developed RCED pharmaceuticals, but no such products have yet reached the marketplace.

VIII. IMPACT OF RCED DELIVERY SYSTEMS ON REGIMEN OPTIMIZATION AND PHARMACODYNAMICS

As a consequence of all these technical developments and the diversity of RCED delivery systems they have spawned, it is now practical to entertain questions about the optimum time course with which a drug should enter the body. That prompts the corollary question of how to define the optimum time course of a drug's concentration in plasma.

Such questions had been of relatively little practical consequence before the advent of practical RCED systems. Now, however, significant choices are increasingly available in the time pattern that the plasma concentration of a drug can be made to follow. This represents new and unfamiliar ground in pharmaceutical product development: it thrusts the definition of a drug's pharmacodynamics to an earlier stage in product development than dosage form design. Previously, pharmacodynamics has not led but followed dosage form design. The selection of a dosage form has usually been made on the basis of manufacturability, in vitro dissolution, and biopharmaceutic considerations related to insuring reproducible extent — but not rate — of drug absorption. Now, however, it is possible to consider changing this order of things: selection of dosage form and drug regimen could be based on pharmacodynamic data that indicate the best temporal pattern for drug concentration in plasma to follow to insure the greatest selectivity of drug action.

Thus, one consequence of the development of RCED delivery systems has been to stimulate the development of pharmacodynamics. In that light, it is useful to contrast the status of pharmacodynamics today with that of pharmacokinetics when it was in a comparable stage of infancy, about 20 years ago. At that time its basic tools (radiochemicals and modern analytical chemical methods) were reaching a critical mass of availability.

Pharmacokinetics rests on a basic physical principle — the conservation of mass — and traces the flux of drug and drug-derived molecules through successive dilutional steps leading to their exit from the body by various routes. In pharmacokinetic models, the physical dimensions of interest are rates and concentrations, which interconvert by the operation of clearance parameters; alternatively, rates and masses are the dimensions of interest, and they interconvert by the operation of time constants or their nonlinear counterparts. Overall, in the physical sense, pharmacokinetic processes are relaxational in character. The nonlinearities that have been encountered in pharmaco-kinetics are almost all aptly described as "soft": they can be linearized by resorting to small perturbations around an operating point, and the concentration of drug in plasma invariably changes in the same direction as the rate of drug administration, irrespective of either the direction or the rate of change of the rate of drug administration.

Pharmacodynamics relates drug concentrations and drug actions. These have to be approached on a case by case basis without the underpinning of a single recognizable, common physical or physiological principle analogous to the role that conservation of mass plays in pharmacokinetics. There is neither anything to conserve nor any other obviously useful general equation that encompasses the ways in which micromoles of a chemical can impinge upon the human organism whose energetic capabilities are in the range of several thousand kilocalories per day. The most apt equations to describe pharmacodynamic phenomena are probably to be found sometimes in integrative or-gan system physiology, sometimes in chemical kinetics, and sometimes in membrane biophysics. As such, of course, it is a tremendous intellectual challenge, and one whose fulfillment will integrate pharmacology with physiology in much richer ways than ever before.

A vivid object lesson in pharmacodynamics is the well-known children's story of "Ferdinand the Bull" — the large, but extraordinarily docile bull that is hurled into a brief but world-class rampage by a microbolus of bee venom; by the time Ferdinand is brought to the bull ring, this pharmacodynamic episode has run its course, and his accustomed docility has returned, to the dismay of the assembled multitude. Equally unpredictable is another possible outcome of a microbolus of bee venom: anaphylactic shock and death.

The disproportionate complexities of pharmacokinetics and pharmacodynamics are suggested by contrasting the simplicity of the clearance parameters that govern inter-conversions between rates and concentrations in pharmacokinetics with the empirical transductive parameters that relate drug concentrations and drug actions in pharma-codynamics. This is an area in which "hard" nonlinearities may be anticipated: dy-namic phenomena that cannot be linearized by resorting to small perturbations in con-centration and whose very direction of response may depend on parameters of concentration change other than simply the direction of change.

Physiological examples of such complex nonlinearities come from fields in which response dynamics have been tested with a variety of temporal patterns of stimulus, an experimental approach that is conspicuously absent in pharmacology. Thus, the ex-amples one may cite are not those of drug actions; this does not prove that the exam-ples do not exist, but only that they have not been systematically sought. Illustrative examples of complex nonlinearities are: the dynamics of ACTH action on adrenocor-tical steroidogenesis,[52] the dynamics of pancreatic insulin secretory responses to glu-cose and various amino acids,[53] the baroreceptor reflex responses to changes in blood pressure,[54] and the dynamics of the pupillary reflex to light.[55] The last-cited example is particularly striking: a sustained light increase causes sustained pupillary constriction; a sustained light decrease causes sustained pupillary dilation; a brief increase in light causes a very brief pupillary constriction, but a brief *decrease* in light also causes brief pupillary *constriction*! Linear models collapse in the face of this kind of nonlinearity, which cannot be linearized and usually becomes relatively more prominent as the site of stimulus perturbations is reduced.

These examples may be colossal red herrings for pharmacodynamics, but they are worth reviewing because they illustrate that particular time patterns of stimulus pres-entation have proven to be especially revealing of important nonlinearities. In the case of the pupillary reflex to light, it was the comparison of upgoing and downgoing brief changes in light intensity. In the case of ACTH action on steroidogenesis, it was the comparison of upgoing and downgoing stepwise changes in ACTH concentration in adrenal arterial blood. Other time patterns of stimulus presentation generated data, but little insight.

If there is a useful generalization to be made from these examples to pharmacodynamics, it comes down to wanting two practical results from pharmacodynamics. The first is regimen optimization—definition of the time course of drug concentration in plasma (or other suitable reference fluid) that will give adequate therapeutic response with the least involvement of extraneous or unwanted biological effects. The second is that no surprising biological effects are triggered during precipitous changes in regimen: during onset or cessation of drug action, changes in concomitant therapy, or changes in physiological/clinical status of the patient. It is useful to recognize that the cessation of drug action can be made precipitous in several ways, besides simply stopping the administration of drug: (1) use of antagonists where they exist, and (2) use of species in which the drug's pharmacokinetic time constants are especially small.

The question of regimen optimization comes down to the selection of protocols to be used in the pharmacodynamic assessment of each drug. The chapter by Fara and Mitchell discusses in detail the evident value of the injection-infusion comparison (IIC) protocol as a logical first step in pharmacodynamic assessment. The IIC protocol was devised orginally by Sikic and his co-workers at the NCI in 1978, and was used to striking advantage in studies on the pharmacodynamics of bleomycin. It has been used by a number of workers in other fields of pharmacology and endocrinology, as noted by Fara and Mitchell.

The IIC protocol is only a first step in what is clearly a new era of pharmacodynamics, driven by the emergent practicability of programming drug concentrations in body fluids. To look 1 or 2 decades ahead, one needs some cognizance of how technological advances from other fields—e.g., analytical chemistry and electronic data processing—have driven pharmacology and therapeutics during the last 2 decades, and specifically how pharmacokinetics has been driven by these advances. As a parallel, it would seem that the bioengineering and pharmaceutical progress in providing programmable control over the rate of drug entry into the body will bring pharmacodynamics into the prominence formerly enjoyed by pharmacokinetics as *the* dynamic field within pharmacology and therapeutics. Pharmacodynamics is inherently much more complex than pharmacokinetics, because of its fundamentally nonlinear character. But since pharmacodynamics deals with "what drugs do to the body", rather than "what the body does to drugs", it goes to the heart of therapeutics and the least-risk use of drugs.

REFERENCES

1. Yum, S. I. and Wright, R. M., Drug delivery systems based on diffusion and osmosis, in *Controlled Drug Delivery*, Vol. 1, Bruck, S. D., Ed., CRC Press, Boca Raton, Fla., 1983, 65.
2. Heilmann, K., Innovations in drug delivery systems, *Curr. Med. Res. Opin.,* 8 (Suppl. 2), 3, 1983.
3. Barry, B. W., Drug delivery systems, *Chemtech,* 13, 38, 1983.
4. Heilmann, K., *Therapeutische Systeme — Konzept und Realisation programmierter Arzneiverabreichung. 2. Uberarbeitete und erweiterte Auflage,* Ferdinand Enke Verlag, Stuttgart, 1982.
5. Zaffaroni, A., Systems for controlled delivery, *Med. Res. Rev.,* 1, 373, 1981.
6. Urquhart, J. and Zaffaroni, A., Assessing drug concentration/effect correlations: implications for research and therapy, in *Pharmacological and Biochemical Properties of Drug Substances,* Vol. 1, Goldberg, M. E., Ed., American Pharmaceutical Association, Washington, D. C., 1981, 477.

7. Martucci, C. P. and Fishman, J., Impact of continuously administered catechol estrogens on uterine growth and luteinizing hormone secretion, *Endocrinology*, 105, 1288, 1979.

8. Fishman, J. and Martucci, C., Biological properties of 16 alpha-hydroxyestrone: implications in estrogen physiology and pathophysiology, *J. Clin. Endocrinol. Metab.*, 51, 611, 1980.

9. Shaw, J. And Urquhart, J., Programmed, systemic drug delivery by the transdermal route, *Trends Pharmacol. Sci.*, 1, 208, 1980.

10. Urquhart, J., Development of the OCUSERT® pilocarpine ocular therapeutic systems — a case history in ophthalmic product development, in *Ophthalmic Drug Delivery Systems*, Robinson, J. R., Ed., American Pharmaceutical Association, Academy of Pharmaceutical Sciences, Washington, D.C., 1980, 105.

11. Urquhart, J., Opportunities for research: methods of drug administration, in Proceedings of the National Academy of Sciences, Institute of Medicine, Conference on Pharmaceuticals for Developing Countries, January 29-31, 1979, 320.

12. Walt, R. P., Kalman, C. J., Hunt, R. H., and Misiewicz, J. J., Effect of transdermally administered hyoscine methobromide on nocturnal acid secretion in patients with duodenal ulcer, *Br. Med. J.*, 284, 1736, 1982.

13. Anonymous, NDA revisions to address elderly drug use issue should include addition of blood level screening in phase II/phase III tests and interaction screens, *FDC Rep.*, 45 (43), 10, 1983.

14. Hendeles, L., Bighley, L., Richardson, R. H., Hepler, C. D., and Carmichael, J., Frequent toxicity from IV aminophylline infusions in critically ill patients, *Drug Intell. Clin. Pharm.*, 11, 12, 1977.

15. Urquhart, J., Rate-controlled drug dosage, *Drugs*, 23, 207, 1982.

16. Hwang, B., Konicki, G., Dewey, R., and Miao, C., GLC determination of ticrynafen and its metabolites in urine, serum, and plasma of humans and animals, *J. Pharm. Sci.*, 67, 1095, 1978.

17. Lowenthal, D. T., Onesti, G., Mutterperl, R., Affrime, M., Martinez, E. M., Kim, K. E., Busby, J., Shirk, J., and Swartz, C., Long-term clinical effects, bioavailability, and kinetics of minoxidil in relation to renal function, *J. Clin. Pharmacol.*, 18, 500, 1978.

18. Deutsch, S. D. and Vandam, L. D., General anesthesia. I. Volatile agents, in *Drill's Pharmacology in Medicine*, 4th ed., DiPalma, J. R., Ed., McGraw-Hill, New York, 1971, 145.

19. Ziser, M., Feezor, M., and Skolaut, M. W., Regulating intravenous fluid flow: controller versus clamps, *Am. J. Hosp. Pharm.*, 36, 1090, 1979.

20. *Physicians' Desk Reference*, 37th Ed., Medical Economics, Oradell, NJ, 1983, 730, 874, 1127, 2065.

21. Yacobi, A., Kartzinel, R., Lai, C. M., and Sum, C. Y., Esmolol: a pharmacokinetic profile of a new cardioselective beta-blocking agent, *J. Pharm. Sci.*, 72, 710, 1983.

22. Lutterman, J. A., Adriaansen, A. A. J., and van't Larr, A., Treatment of severe diabetic ketoacidosis: a comparative study of two methods, *Diabetologia*, 17, 17, 1979.

23. Salzman, E. W., Deykin, D., Shapiro, R. M., and Rosenberg, R., Management of heparin therapy, *N. Engl. J. Med.*, 292, 1046, 1975.

24. Sikic, B. I., Collins, J. M., Mimnaugh, E. G., and Gram, T. E., Improved therapeutic index of bleomycin when administered by continuous infusion in mice, *Cancer Treat. Rep.*, 62, 2011, 1978.

25. Prestayko, A., Comis, R. L., Daskal, Y., Samuels, M. L., and Sikic, B. I., Bleomycin-associated Pulmonary Toxicity, Bristol Laboratories, Syracuse, N.Y., 1979.

26. CIBA Pharmaceuticals, *Medicine by Osmosis: Acutrim* [promotional brochure], August 1983.

27. Theeuwes, F., Drug delivery systems, *Pharmacol. Ther.*, 13, 149, 1981.

28. Lokich, J. and Ensminger, W., Ambulatory pump infusion devices for hepatic artery infusion, *Semin. Oncol.*, 10, 183, 1983.

29. Buchwald, H., Rohde, T. D., Schneider, P. D., Varco, R. L., and Blackshear, P. J., Long-term, continuous intravenous heparin administration by an implantable infusion pump in ambulatory patients wih recurrent venous thrombosis, *Surgery*, 88, 507, 1980.

30. Kleinjans, J. C. S., Stimulation of Renal Adrenergic Mechanisms as a Model for the Development of Hypertension, Dissertation, State University of Limburg, Netherlands, 1983.

31. Smits, J. F. M., Kasbergen, C. M., van Essen, H., Kleinjans, J. C., and Struyker-Boudier, H. A. J., Chronic local infusion into the renal artery of unrestrained rats, *Am. J. Physiol.*, 244, H304, 1983.

32. Kleinjans, J. C. S., Smits, J. F. M., Kasbergen, C. M., Vervoort-Peters, H. T. M., and Struyker-Boudier, H. A. J., Blood pressure response to chronic low-dose intrarenal noradrenaline infusion in conscious rats, *Clin. Sci.*, 65, 111, 1983.

33. Weeks, J. R., A method for administration of prolonged intravenous infusion of prostacyclin (PGI₂) to unanesthetized rats, *Prostaglandins*, 17, 495, 1979.

34. Myers, R. D., Ed., *Methods in Psychobiology: Advanced Laboratory Techniques in Neuropsychology and Neurobiology*, Vol. 3, Academic Press, New York, 1977, 315.

35. Rose, S. and Nelson, J., A continuous long-term injector, *Aust. J. Exp. Biol. Med. Sci.*, 33, 415, 1955.

36. Urquhart, J., Davis, J. O., and Higgins, J. T., Jr., Effects of prolonged infusion of angiotensin II in normal dogs, *Am. J. Physiol.*, 205, 1241, 1963.

37. Urquhart, J., Davis, J. O., and Higgins, J. T., Jr., Simulation of spontaneous secondary hyperaldosteronism by intravenous infusion of angiotensin II in dogs with an arteriovenous fistula, *J. Clin. Invest.*, 43, 1355, 1964.

38. Folkman, J. and Long, D. M., The use of silicone rubber as a carrier for prolonged drug therapy, *J. Surg. Res.*, 4, 139, 1964.

39. Theeuwes, F. and Yum, S. I., Principles of the design and operation of generic osmotic pumps for the delivery of semisolid or liquid drug formulations, *Ann. Biomed. Eng.*, 4, 343, 1976.

40. Urquhart, J., Fara, J. W., and Willis, K. L., Rate-controlled delivery systems in drug and hormone research, *Annu. Rev. Pharmacol. Toxicol.*, 24, 199, 1984.

41. Richardson, K. T., Ocular microtherapy: membrane-controlled drug delivery, *Arch. Ophthalmol.*, 93, 74, 1975.

42. Pharriss, B. B., Clinical experience with the intrauterine progesterone contraceptive system, *J. Reprod. Med.*, 20, 155, 1978.

43. Newton, J., Szontagh, F., Lebech, P., and Rowe, P. J., A collaborative study of the progesterone intrauterine device (PROGESTASERT®), *Contraception*, 19, 575, 1979.

44. Spangler, D. L., Kalof, D. D., Bloom, F. L., and Wittig, H. J., Theophylline bioavailability following oral administration of six sustained-release preparations, *Ann. Allergy*, 40, 6, 1978.

45. Theeuwes, F., Evolution and design of "rate controlled" osmotic forms, *Curr. Med. Res. Opin.*, 8 (Suppl. 2), 20, 1983.

46. Rhymer, A. R., Sromovsky, J. A., Dicenta, C., and Hart, C. B., "Osmosin": a multi-centre evaluation of a technological advance in the treatment of osteoarthritis, *Curr. Med. Res. Opin.*, 8 (Suppl. 2), 62, 1983.

47. Muller, P., Imhof, P. R., Burkart, F., Chu, L. C., and Gerardin, A., Human pharmacological studies of a new transdermal system containing nitroglycerin, *Eur. J. Clin. Pharmacol.*, 22, 473, 1982.

48. Chien, Y. W., Transdermal controlled-release drug administration, in *Drugs and the Pharmaceutical Sciences*, Vol. 14, Swarbrick, J., Ed., Marcel Dekker, New York, 1982, 149.

49. Mroczek, W. J., Ulrych, M., and Yoder, S., Weekly transdermal clonidine administration in hypertensive patients, *Clin. Pharmacol. Ther.*, 31, 252, 1982.

50. Theeuwes, F., Swanson, D., Wong, P., Bonsen, P., Place, V., Heimlich, K., and Kwan, K. C., Elementary osmotic pump for indomethacin, *J. Pharm. Sci.*, 72, 253, 1983.

51. Committee on Safety Medicines, OSMOSIN (controlled release indomethacin), *Curr. Prob.*, 11, 1, 1983.

52. Urquhart, J., Fourteenth Bowditch Lecture. Bloodborne signals: the measuring and modelling of humoral communication and control, *Physiologist*, 13, 7, 1970.

53. Bergman, R. N. and Urquhart, J., The pilot gland approach to the study of insulin secretory dynamics, *Rec. Prog. Horm. Res.*, 27, 583, 1971.

54. Lamberti, Jr., J. J., Urquhart, J., and Siewers, R. D., Observations on the regulation of arterial blood pressure in unanesthetized dogs, *Circ. Res.*, 23, 415, 1968.

55. Clynes, M., The non-linear biological dynamics of unidirectional rate sensitivity illustrated by analog computer analysis, pupillary reflex to light and sound, and heart rate behavior, *Ann. N.Y. Acad. Sci.*, 98, 806, 1962.

Chapter 2

CONTROLLED AND RATE-CONTROLLED DRUG DELIVERY; PRINCIPAL CHARACTERISTICS, POSSIBILITIES, AND LIMITATIONS

F. W. H. M. Merkus

TABLE OF CONTENTS

I. INTRODUCTION

The field of research into and clinical applications of controlled drug delivery is growing very rapidly. A good illustration of this is the number of pharmaceutical patents issued per year in the area of controlled drug delivery research. This number has been increasing steadily since the early 1970s, with a total of about 1200 to 1400 patents over the period 1958 to 1978.[1]

The main objective of pharmaceutical and pharmacological research is the finding of chemical compounds with favorable therapeutic properties and only relatively low risks of adverse effects. Nevertheless, one of the major problems of the pharmaceutical industry today is the limited number of new chemical entities which have been approved for marketing in the U.S. and European countries in recent years. For instance, in the mid-1950s, about 40 new drugs were introduced in the U.S. with a total annual research and development (R & D) budget of $100 million, while in 1975, pharmaceutical companies in the U.S. spent $1 billion on R & D, but produced only 7 new drugs.[2]

Recently, a study of innovation and trends in new drug development was conducted by seven U.K.-owned research-based pharmaceutical companies using a comprehensive questionnaire completed for all new chemical entities (NCEs) evaluated in man between 1964 and 1980. This investigation has analyzed the annual rate of entry of new drugs into clinical testing over this period, the fate of these drugs either in their marketing or in clinical research, and the reasons for this outcome. About 50 NCEs were marketed by these companies between 1964 and 1980, and the success rate as measured by the ratio of new drugs taken into man to those marketed, was 6:1. During this period, the total development time increased from 4 1/2 years for drugs marketed between 1964 and 1968 to more than 11 years for 1976 to 1980; in this time there was a corresponding decrease in the effective patent life from nearly 13 years to 6 1/2 years.[3]

Nowadays, instead of the traditional constant search for new pharmacologically active agents, the strategy of many pharmaceutical companies and research institutes is focusing on the development of new drug formulations which achieve an optimal therapeutic effect not solely on the basis of the drug itself, but also on the basis of principals of release and absorption. In the traditional dosage forms and the so-called sustained-release preparations, the drug input into the body is specified by the *amount* of the drug. Nowadays, there are dosage forms that are specified by the *rate* at which they deliver the drug. Rate-controlled drug delivery offers very promising perspectives to pharmacological and therapeutic applications and industrial product development.[4]

Research in the field of drug delivery is multidisciplinary: it brings together many aspects of pharmaceutical technology, pharmaceutics, biopharmaceutics, pharmacokinetics, pharmacodynamics, and clinical pharmacology. The flow diagram in Figure 1 shows the path followed by a drug administered in conventional or controlled delivery formulation to the receptor site, classified according to the major disciplines in pharmaceutical and pharmacological sciences.

II. HISTORICAL BACKGROUND

The majority of drugs (70 to 80%) are taken orally, mostly as plain tablets, coated tablets, or capsules. In the late 1940s and early 1950s, sustained-release formulations appeared in clinical practice as a new application form in which the product was intended to improve therapy by slowing down the rate of release, increasing the duration of action, and reducing the required frequency of drug administration.

The evolution of oral dosage forms, which has culminated in the 1970s in the development of very sophisticated prolonged release dosage forms and an oral osmotic-

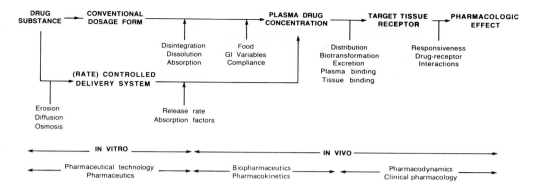

FIGURE 1. Flow diagram showing the path followed by an oral drug, administered in either conventional or controlled-delivery formulations to its site of therapeutic action.

release product, Oros®, may be traced back directly to a dramatic demonstration made 100 years ago by a German dermatologist, Paul G. Unna.[5] He showed at a meeting of the Hamburg Medical Society on June 24, 1884 that a keratin coating could protect pills intended for the intestine as they passed through the acidic pH of the stomach. By the end of the 19th century, the many and in a certain sense, obsolete and exotic dosage forms of earlier centuries had disappeared entirely, and only a few elixirs and troches were still in use. Pills, powders, solutions, mixtures, tinctures, and spirits were the common oral dosage forms of the day. In the early 1900s, the first tablets were introduced on a large scale in medicine.

In general, tablets are prepared by compression (Latin: tabulae compressae) using tablet machines capable of exerting great pressure to compact the powdered or granulated tableting material through the use of various shaped punches. We now use in therapy normal compressed tablets, multiple compressed tablets, sugar-coated, enteric-coated, and film-coated tablets.

In the 1960s and 1970s, many pharmaceutical companies marketed sustained-release oral dosage forms. This type of dosage form is commonly referred to by a designation such as "sustained, depot, prolonged, delayed, retard, slow, timed, gradual" as adjectives, with the nouns "release" or "action". These dosage forms have been used now for about 25 years to enhance the duration of action and to improve patient compliance. Usually the rate of release decreases with time in almost all products, although some new systems appear to release a large part of the drug at a constant rate.

Although the oral application of drugs in therapy is the most important, there are also other routes of drug entry into the body involving prolonged action formulations which can be roughly classified as oral, ocular, transdermal, rectal, intravaginal, intrauterine, and parenteral. There exists a vast literature regarding the investigations of the many prolonged release preparations in volunteers and patients. In 1978, Ballard[6] summarized the reports over the period 1962 to 1978 on human clinical trials involving various types of oral formulations which are claimed to have a prolonged action (Table 1). Also, many monographs and symposium books have been published in the past years providing numerous examples of novel drug formulations.[2,7-10]

III. PHARMACOKINETICS, CONTROLLED DELIVERY, AND SELECTIVITY OF ACTION

Drugs at the present time are usually amorphous or crystalline powders (or sometimes liquids) with a well-defined chemical and physical identity. With a few exceptions, however, all drugs are administered not in their pure state, but as a drug product

Table 1

**EXAMPLES OF DRUGS OF WHICH ORAL
SUSTAINED ACTION PRODUCTS HAVE
BEEN FORMULATED AND TESTED IN
HUMANS BETWEEN 1962—1978**

Acetazolamide	Isoniazid
Alprenolol	Isoproterenol
Aminophylline	Isosorbide dinitrate
Amitryptiline	Lithium sulfate
Amphetamines	Nicotinic acid
Aspirin	Nitroglycerin
Chlorpromazine	Papaverine HCl
Dextropropoxyphene HCl	Pentraerythritol tetranitrate
Dicyclomine HCl	Phendimetrazine tartrate
Diethylpropion HCl	Potassium chloride
L-dopa	Procainamide HCl
Fenfluramine	Quinidine bisulfate
Ferrous sulfate	Tetracycline HCl
L-hyoscyamine	Theophylline
D-isoephedrine	Xanthinol nicotinate

Adapted from Ballard, B. E., *Sustained and Controlled Drug Delivery Systems*, Robinson, J. R., Ed., Marcel Dekker, New York, 1978, 1.

in a pharmaceutical formulation. Therefore, the therapeutic efficacy and therapeutic index (ratio of LD_{50} to ED_{50}) of a drug product is not defined by the physicochemical characteristics of the drug substance and its pharmacokinetic properties. The presentation of the drug to the patient affects greatly the clinical usefulness and efficacy of a certain treatment.

It is well recognized now that a particular rate of delivery of a drug may elicit very specific pharmacological effects. For instance, pilocarpine delivery at a very low rate to the eye produces ocular hypotension, while at higher rates of delivery it may cause miosis, myopia, and even systemic effects. Another often used example is scopolamine, which causes only mild bradycardia at a low delivery rate, prevents motion sickness at a slightly higher rate, but induces systemic side effects (dry mouth, tachycardia, drowsiness) at higher rates of delivery. The relation between dose and effects of drugs is best illustrated by the dose-response curve. Figure 2 shows this relation for the drug dose (Panel A) or serum level (Panel B) and both benefits and side effects, as presented recently by Goldman.[12]

If the drug is theophylline, for example, the benefit may be optimal bronchodilation in an asthmatic patient, whereas the side effects may be nausea, insomnia, tremor, and convulsions. When beneficial and side effects are widely separated in this dose-response relation (large therapeutic index) then there is obviously no need for careful dosage adjustments in individual patients. But in the case of a drug such as theophylline, dosing is a serious problem. A plasma concentration range of 10 to 20 mg/ℓ (55 to 110 μmol/ℓ, is generally considered to be optimal in both children and adults, although lower levels are also beneficial in milder asthmatic patients and neonates. Theophylline's elimination half-life varies between 3 to 12 hr in adults and 1.5 to 8 hr in children so that very frequent dosing is needed (especially in children and also adults with a short elimination half-life) to keep the plasma level in the "therapeutic range". Therefore, in the case of theophylline and many other drugs with a narrow therapeutic range (see Table 2) we seek a dose and a dosage form that will provide the drug concentration in a patient that yields the best compromise between beneficial and adverse

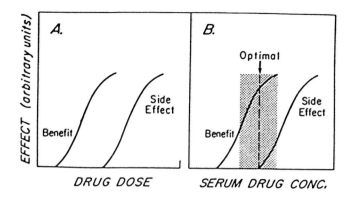

FIGURE 2.   Relation between drug dose (Panel A) or serum concentration (Panel B) and both benefits and side effects. Panel B indicates the optimal serum drug concentration by a dotted line and its variation during the dosage interval as a shaded area. (From Goldman, P., *N. Engl. J. Med.*, 307, 286, 1982. With permission.)

Table 2
THERAPEUTIC PLASMA
CONCENTRATION RANGES
FOR SELECTED DRUGS

Drug	Range
Carbamazepine	3—8 mg/l
Digitoxin	15—30 µg/l
Digoxin	1—2.5 µg/l
Disopyramide	2.5—5 mg/l
Ethosuximide	40—80 mg/l
Gentamicin (adults)	5—10 mg/l
Gentamicin (neonates)	3—6 mg/l
Lidocaine	1.5—6.0 mg/l
Lithium	3.5—10.5 mg/l
Phenytoin	5—15 mg/l
Primidone	5—15 mg/l
Procainamide	4—8 mg/l
Quinidine	2—5 mg/l
Salicylates	200—300 mg/l
Theophylline (adults)	10—20 mg/l
Theophylline (neonates)	5—10 mg/l
Valproate	40—80 mg/l

effects. This ideal drug concentration is represented by the dotted line in Figure 2 (Panel B). By controlled delivery, we try to maintain that drug concentration. Table 3 lists a number of drugs and hormones whose selectivity of action is enhanced when the agent is delivered in an actual or approximate rate-controlled fashion.

IV. DEFINITIONS OF CONTROLLED DRUG DELIVERY

It is pertinent to ask what controlled delivery really means, because the terminology in the dosage form field is chaotic. The term "controlled" denotes the incorporation into the dosage form of physicochemical mechanisms that hold in vivo drug release, expressed as a function of time, within specific bounds of rate and duration. This

Table 3
EXAMPLES OF AGENTS WHOSE
SELECTIVITY OF THERAPEUTIC OR
PHYSIOLOGICAL ACTION IS
RELATED TO THE RATE OF
ADMINISTRATION[11]

Acetazolamide	Heparin
Adrenocorticotropic hormone	Hydrochlorothiazide
Angiotensin II	Insulin
Bleomycin	Methoxyflurane
Chlordiazepoxide	Minocycline
Clonidine (added)	Morphine
Cytosine arabinoside	Nitrofurantoin
Diethylcarbamazine	Nitroglycerin
Diphenhydramine	Nitroprusside
Dopamine	Norepinephrine
Estradiol	Parathyroid hormone
Ether	Phenacetin
Furosemide	Pilocarpine
Glucagon	Scopolamine
Gonadotropin-releasing	Vasopressin
hormone (GnRH)	

definition by Urquhart[11] was extended by him using a "checklist of performance expectations for controlled-release pharmaceuticals".

- Release drug in vivo according to a pharmacokinetically rational rate or rate program (predictable time sequence of rates), predictable from in vitro test methods.
- Maintain plasma and biophase concentrations of drug within the therapeutically desirable range with minimal intrapatient fluctuation, noting that the ideal therapeutic concentration range for some drugs may have circadian or other variations of constancy, thus calling for a complex rate program rather than a single, fixed rate.
- Optimize the selectivity of drug action, i.e., minimize the number of side effects and, when they occur, their severity and incidence.
- Provide predictable, extended duration of drug action.
- Minimize the inconvenience of remedication.
- Reduce disincentives to regimen compliance.
- Rationalize the combination, in a single dosage form, of drugs that have complementary therapeutic actions, but are pharmacokinetically dissimilar, by releasing each drug at its respective optimum rate, both for the same duration.
- Stimulate innovation in the therapeutic use of drugs and improving research methods in pharmacodynamic, chronic toxicity and pharmacokinetic studies.

In the same publication, Urquhart also offered a terminology pertaining to systemic controlled release pharmaceuticals. *Controlled release*: the form releases the drug (in vitro) as predicted by physicochemical mechanisms, believed to be operating in physiological in vitro test conditions. *Rate-controlled*: the form releases the drug (in vivo) as predicted from physiological in vitro test conditions. *Rate-controlling*: the rate and extent of absorption of the drug occurs in humans as predicted from the rate and extent of drug release. The rate is called "specified" if after peer and regulatory review the correlations between release rate and absorption rate are definitive.

Also, another definition of "controlled drug release" is used: "It is the phasing of drug administration to the needs of the condition at hand so that an optimal amount of drug is used to cure or control the condition in a minimum time".[9] In some situations, this might mean that the drug is delivered more promptly for a short period and sometimes it would mean prolongation of drug levels. In the latter case, usually terms such as "prolonged" or "sustained" release are employed. This designates only one aspect of "controlled" release; namely, the production of protracted levels of drug. All presently available sustained release preparations offer some degree of "controlled" release, but the control is incomplete. A few drug delivery systems, indeed, release drugs at a zero-order rate. Many investigational or commercially available formulations for oral use have promising release rate properties but not a real (rate) controlled drug delivery.

Most clinical investigations regarding (rate-) controlled and prolonged release oral drug products show the problems involved in designing good drug delivery systems, including for instance, the problem of the intra- and interindividual variation in gastric emptying and transit-time along the gastrointestinal tract, which often causes a variable and unreliable absorption after oral administration.

When reviewing the available controlled delivery formulations, it is appropriate to summarize some ideal attributes of a drug delivery system.[13]

A good delivery system is

- Capable of controlled delivery rates to accommodate the pharmacokinetics of various drugs (flexible programming)
- Capable of precise control of a constant delivery rate (precise programming)
- Not highly sensitive to physiological variables, such as:

  - Gastric motility and emptying
  - pH, fluid volume, and content of the gut
  - Presence/absence or concentration of enzymes
  - State of fasting and type of food present
  - Physical position and activity of subject
  - Individual variability
  - Disease state

- Based on physicochemical principles
- Capable of a high order of drug dispersion (the ultimate is molecular in scale)
- Maintaining or enhancing drug stability
- Applicable to a wide range and variety of drugs
- One in which the "controlling" mechanism adds little mass to the dosage form

The enumeration of ideal properties of drug delivery systems facilitates the description and comparison of their characteristics, possibilities, and limitations.

A principal difference between the mechanisms of rate-controlled drug delivery divides the available systems into two groups: *(1) open-loop delivery systems and (2) closed-loop delivery systems* (see Figures 3 and 4).[14] The therapeutic system (platform) contains a drug reservoir, an energy source, and in more sophisticated systems, a therapeutic program governing the amount of drug passing the rate-controlling mechanism. In the open-loop system, the drug is delivered to the human body without any influence on or feedback from the therapeutic effect. In the closed-loop systems, on the other hand, the pharmacokinetic process is fed back to the therapeutic program by using a very sensitive sensor in the biological environment which is capable of sending signals to the delivery program. A good example of the closed-loop (infusion) systems

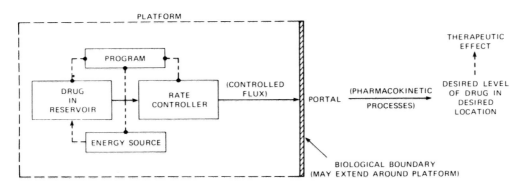

FIGURE 3.   Schematic representation of an open-loop controlled delivery system. (From Yates, F. E. et al., *Advances in Biomedical Engineering*, Brown, J. H. and Dickson, J., III, Eds., Academic Press, New York, 1975, 1. With permission.)

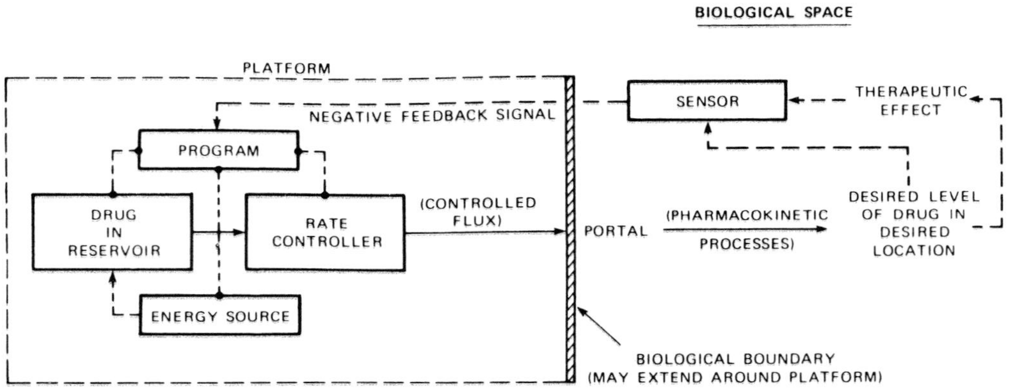

FIGURE 4.   Schematic representation of a closed-loop controlled delivery system (From Yates, F. E. et al., in *Advances in Biomedical Engineering*, Brown, J. H. and Dickson, J., III, Eds., Academic Press, New York, 1975, 1. With permission.)

has been developed for diabetes treatment in which the drug (insulin) delivery is dependent on the glucose level within the systemic circulation (see Chapter 6 by Pickup and Stevenson).

At present, the large majority of available drug delivery systems belong to the open-loop systems. Many innovative (and pseudoinnovative) formulations have been developed in the past 15 years. In the next section, this group of open-loop delivery systems will be discussed and classified.

V. CLASSIFICATION AND PRINCIPAL CHARACTERISTICS OF CONTROLLED DRUG DELIVERY

Research into and practical applications of novel drug delivery systems is characterized by a multidisciplinary approach. As a consequence, the nomenclature and classification of these systems is based on the physicochemical properties, *pharmaceutical* formulation, or *clinical* application of these dosage forms. In this section, an attempt will be made to classify the presently available systems accordingly (see Tables 4, 5, and 6).

Table 4
PHYSICOCHEMICAL CLASSIFICATION OF DRUG DELIVERY SYSTEMS

1. Pumps (i.v. infusion, osmotic pump)
   Mechanism: gravity, pump, osmosis
   Zero-order release: yes
2. Diffusional systems
   Mechanism: diffusion through polymer matrix or
      polymer membrane
   Zero-order release: only by using a rate-controlling
      membrane or a matrix of special geometry
3. Bioerodible systems
   Mechanism: bioerosion of polymer containing drug or
      drug-polymer complex
   Zero-order release: difficult to achieve
4. Combination of diffusional and bioerodible systems
   Mechanism: bioerosion and diffusion
   Zero-order release: possible, but difficult to achieve

Table 5
PHARMACEUTICAL CLASSIFICATION OF DRUG DELIVERY SYSTEMS

1. Pumps (i.v. infusion, osmotic pump)
   Mechanism: gravity, pump, osmosis
   Zero-order release: yes
2. Reservoir (capsule-type) system (surrounded
   by polymer membrane)
   Mechanism: diffusion
   Zero-order release: possible (using rate-
      controlling membrane)
3. Matrix (monolithic) system (porous or nonporous)
   Mechanism: diffusion through matrix or bioerosion
   Zero-order release: only possible with matrix of special geometry
4. Sandwich system (reservoir included in matrix
   system or matrix system surrounded by rate-
   controlling membrane)
   Mechanism: diffusion
   Zero-order release: possible (see 2 and 3)

Table 6
CLINICAL CLASSIFICATION OF DRUG DELIVERY SYSTEMS

1. Ocular
2. Oral
3. Intravaginal, intrauterine
4. Rectal
5. Parenteral (i.m., i.v., s.c.)
6. Transdermal

A. Pumps

The best known form of a controlled delivery of drugs is by an intravenous infusion that is constantly monitored by a pump or drop counter which acts as the rate-controlling element. If the pump and infusion fluid are compact, there are two possibilities for a controlled delivery system: a system which can be worn externally by ambulatory patients (e.g., releasing insulin) or a system which can be implanted under the skin to perfuse specific organs with certain drugs (e.g., cytostatic agents). The driving force to deliver the drug is either gravity or a pump. Infusaid® is an example; this is a pump, the size of a hockey puck, which can be implanted easily in the abdomen. The pump is a disc made of titanium, divided inside into two chambers. The bottom compartment contains a fluorocarbon propellant that exerts a constant pressure. The drug, in the upper chamber, is pushed by the propellant into a catheter inserted in a vein or artery. The upper chamber can be refilled as needed by means of a syringe without much discomfort to the patient. Two other examples, the miniature osmotic pump for oral administration and the multipurpose (generic) osmotic pump, will be discussed in Sections F and H, respectively.

B. Reservoir Systems

Reservoir systems (also called capsule-type systems) consist of a reservoir of drug encapsulated and surrounded by a polymer membrane. Diffusion of the drug through the polymer is the rate-limiting step. It remains constant (zero-order release) as long as the concentration outside the system is negligibly small compared with the inside (saturated solution) and the membrane characteristics remain constant. Ethylene-vinyl-acetate (EVAc), hydrogels, and silicone rubbers are used as polymers. Examples of this system are Ocusert®, Progestasert®, and some transdermal systems, all developed by ALZA. To obtain a saturated solution over a long period within the reservoir, the drug is generally loaded to a level far exceeding the solubility. A disadvantage, therefore, could be the risk of toxic reactions due to an overdose when the system is ruptured.

C. Matrix Systems

In a matrix system, the drug is homogeneously dispersed as discrete crystals or solid particles in the matrix material. Drug particles, when mixed in a suitable thermoplastic polymer or cross-linkable elastomeric material, partly dissolve in the matrix. Polymeric matrix systems were first believed to be unsuitable for the delivery of macromolecules such as polypeptides. This was because most macromolecules (molecular weight > 600) were too large to diffuse through the polymer chains. Now, porous matrices are also available for controlled delivery of polypeptides and other macromolecules.

Usually, excess drug is added (remaining undissolved) to obtain sufficient drug for a prolonged release. Diffusion of the drug through the polymer is (also) in matrix systems the rate-limiting step, but the release rate decreases with time. The drug can elute out of the matrix, first by dissolution and second by diffusion through the polymer. The drug molecules at the surface of the matrix are the first to be eluted, and after the surface layer becomes exhausted, the inner layer then begins to be depleted. As more drug particles elute out of the matrix, the drug depletion zone becomes larger and the thickness of the polymer to be passed by the drug becomes greater. The release rate is not zero-order but proportional to the square root of time.

The reader is referred to References 15 to 18 for a description of the release kinetics from matrices under various conditions and geometries. It is very interesting to note that it is possible to get a zero-order release of the drug by altering the geometry of the matrix. An appropriate shape of the matrix, according to Langer and co-workers,[19-21] is that of a hemisphere (Figure 5). The hemisphere is coated with an impermeable barrier everywhere except in a small aperture drilled in the center of the circular face. All release is through the aperture. The use of hemispheres to produce zero-order release rates for peptides has been studied experimentally and Figure 6 shows indeed that bovine serum albumin is released in vitro at a constant rate from an hemisphere.[19] Also, in vivo studies have been conducted in which insulin from an hemispheric matrix

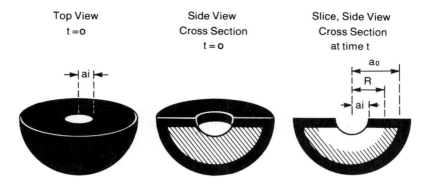

Top View
t = o

Side View
Cross Section
t = o

Slice, Side View
Cross Section
at time t

FIGURE 5. Diagram of an inwardly-releasing hemisphere; a_i is the inner radius, a_o is the outer radius, and R is the distance to the interface between the dissolved region (white area) and the dispersed zone (diagonal lines). Black represents laminated regions through which release cannot occur. (From Hsieh, D. S. T. et al., *J. Pharm. Sci.*, 72, 17, 1983. With permission.)

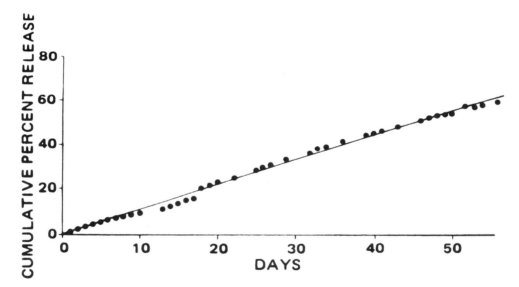

FIGURE 6. Cumulative release of bovine serum albumin vs. time. The matrix was made of ethylene-vinyl acetate copolymer and bovine serum albumin. Standard error of the mean of the cumulative release at each time point was within 12%. (From Hsieh, D. S. T. et al., *J. Pharm. Sci.,* 72, 17, 1983. With permission.)

implanted into diabetic rats was released constantly over 100 days.[21] Other potentially clinically important polypeptides can also be released constantly using this system.

In *bioerodible (= biodegradable) matrix systems*, the drug is also distributed homogeneously through the matrix. Polymers used are, for instance, copolymers of lactic acid and glycolic acid and polypeptides of glutamic acid and leucine. The degradation of the polymer or polymer-drug conjugate is a continuous process, thereby releasing the drug proportional to the square root of time. Zero-order release may be achieved if the area of drug delivery maintains a constant value during the whole release period. This can be accomplished theoretically by using a special geometric shape, such as the slab form.

Bioerodible pellet-type drug delivery systems for subcutaneous administration of

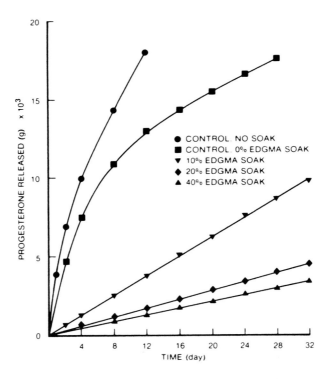

FIGURE 7.   Progesterone release from a polymeric delivery system comprising progesterone dispersed in a polyhydroxyethyl methacrylate (p-HEMA) matrix. The 9.1% progesterone HEMA devices were soaked in varying concentrations of ethylene glycol dimethacrylate (EGDMA) for 4 hr and exposed to UV light for 3 hr. (From Lee, E. S. et al., *J. Membr. Sci.,* 7, 293, 1980. With permission.)

narcotic antagonists, contraceptives, and antimalarials received a great deal of attention from governments and also WHO, but these products are still in the experimental phase. For a review of polymers, their physicochemical properties and application in delivery systems, the reader is referred to References 22 and 23.

One class of polymers, hydrogels, deserves special attention.[24] The manufacturing of reservoir and matrix systems of, for example, synthetic polyhydroxethyl methacrylate (p-HEMA) is relatively easy. Some methods are available to achieve zero-order release of drugs from a device, using a rate-controlling hydrogel membrane surrounding a drug reservoir or a drug within a matrix system. As stated before, the release rate of drugs from a matrix declines continuously proportional to the square root of time. After soaking an acrylate polymeric (p-HEMA) matrix (containing, e.g., progesterone) in different concentrations of ethylene glycol dimethacrylate (EGDMA), followed by irradiation with UV light to achieve a cross-linking effect, an almost perfect rate-controlled membrane is formed within the surface of the matrix. Drug release from such systems can be fairly steady and depends on soaking time, cross-linking solution concentration, and UV irradiation time (Figure 7).[25]

A simplified scheme of the main properties of reservoir and matrix systems can be found in Table 7. Besides reservoir and matrix systems, some investigators developed *sandwich-type systems for controlled drug delivery*, characterized by a combination of the constant release kinetics of the reservoir-type delivery and the mechanical superiority of the matrix system. In the next sections (E to I) examples of all these systems will be described.

Table 7

SIMPLIFIED SCHEME OF SOME DRUG DELIVERY SYSTEMS

System	Reservoir	Matrix		
		Nonporous small molecules	Porous large molecules	Bioerodible
Release mechanism	Diffusion Fick's first law	Diffusion Fick's second law		Bioerosion and diffusion simultaneously
Geometry	Constant	Constant	About constant	Decreasing
Zero-order release	Yes	No; only possible with special geometry		No

A very promising, new mechanism for zero-order drug release was described recently, namely the *swelling controlled drug delivery*. Because no successful pharmaceutical formulation of this type is yet known from clinical practice, only a reference to a recent survey of the literature is made here.[26]

D. Carrier-Mediated Drug Delivery and Magnetic Systems

The use of carrier systems to deliver drugs to specific areas in the body has been the subject of intensive research. The carrier can be used, theoretically, to transport the drug to the target tissue or to release the drug in the target area at an optimal rate. One system that has attracted much attention is the use of *liposomes*. In the past decade, a lot of potential applications for liposomes have been studied, as can be derived from recent reviews.[27,28]

Liposomes are phospholipid bilayer vesicles consisting of alternating aqueous layers containing the drug and lipid bilayers. Liposomes have a bilayer structure which resembles natural cell membranes. The phospholipid content of the liposome membrane is very similar to that of naturally occurring cells with lipid exchange actually occurring between the liposomes and the natural cell membrane. Liposomes are completely biocompatible. In the early 1970s, research began to focus on liposomes as drug delivery systems because it was realized that drugs could be incorporated in the aqueous spaces between the lipid bilayers. Liposomes are capable of maintaining the drug trapped within the bilayers until they reach the desired target site. Targets which are available to the liposome drug delivery system are phagocytic cells which are capable of internalizing the lipid particles by phagocytosis. Originally, it was thought that liposomes would be ideal for targeting cytotoxic agents to neoplasms while at the same time reducing the toxic systemic side effects. Although some interesting results have been obtained in cancer therapy, liposomes generally have failed to be a useful method for delivery of drugs in vivo. Perhaps the use of magnetically responsive antineoplastic drug carriers, prepared using either a lipid (for water-insoluble drugs) or a protein carrier (for water-soluble drugs) may have clinical relevance in future cancer therapy.[29]

However, there have been some promising results in liposome targeting to the liver. The use of a liposome delivery system to deliver antimonial compounds to the liver to treat leishmaniasis, a parasitic disease of the liver, has provided an example of the benefits obtainable with specific drug targeting.[28] In this case, the dose of the antimony compound has been reduced by a factor of 800 with a resulting elimination of the side effects usually associated with antimony therapy. A liposome drug delivery system is expected to be marketed soon. Another liposome drug delivery system has also been shown to be useful in targeting acetylcysteine to the parenchymal cells of the liver to treat acute acetaminophen overdose in mice.[28]

Langer and co-workers[21] were the first group to disperse *magnetic particles within a*

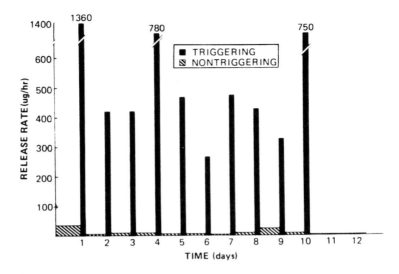

FIGURE 8.   Magnetic modulation of bovine serum albumin release. Prior to triggering, the pellets were prereleased for 1 day. The pellets were triggered for 5 hr, followed by nontriggering for 19 hr. The cycle of triggering and nontriggering was repeated daily. ■ = The quantity of BSA release during the magnetic modulation period; ⊠ = the quantity of BSA released during the nontriggering period. (From Siegel, R. A. and Langer, R., *Pharm. Res.*, 1, 1, 1984. With permission.)

matrix system. For many polypeptide hormones, a constant drug release is probably not desirable. Insulin, for example, should be released constantly, but supplemented by an increase near mealtime to control higher glucose levels. A system containing small magnetic beads has been developed in which the release rate can be controlled by application of an oscillating magnetic field.

When exposed to the magnetic field, polymer matrices released up to 30 times more drug and release rates returned to normal when the magnetic field was discontinued (Figure 8). While the mechanism of release is still under study, one possibility is that the magnetic field increases release rates because the beads alternately compress and expand the matrix pores, thereby "squeezing" out more drug. Such factors as magnetic field strength, magnetic field orientation, and the frequency of oscillation all influence the degree of modulation. The magnetic controlled release systems could perhaps be used to increase insulin delivery at desired times, such as after a meal (perhaps by placing the implant under the skin of the wrist and designing a triggering device in the form of a special watch). Other polypeptide hormones that are produced in a time-dependent manner by the body may also be amenable to improved therapeutic efficiency by using modulated delivery systems.

These proposals and experiments are very interesting and suggestive of more potential applications in the future.

In the next sections, a large number of controlled delivery systems are described according to a classification of clinical applications (see Table 6).

E. Ocular Controlled Drug Delivery

Drugs are applied to the eye for a local effect of the medication on either the surface or the interior of the eye. Most frequently aqueous solutions as eyedrops are employed; but suspensions and ophthalmic ointments are also quite common in practice. This type of treatment of the eye is simple in the sense that the drug is delivered almost

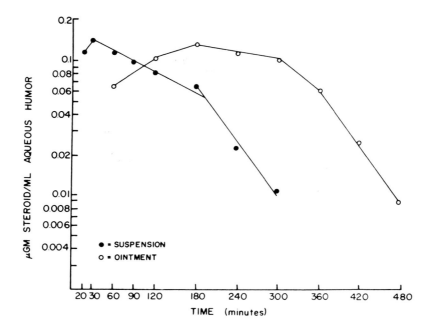

FIGURE 9. Fluorometholone concentration in rabbit aqueous humor following top-ical dosing with a 0.1% aqueous suspension and a 0.1% ointment. Each data point is based on at least 8 eyes and the standard error of the mean is less than 10%. (From Sieg, J. W. and Robinson, J. R., *J. Pharm. Sci.*, 64, 931, 1975. With permission.)

directly to the target tissue. An important drawback inherent to most eye preparations is the extensive drug loss after application. The removal of drugs from the eye is so efficient that it is no exception when actually only a few percent of the applied drug penetrates the eye. A great part of the medication is diluted immediately by the resident tears and second, the tear chamber can only hold 10 to 20 $\mu\ell$ of each eyedrop applied, which is normally 50 $\mu\ell$. A very large part of the ocular medication is rapidly drained away by a constant tear flow (especially in the inflamed eye) and by the lacrimal-nasal drainage. The latter drainage system frequently causes systemic side effects of drugs because the drained drug is absorbed in the gastrointestinal tract. Tear turnover strongly contributes to drug dilution. Tears in the human eye are continuously being replaced at a rate of about 15%/min. Consequently, a second and very serious draw-back of the conventional ocular drug preparations is the need for very frequent appli-cations in order to achieve a steady-state drug level in the target tissue. There exists no doubt that suspensions and ointments do prolong the contact time of a drug with the eye tissues. A good example of the aqueous humor drug concentration time profile comparing 0.1% fluorometholone ointment and suspension is given in Figure 9. The release of fluorometholone from the ointment is prolonged, resulting in a sustained action and improved local drug bioavailability.[30]

The efficacy of a drug is improved by prolonging its contact with the ocular tissue. Therefore, viscosity-enhancing agents in eye drops or ointment bases are chosen to sustain drug effects of ocular drug preparations.

A promising development in the ocular drug therapy is the Ocusert®, an ocular insert unit for the controlled delivery of pilocarpine. The system fits into the cul-de-sac of the eye (Figure 10) and delivers pilocarpine at a rate of 20 μg/hr (Pilo-20) or 40 μg/ hr (Pilo-40) for 7 days. Each unit consists of a pilocarpine core surrounded on each side by a flexible, biocompatible, ethylene-vinyl acetate (EVAc) membrane. After

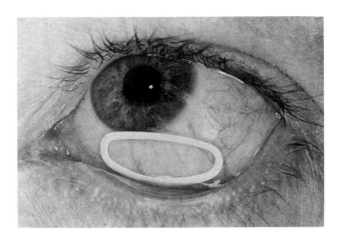

FIGURE 10. Ocular therapeutic system (Ocusert®) which releases pilocarpine continuously at a constant rate for 7 days for the relief of intraocular pressure.

placement of the Ocusert® into the eye, the pilocarpine molecules permeate through the EVAc membrane at a zero-order rate, as described already for reservoir systems, assuming that the diffusion and partition coefficient of the drug in the membrane are constant and that infinite sink conditions are maintained in the ocular fluid. Thus the drug release should remain constant until the drug concentration in the reservoir drops off below the drug saturation concentration. In vivo, this system has proven to release pilocarpine over a 7-day period at a rate that correlates well with the in vitro values.[31] The sustained control of ocular pressure by pilocarpine is achieved by the Ocusert® system with a total dose of pilocarpine that is much lower than that required using conventional eye drops and also with a lower incidence of local and systemic side effects.

It may be possible in therapy to administer also other ophthalmic drugs by this zero-order release principle. Possible candidates could be the beta-adrenergic blocker timolol and the sympathicomimetic drug epinephrine. In the area of ophthalmic drug delivery, Ocusert® has proven an excellent rate controlled drug delivery system, but it is not very well accepted by the patient. Perhaps bioerodible systems, the use of liposomes, or ocular bioadhesives may improve patient acceptance, but probably these systems do not show a zero-order release.

F. Oral Controlled Drug Delivery

Already in the early 1950s, an advanced oral sustained-release drug formulation was introduced under the name Spansule® (Smith, Kline and French). It consisted of hundreds of small medicated pellets in a gelatin capsule. In fact, there were several groups of pellets. One group was uncoated serving as the primary dose and the other groups were coated with lipid membranes of different thicknesses.

Numerous other types of oral drug delivery systems, designed to sustain the release and prolong the action of the active agent, have been developed over the past 30 years. The reasons for marketing these products include a reduction in unnecessary fluctuations in plasma drug concentration and thus avoidance of side effects and a better patient compliance due to a simplified dosage schedule. Conventional sustained oral delivery systems in clinical use today are usually of two types: matrix embedded drug systems and encapsulated products with a disintegrating or nondisintegrating coating.[32]

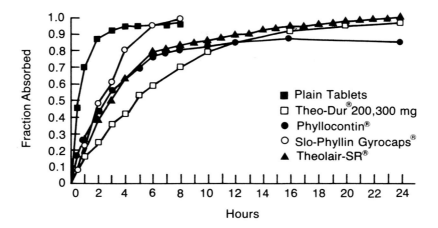

FIGURE 11. Comparison of the rate and extent of absorption of theophylline from plain tablets and selected slow-release formulations with international distribution following single doses in adult volunteers. Data were obtained from groups of healthy adult volunteers given single doses of the formulation examined and an appropriate reference formulation. The fraction of the dose absorbed was computed by calculating the amount of drug that reached the systemic circulation and dividing by the amount ingested (from Weinberger, M. and Hendeles, L., *Sustained Release Theophylline*, Merkus, F. W. H. M., Ed., Excerpta Medica, New York, 1983, 155. With permission.)

The matrix can be of inert or noninert bioerodible material. Enteric coating is the oldest way of sustaining drug delivery. It protects the drug from degradation in the acidic gastric environment and it postpones the process of disintegration of the dosage form and dissolution of the active compound. Cellulose acetate phthalate (CAP) and a few other polymers have been widely used in the past as coating material, offering a reliable enteric coating. At a pH greater than 4, as in the intestine, the CAP coating changes by ionization of the phthalate moiety, expansion of the coating, and penetration of intestinal fluid, resulting in leaching of the drug from the dosage form. The use of CAP does not really contribute to a continuous release of the active agent. Once the coating material has dissolved, the disintegration, dissolution, and absorption is identical with that of the plain tablets (first-order release), but this process is delayed by a time period equal to the transit time of the product from the mouth to the intestine and by the dissolution time for the coating. The transit time is largely dependent on the stomach emptying rate, which depends on concomitant food and/or fluid intake, size of the drug product (single or multiple units), posture of the patient, and some other factors. Large "single-unit" dosage forms indeed show long and variable gastrointestinal transit times. Reproducible gastric emptying rates can be achieved by "multiple-unit" delivery systems.[33] It has been suggested that the density of the pellets ("subunits") may also play a substantial role in the transit time. By using pellets of different composition and density and by varying the thickness or the composition of the (successive) pellet coatings, it is possible to get a continuous release of the drug. Coated pellets can be incorporated in capsules, compressed in tablets, or even embedded in a matrix. A good example of a clinically well-accepted oral sustained release product is Theo-Dur®. This product shows a zero-order in vitro release that was reasonably approximated in vivo (Figure 11).[34,35] A Theo-Dur® tablet consists of many small cores (containing a sugar particle surrounded by theophylline, wax, and CAP layers), embedded in a theophylline-containing granulated matrix, serving as the initial dose. One tablet of 300 mg contains 195 mg theophylline in the cores and 105 mg in the matrix.

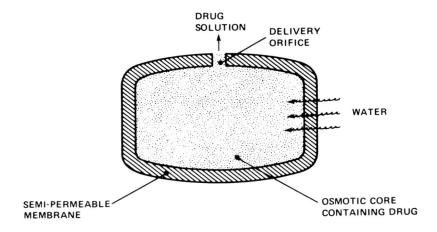

FIGURE 12.   Elementary osmotic pump cross section. (From Theeuwes, F., *J. Pharm. Sci.,* 64, 1987, 1975. With permission.)

Generally, the optimal form of oral drug delivery is undoubtedly the product that delivers the drug according to a true zero-order profile. A very interesting well-documented product is the Oros® tablet based on the principles of an elementary osmotic pump (EOP) to deliver drugs at a constant rate.[36] The elementary osmotic pump for oral use consists of an osmotically active core, including the drug, surrounded by a rate-controlling, semipermeable membrane with an exit port made by an automated laser or high-speed drill. Rate-controlled drug delivery depends on two factors: water permeability of the semipermeable membrane and the osmotic pressure of the core material. When exposed to an aqueous environment in the gastrointestinal tract, the drug core imbibes water at a rate determined by the properties of the membrane and the osmotic activity of the core. Since the rigid membrane holds the tablet's internal volume constant, the internal pressure can be released only by the exit of the drug solution through the orifice. The device delivers, in any time interval, a volume of saturated drug solution equal to the volume of water imbibed. As long as excess solute remains within the device, the rate of solute delivery by the system is constant, the emerging solution remains saturated, and the osmotic pressure gradient across the membrane remains constant. As excess solid is exhausted, the concentration of solute falls below the saturation level, causing the delivery rate to decline in a parabolic pattern — and to reach zero when the osmotic pressure gradient across the membrane vanishes. The cross section and a demonstration model of an elementary osmotic pump is shown in Figures 12 and 13.

The first commercial product containing indomethacin was recently introduced in clinical practice in many countries, but due to ulcerogenic effects in a small number of patients, the product was withdrawn from the market. The Oros® system as a single unit dosage form apparently delivered the drug at a fixed spot in the gastrointestinal tract. There are limitations to the applicability of the Oros® tablet for drugs with a low solubility. The latest development in osmotic pump drug delivery is a version which is suitable for insoluble or excessively soluble drugs ("push-pull pump").[37]

Recently, an interesting oral drug delivery system was introduced based on the principle of a prolonged gastric residence, called "hydrodynamically balanced" system (Figure 14).[38] The product consists of a gelatin capsule designed to "float" on the gastric juice. The capsule remains in the stomach for 4 to 10 hr, slowly releasing the drug into the gastrointestinal tract. The "floating" capsule is a new approach to the problem of how to increase the retention time of a drug in the part of the gastrointes-

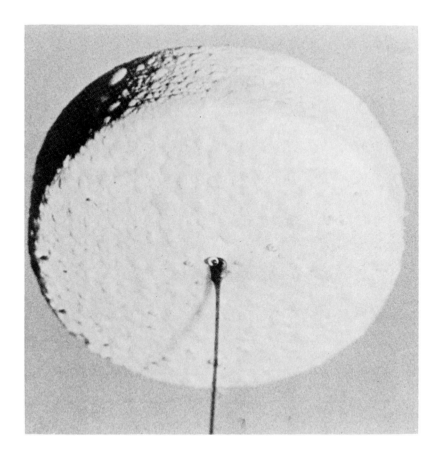

FIGURE 13.   Demonstration model of an Oros® tablet (courtesy of Merck Sharp & Dohme, The Netherlands).

tinal tract, where the drug should be released or is best absorbed. It will undoubtedly be followed by other formulations, intended to a ''positioned release'' of the active compound.

G. Intrauterine and Intravaginal Controlled Drug Delivery

Contraceptive pills and intrauterine contraceptive devices (IUD) are the most effective methods of contraception currently available. IUDs are sometimes nonmedicated, but commonly are medicated and in the latter case serve as a delivery system for antifertility agents such as copper (e.g., Cu-7®, Multiload Cu 250®) or progesterone (e.g., Progestasert®). It is estimated that world-wide about 15 million women currently use IUDs.[2]

A Cu-7® IUD is a polypropylene plastic device, shaped as the number 7, with 89 mg of copper wire wound around the vertical limb, giving an effective copper surface of 200 mm². A mean daily dose of about 10 μg Cu is released *in utero* for about 3 years. Also, T-formed copper devices are available (e.g., Cu 250®). The Progestasert® continuously applies progesterone to the uterine lumen in an amount of 65 μg per day for about 1 year (see Figure 15).

The progesterone release from this device is principally similar to the release of drug from the Ocusert® system. Progesterone is dispersed in a reservoir vehicle, from which it diffuses through the EVAc polymeric membrane at a constant rate (Figure 16).[39]

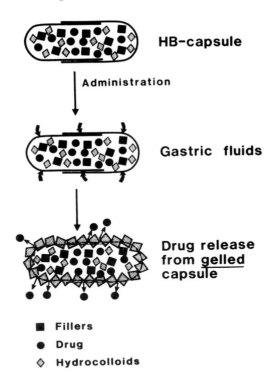

HB-capsule

Administration

Gastric fluids

Drug release from gelled capsule

■ **Fillers**

● **Drug**

◇ **Hydrocolloids**

FIGURE 14.   Working principle of the hydrodynamically balanced capsule. The hard gelatine capsule contains a special formulation of hydrocolloids which swell into a gelatinous mass upon entering of gastric fluids (From Bogenteft, C., *Pharm. Int.*, 3, 366, 1982. With permission.)

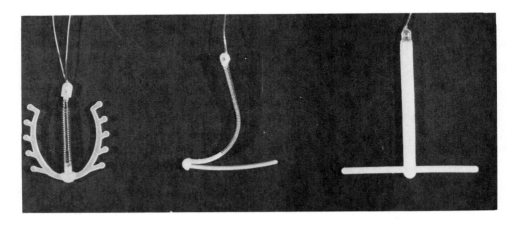

FIGURE 15.   Progestasert®, Cu-7® and Multiload Cu 250®.

An intrauterine device has some clinically important advantages over the conventional hormonal contraceptive pills. The contraceptive effects are confined only to the uterus. There is no need for daily self-medication thus avoiding the risk of patient noncompliance and there are no hormonal systemic side effects.

From the use of intravaginal suppositories, tablets, and capsules, we know that

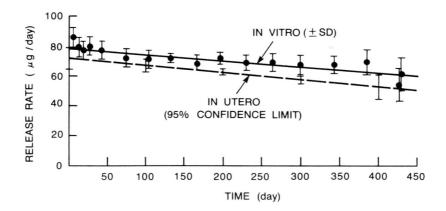

FIGURE 16. Comparison of in vitro and in vivo release rates from the Progestasert® system. (From Chandrasekaran, S. K. et al., *J. Membr. Sci.*, 3, 271, 1978. With permission.)

many drugs are absorbed quite well by the vaginal epithelium. Using the vagina as the route of administration for contraceptive agents has two advantages: (1) the possibility of self-insertion and removal and (2) a continuous release of the drug, thus improving patient compliance. Good examples of a controlled-release vaginal drug delivery system are a vaginal ring fabricated from a silicone elastomer containing medroxyprogesterone acetate (MPA), an effective contraceptive agent and sandwich-type vaginal rings, containing gestagen and estrogen simultaneously.[2]

Also, controlled-release systems for vaginal application of prostaglandins to induce abortion have been successfully tested.

H. Rectal Controlled Drug Delivery

The rectal route of drug administration is sometimes chosen for therapeutic reasons and as an interesting route of drug administration for clinical pharmacological studies.[40] Rectal drug administration offers obvious advantages in cases of nausea and vomiting or unconsciousness of the patient. Rectal drug delivery and absorption are not dependent on the presence of food, gastric emptying rate, or intestinal transit time. Also, contact with digestive fluids of the upper GI tract is avoided, thereby preventing some drugs from decomposing or forming toxic metabolites. Finally, "first-pass" elimination of high clearance drugs may be partly avoided, because the upper part of the rectal venous blood supply is connected with the portal system, whereas the lower part is directly connected with the systemic circulation. Nevertheless, there are two important drawbacks of the rectal route of drug administration: the lack of patient acceptance and the removal of the delivery system by defecation.

The mechanism of drug absorption from the rectum is probably no different from that in the upper part of the GI tract, despite the fact that the anatomy, physiology, pH, and fluid content differ substantially. Although rectal absorption of drugs from aqueous and alcoholic solutions may occur rapidly, the absorption from suppositories is slower and dependent on the suppository base and physicochemical drug factors. When a drug is presented in solution, absorption is only a problem when the drug is too polar (e.g., quaternary ammonium compounds) so that membrane passage is a limiting factor.

Breimer and co-workers[41-45] recently applied the Osmet® drug delivery system (developed by ALZA) for rectal drug administration in human volunteers (Figure 17).[46] It is a "generic" osmotic pump, fabricated empty and preprogrammed to deliver a total

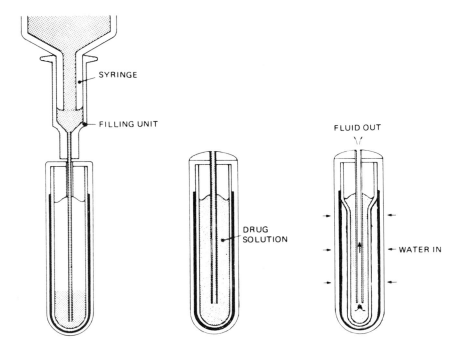

FIGURE 17.   Schematic representation of the filling and operation of the osmotic pump.

volume of 2 mℓ in 24 to 40 hr. The system is slightly larger than a normal suppository for an adult. The pump has a reservoir, surrounded by an osmotic driving agent, encapsulated in a semipermeable membrane; the membrane serves as a rigid housing and contains an orifice for delivery of drug solution or suspension. Using a blunted needle (filling tube), the investigator fills the system through the orifice with the drug solution or suspension to be investigated. After filling, insertion of a flow moderator is desirable so that uncontrolled loss of drug through the orifice is prevented. In operation the osmotic agent imbibes water across the semipermeable membrane to displace an equal volume of drug formulation from the reservoir. Preincubation in an aqueous medium is required for about 16 hr. The system should be inserted into the rectum with the orifice pointing to the anus (downwards) in order to prevent dumping effects.

The system was tested in volunteers with antipyrine and theophylline, obtaining constant plasma concentrations comparable to those during an i.v. infusion. Furthermore, the system was used in several clinical pharmacological studies (e.g., with propranolol, lidocaine, triazolam, nifedipine).[40-45] The same group studied also the drug release characteristics of a cylindrical hydrogel preparation as a rectal delivery system using model drugs like antipyrine and theophylline. The use of the several delivery systems for rectal administration will probably be limited to treatments of short duration, but the generic osmotic pump offers an excellent tool to study toxicity, pharmacodynamics, and kinetics of drugs under steady-state conditions.

I. Parenteral Controlled Drug Delivery

Three pharmaceutical formulation approaches are applied to the development of parenteral controlled drug delivery or sustained drug release from the injection site:

1. Chemical approach, by making water-insoluble drug derivatives (''prodrugs'') like esters, complexes, salts

2. Pharmacological approach, by coadministration of vasoconstrictors
3. Pharmaceutical approach, by using, for instance, viscous vehicles, hydrophobic vehicles (vegetable oils), thixotropic suspensions, crystalline suspensions, encapsulation within polymeric material (microcapsules), or dispersion (or solution) of a drug in a polymer (microspheres)

The benefit of parenteral controlled drug delivery via intramuscular and subcutaneous injection or by implantation lies primarily in the achievement of a constant and prolonged therapeutic drug level with a reduced frequency of injections and an improved patient compliance. At the current state of development, none of the parenteral drug delivery formulations is capable of delivering drugs completely according to zero-order kinetics, but a lot of products show a sufficiently constant release over a period of weeks or even months. In modern pharmacotherapy, numerous injectable depot formulations are used, such as procaine penicillin G suspensions, medroxyprogesterone acetate suspensions, fluphenazine-, haloperidol-, and nandrolone decanoate in oleaginous solutions and insulin-Zn suspensions. For an historical overview of parenteral drug formulations, the reader is referred to Reference 6.

The physicochemical mechanisms of drug release from parenteral depot formulations can be summarized as follows:

- Drug esters, complexes and salts, dissolved or suspended in oleaginous or aqueous vehicles: bioerosion, dissociation, dissolution, diffusion
- Drugs encapsulated in polymeric material: bioerosion, dissolution, diffusion
- Drugs suspended in oleaginous or aqueous vehicles: dissolution, diffusion

A few examples of depot formulations will be described here. With solutions in oil, the absorption rate depends on the partitioning of the drug, the dissolution or degradation of the vehicle, the diffusion rate of the drug in the oil and in the tissue fluid, the rate of permeation of vascular membranes, and the vascularity around the injection site. A prolonged release of a drug can be achieved for a period ranging from a few days to several months by using solutions in oil, e.g., of hormones or antipsychotic drugs. In Figure 18, the mean plasma levels of haloperidol decanoate depot injections are given after five monthly injections.[47]

When injecting a suspension in oil, the same factors are controlling drug absorption, but additionally the dissolution rate of the drug in the oil and in the surrounding tissue fluid plays an important role. After injection of an aqueous suspension, drug absorption depends on the dissolution rate of the drug in the tissue fluid, the diffusion rate, the permeation of capillary membranes, and the vascularity and perfusion rate at the injection site. Injectable suspensions in vegetable oil are less frequently used today. One of the few examples is the injectable suspension of procaine penicillin G, but these injections have been almost entirely replaced by the more convenient aqueous suspensions. Oily vehicles have the disadvantage of remaining in the tissue as small, multiple cysts of clear oil, long after absorption of the active drug. Aqueous media are more compatible with physiological conditions and have the advantage of avoiding or at least minimizing the deposition in the body of foreign material. Aqueous injections usually cause less pain to the patients. Therefore, our research group[48-52] preferred the use of an aqueous medium in the development of a depot dapsone (DDS) injection in the chronic treatment of leprosy patients. In Figure 19, a representative curve of DDS (and the monoacetyl-metabolite MADDS) is given after administration of 900 mg of a sustained release i.m. injection showing an almost constant serum level of dapsone for 4 weeks, although DDS itself has an elimination half-life of about 24 hr.

Very little is known about the intramuscular absorption characteristics and kinetics

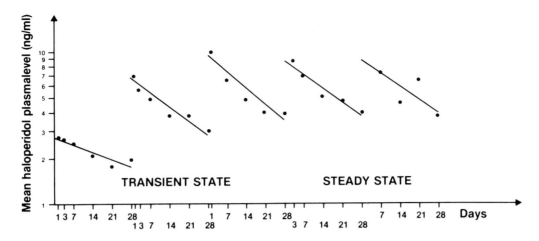

FIGURE 18.   Haloperidol plasma levels converted according to a 100-mg dose during the first 5 months with haloperidol decanoate. (From Reyntjens, A. J. M. et al., *Int. Pharmacopsychiatry,* 17, 238, 1982. With permission.)

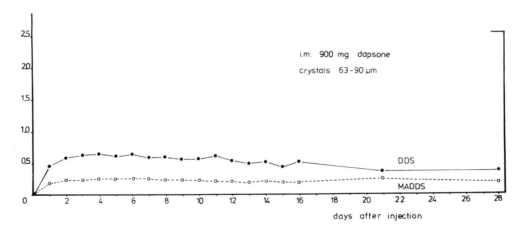

FIGURE 19.   Representative serum level curve of DDS and MADDS (µg/mℓ) during 28 days after i.m. injection of 900 mg dapsone crystals, 63 to 90 µm in an aqueous medium. (From Modderman, E. S. M. et al., in *Controlled Release Delivery Systems,* Marcel Dekker, New York, 1983, 199. With permission.)

of practically water-insoluble drugs from aqueous suspensions. Drug absorption is dependent on the initial drug concentration, injection volume, drug solubility, particle size, and the type or concentration of a macromolecular dispersing agent. With drugs of low solubility (<0.3%) the dissolution rate becomes the absorption rate limiting step. The dissolution rate of a drug can be influenced by several factors: particle size, crystallization form, viscosity of the vehicle, and injection site.[53]

Generally, duration of action is proportional to the particle size, but the size of the particles is restricted by injectability problems. The upper limit is approximately 100 µm, but this also depends on the shape of the particles and the diameter of the injection needle. The crystallization form used is another important aspect. Many drugs show polymorphism and the different crystallization forms often show different dissolution rates.

An increase in the viscosity of the suspension vehicle has two main effects. First, an

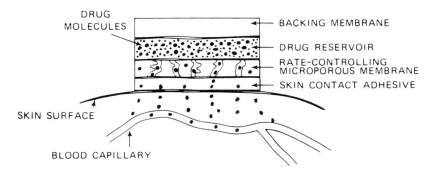

FIGURE 22. Diagram of a transdermal therapeutic system. The drug is stored in a reservoir from which it diffuses with a constant rate through a rate-controlling membrane.

the drug. The TTS-scopolamine delivers scopolamine at a rate lower than even the least permeable part of the human skin can absorb. So the system and not the skin controls the rate of drug absorption in the blood. The release kinetics are similar to those in the Ocusert® and Progestasert®. Besides scopolamine, nitroglycerin is also widely used in the present time in several controlled release transdermal systems.

In fact, nitroglycerin is an ideal candidate for this application, because it has a very short half-life (a few minutes). It passes easily through the skin and it undergoes extensive first-pass metabolism after oral administration. Topical application of a nitroglycerin ointment is not very practical and the absorption is variable. Sublingual tablets are very short-acting with large fluctuations in nitroglycerin plasma levels.

Three systems for transdermal nitroglycerin delivery are used at present: (1) a reservoir system, (2) a matrix system, and (3) a sandwich-type system. The differences between these systems in the approach to get a transdermal delivery of nitroglycerin are quite essential.[59] In the Transderm-Nitro® (Ciba) product, nitroglycerin is stored in a reservoir from which it diffuses through a rate-controlling membrane (EVAc) to the absorption site, providing a constant release of the drug (Figure 22). In Nitro-Dur® (Key), nitroglycerin is uniformly dispersed throughout a polymeric matrix through which slow diffusion of the drug occurs to the absorption site (Figure 23). The third system, Nitrodisc® (Searle), is a combination (sandwich-system) of the reservoir system and the matrix-type drug delivery system. This system is called by Searle a microsealed drug delivery system (MDD), in which nitroglycerin is dispersed throughout a solid polymer (matrix) in microcompartments serving as tiny reservoirs.[2] The drug can elute out of the MDD by first dissolution in the liquid of the reservoir, partition, and then diffusion through the polymer matrix. Recently, a new transdermal system for nitroglycerin was introduced (Deponit®).[60]

There is no consensus among experts that all systems offer real zero-order release of the drug. If the skin acts as a "perfect sink" then zero-order release is only achievable if the system contains a rate-controlling delivery mechanism such as, for instance, a rate-controlling membrane which exactly delivers the amount of the drug that is accepted by the skin. On the other hand, the great influence of the skin as the rate-limiting step in nitroglycerin absorption rather than the system's controlled delivery mechanism of nitroglycerin was recently stressed by many authors.[59-61]

In a randomized crossover study, for instance, two patches of Transderm-Nitro® (each patch = 25 mg nitroglycerin over 10 cm²) or two patches of Nitrodisc® (each patch = 16 mg nitroglycerin over 8 cm²) were applied for 24 hr on the chest of 16 adult healthy male subjects. (For product labeling see Table 8.) The mean ± SD in vivo release from each Nitrodisc® and Transderm-Nitro® was 5.4 ± 2.0 mg and 6.2 ± 1.7

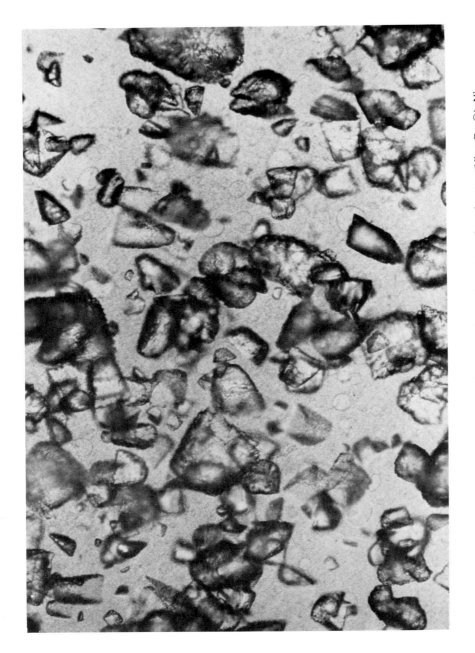

FIGURE 23.   Cross-section under the microscope of a matrix-type transdermal system (Nitro-Dur®). Nitroglycerin (a mixture with lactose) is uniformly dispersed throughout a polymer matrix. Lactose (see large crystals) is used as carrier for the nitroglycerin solution. (Magnification × 200.)

Table 8
COMPARISON OF TRANSDERMAL NITROGLYCERIN PRODUCTS

Product	Manufacturer	Surface area (cm²)	Nitroglycerin content (mg)	Nitroglycerin delivered in vivo (mg/24 hr)
Transderm-Nitro® 5	Ciba	10	25	5.0
Transderm-Nitro® 10	Ciba	20	50	10.0
Nitro-Dur® 5	Key	5	26	2.5
Nitro-Dur® 10	Key	10	51	5.0
Nitro-Dur® 15	Key	15	77	7.5
Nitro-Dur® 20	Key	20	104	10.0
Nitrodisc® 5	Searle	8	16	5.0
Nitrodisc® 10	Searle	16	32	10.0
Deponit® 5	Sanol Schwarz	16	16	5.0
Deponit® 10	Sanol Schwarz	32	32	10.0

mg, respectively.[59] Furthermore, a weak but statistically significant correlation was found between the total amount of drug released in vivo from Nitrodisc® and from Transderm-Nitro®. Bioavailability studies summarized by Chien[2], with two units of 10 cm² Transderm-Nitro® (reservoir) system, one unit of 20 cm² Nitro-Dur® (matrix) system, and one unit of 16 cm² Nitro disc® (MDD) system demonstrated that all systems maintain a mean steady state plasma level of nitroglycerin of about 0.2 to 0.3 ng/mℓ for over 24 hr.

Although the transdermal delivery systems of drugs like scopolamine, nitroglycerin, clonidine, and estradiol, can play an important role in future pharmacotherapy, a major constraint of this new application is the need for drugs that are pharmacologically potent in doses of only a few mg/day. The number of potential candidates is therefore limited.

VI. LIMITATIONS OF CONTROLLED DRUG DELIVERY

The substantial rise in the research costs of developing new chemical entities has given impetus to the development of new drug delivery systems as good alternatives in the finding of new and better drug products.

Conventional dosage forms in some cases produce large fluctuations in drug concentrations in the blood, causing subtherapeutic levels or toxic effects of some drugs. Although it is, in general, impossible to obtain a true rate-controlled drug delivery with most of the present oral dosage forms (except the osmotic pump system), there are products with a reasonable sustained release profile. The summation of the initial dose together with the maintenance doses released from such a product may produce a plasma concentration curve that imitates a zero-order release profile. Some slow-release preparations have been created only for commercial reasons and not to answer any valid therapeutic need.[62] For other drugs, the difference in clinical effectiveness between good conventional products and new controlled release products is negligible. The difference in cost between those products is a limitation for the new products, because they are usually more expensive per unit of dose.

Accidental or suicidal intoxications with sustained release products present sometimes special treatment problems. Slow release of a drug from a large amount of tablets in the gastrointestinal tract may extend the absorption over many hours. On the other hand, immediate release of the drug through failure of the "controlled" release principle may subject the body to extremely high doses of a potentially dangerous drug.

For oral drugs which are subject to metabolic degradation in the intestinal wall, a sustained or rate-controlled drug delivery in the gastrointestinal tract may cause a greater degree of enzymatic breakdown by the large increase in contact time of drug and intestinal epithelium. On some occasions, single-unit controlled release products containing drugs with ulcerogenic properties (KCl, indomethacin) may develop deep ulcers in the gastrointestinal tract.

Because of the interpatient variability of drug absorption, gastric emptying, and transit time in the small intestine, the reliability of prolonged release products is improved when the release rate is independent from patient factors. This is hardly the case in most products. Also, alterations in gastrointestinal physiology due to a number of disease states seriously affect the release of a drug in some controlled drug delivery systems. Another important limitation of some oral products is the relatively brief transit time of most drug products through the gastrointestinal tract (approximately 12 hr).

It is good to keep in mind that drug quantities released from a controlled delivery device are not automatically equal to the drug concentration in plasma. Apart from interindividual differences in transit rate and in absorption, there are also, for instance, large intraindividual variations in blood flow in the absorption area, differences in first-pass effect, and small fluctuations due to individual activities like eating, sleeping, and physical activity.

Mechanical pumps, although valuable adjuncts in therapy, have limitations because of their relative bulkiness, need for surgical removal, and relatively high cost. In contrast to some mechanical or osmotic devices, the advantages of bioerodible delivery systems are the elimination of the need for surgical removal, their small size, and potential low cost. Nevertheless, there is a risk that bioerodible products (and their degradation products) may be toxic (carcinogenic, immunogenic, or teratogenic).

Reservoir systems containing a rate-controlling membrane and loaded with excess drug within the membrane may lead to a rapid release of an overdose due to a tear or break in the membrane.

Treatment of patients with transdermal systems may lead to allergic skin reactions.

Despite these limitations, technology in the field of controlled drug delivery is moving forward at a rapidly accelerating pace, leading to new products and helping to overcome most of the limitations which at present accompany some of the controlled drug delivery systems. It is the author's view that future developments and especially clinical acceptance of new drug delivery systems will move forward step by step and will strongly need the close multidisciplinary collaboration of biomedical engineering, pharmacological, pharmaceutical, and clinical scientists.

ACKNOWLEDGMENT

The author wishes to thank Dr. Jan Zuidema and Dr. Ellen Modderman for fruitful discussions and close cooperation in the field of the development of parenteral drug delivery systems. The excellent secretarial work in preparing this manuscript of Miss Brigitte Bessems is gratefully acknowledged.

Some investigations presented in this chapter (References 48 to 52 and 55) received financial support from the chemotherapy of leprosy (THELEP) component of the UNDP/World Bank/WHO Special Programme of Research and Training in Tropical Diseases.

REFERENCES

1. Chandrasekaran, S. K., Wright, R. M., and Yuen, M. J., Controlled release, status and future prospects, in *Controlled Release Delivery Systems,* Roseman, T. J. and Mansdorf, S. Z., Eds., Marcel Dekker, New York, 1983, 1.
2. Chien, Y. W., *Novel Drug Delivery Systems, Fundamentals — Developmental Concepts — Biomedical Assessments,* Marcel Dekker, New York, 1982.
3. Walker, S. R., Ravenscroft, M. K., and Wardell, W., Trends in the development of new drugs by U.K. owned pharmaceutical companies (1964—1980), Second World Conference on Clinical Pharmacology and Therapeutics, Abstract 180, Washington D.C., 1983.
4. Struyker-Boudier, H. A. J., Rate-controlled drug delivery: pharmacological, therapeutic and industrial perspectives, *Trends Pharmacol. Sci.,* 3, 162, 1982.
5. Helfand, W. H. and Cowen, D. L., Evolution of a revolutionary oral dosage form, *Pharm. Int.,* 2, 393, 1982.
6. Ballard, B. E., An overview of prolonged action dosage forms, in *Sustained and Controlled Drug Delivery Systems,* Robinson, J. R., Ed., Marcel Dekker, New York, 1978, 1.
7. Bruck, S. D., Ed., *Controlled Drug Delivery,* Vol. I and II, CRC Press, Boca Raton, Fla., 1983.
8. Juliano, R. L., Ed., *Drug Delivery Systems,* Oxford University Press, New York, 1980.
9. Robinson, J. R., Ed., *Sustained and Controlled Release Drug Delivery Systems,* Marcel Dekker, New York, 1978.
10. Roseman, T. J. and Mansdorf, S. Z., Eds., *Controlled Release Delivery Systems,* Marcel Dekker, New York, 1983.
11. Urquhart, J., Performance requirements for controlled-release dosage forms: therapeutical and pharmacological perspectives, in *Controlled-Release Pharmaceuticals,* Urquhart, J., Ed., American Pharmaceutical Association, Academy of Pharmaceutical Sciences, Washington, D.C., 1981, 1.
12. Goldman, P., Rate-controlled drug delivery, *N. Engl. J. Med.,* 307, 286, 1982.
13. Banker, G. S., Drug products: their role in the treatment of disease, their quality and their current and future status as drug delivery systems, in *Modern Pharmaceutics,* Banker, G. S. and Rhodes, C. T., Eds., Marcel Dekker, New York, 1979, 1.
14. Yates, F. E., Benson, H., Buckles, R., Urquhart, J., and Zaffaroni, A., Designs for improved therapy through controlled delivery of drugs, in *Advances in Biomedical Engineering,* Brown, J. H. and Dickson, J., III, Eds., Academic Press, New York, 1975, 1.
15. Guy, R. H. and Hadgraft, J., Calculations of drug release rates from cylinders, *Int. J. Pharm.,* 8, 159, 1981.
16. Chandrasekaran, S. K. and Hillman, R., Heterogeneous model of drug release from polymeric matrix, *J. Pharm. Sci.,* 69, 1311, 1980.
17. Lee, P. I., Diffusional release of a solute from a polymeric matrix: approximate analytical solutions, *J. Membrane Sci.,* 7, 255, 1980.
18. Baker, R. W. and Lonsdale, H. K., Controlled release: mechanisms and rates, in *Controlled Release of Biologically Active Agents,* Tanquary, A. C. and Lacey, R. E., Eds., Plenum, New York, 1974, 15.
19. Hsieh, D. S. T., Rhine, W. D., and Langer, R., Zero-order controlled-release polymer matrices for micro- and macromolecules, *J. Pharm. Sci.,* 72, 17, 1983.
20. Hsieh, D. S. T. and Langer, R., Zero-order drug delivery systems with magnetic control, in *Controlled Release Delivery Systems,* Roseman, T. J. and Mansdorf, S. Z., Eds., Marcel Dekker, New York, 1983, 121.
21. Siegel, R. A and Langer, R., Controlled release of polypeptides and other macromolecules, *Pharm. Res.,* 1, 1, 1984.
22. Fankhauser, P., Kunststoffe für Arzneimittelabgabesysteme, *Acta Pharm. Technol.,* 28, 311, 1982.
23. Pitt, C. G. and Schindler, A., Biodegradation of polymers, in *Controlled Drug Delivery* (Vol. I), Bruck, S. D., Ed., CRC Press, Boca Raton, Fla., 1983, 53.
24. Kim, S. W., Hydrogels as drug delivery system, *Pharm. Int.,* 4, 90, 1983.
25. Lee, E. S., Kim, S. W., Kim, S. H., Cardinal, J. R., and Jacobs, H., Drug release from hydrogel devices with rate controlling barriers, *J. Membr. Sci.,* 7, 293, 1980.
26. Korsmeyer, R. W and Peppas, N. A., Macromolecular and modeling aspects of swelling-controlled systems, in *Controlled Release Delivery Systems,* Roseman, T. J. and Mansdorf, S. Z., Eds., Marcel Dekker, New York, 1983, 77.
27. Gregoriadis, G., Liposomes as drug carriers, *Pharm. Int.,* 4, 33, 1983.
28. Banker, G. S., Anderson, N. R., and Kildsig, D. O., The future of pharmacotherapeutics; trends in drugs, dosage forms and drug delivery, *Pharm. Int.,* 4, 9, 1983.
29. Widder, K. J., Senyei, A. E., and Sears, B., Experimental methods in cancer therapeutics, *J. Pharm. Sci.,* 71, 379, 1982.

30. Sieg, J. W. and Robinson, J. R., Vehicle effects on ocular bioavailability. I. Evaluation of fluor-metholone, *J. Pharm. Sci.,* 64, 931, 1975.

31. Chandrasekaran, S. K., Benson, H., and Urquhart, J., Methods to achieve controlled drug delivery, in *Sustained and Controlled Drug Delivery Systems,* Robinson, J. R., Ed., Marcel Dekker, New York, 1978, 557.

32. Bogentoft, C. and Sjogren, J., Controlled release from dosage forms, in *Towards Better Safety of Drugs and Pharmaceutical Products,* Breimer, D. D., Ed., Elsevier/North Holland, New York, 1980, 229.

33. Bechgaard, H., Critical factors influencing gastrointestinal absorption; what is the role of pellets, *Acta Pharm. Technol.,* 28, 149, 1982.

34. Weinberger, M. and Hendeles, L., The importance of the absorption characteristics of theophylline in clinical practice, in *Sustained Release Theophylline,* Merkus, F.W.H.M., Ed., Excerpta Medica, New York, 1983, 155.

35. Cabana, B., Bioequivalence and in vitro testing of drug formulations, in *Towards Better Safety of Drugs and Pharmaceutical Products,* Breimer, D. D., Ed., Elsevier/North Holland, New York 1980, 301.

36. Theeuwes, F., Elementary osmotic pump, *J. Pharm. Sci.,* 64, 1987, 1975.

37. Theeuwes, F., Oral dosage form design: status and goals of oral osmotic systems technology, *Pharm. Int.,* 5, 293, 1984.

38. Bogentoft, C., Oral controlled-release dosage forms in perspective, *Pharm. Int.,* 3, 366, 1982.

39. Chandrasekaran, S. K., Capozza, R., and Wong, P. S. L., Therapeutic systems and controlled drug delivery, *J. Membr. Sci.,* 3, 271, 1978.

40. Breimer, D. D., De Leede, L. G. J., and De Boer, A. G., New drug delivery systems as tools in clinical pharmacology, Proceedings Second World Conference on Clinical Pharmacology and Therapeutics, 1983, in press.

41. De Leede, L. G. J., De Boer, A. G., and Breimer, D. D., Rectal infusion of antipyrine with an osmotic delivery system, *Biopharm. Drug Dispos.,* 2, 131, 1981.

42. De Boer, A. G., Moolenaar, F., De Leede, L. G. J., and Breimer, D. D., Rectal administration: clinical pharmacokinetic considerations, *Clin. Pharmacokinet.,* 7, 285, 1982.

43. De Leede, L. G. J., De Boer, A. G., Van Velzen, S. L., and Breimer, D. D., Zero-order rectal delivery of theophylline in man with an osmotic system. *J. Pharmacokinet. Biopharm.,* 10, 525, 1982.

44. De Leede, L. G. J., Hug, C. C. Jr., De Lange, S., De Boer, A. G., and Breimer, D. D., Rectal and intravenous infusion of propranolol to steady-state: Kinetics and β-receptor blockade, *Clin. Pharmacol. Ther.,* 35, 148, 1984.

45. De Leede, L. G. J., Ph.D. thesis, University of Leyden, 1983.

46. Eckenhoff, B. and Yum, S. I., The osmotic pump, novel research tool for optimizing drug regimens, *Biomaterials,* 2, 89, 1981.

47. Reyntjens, A. J. M., Heykants, J. J. P., Worstenborghs, R. J. H., Gelders, Y. G., and Aerts, T. J. L., Pharmacokinetics of haloperidol decanoate, *Int. Pharmacopsychiatry,* 17, 238, 1982.

48. Modderman, E. S. M., Huikeshoven, H., Zuidema, J., Leiker, D. L., and Merkus, F. W. H. M., Intramuscular injection of dapsone in therapy for leprosy: a new approach, *Int. J. Clin. Pharmacol. Ther. Toxicol.,* 20, 51, 1982.

49. Modderman, E. S. M., Merkus, F. W. H. M., Zuidema, J., Huikeshoven, H., and Leiker, D. L., Controlled release of dapsone by intramuscular injection, in *Controlled Release Delivery Systems,* Roseman, T. J. and Mansdorf, S. Z., Eds., Marcel Dekker, New York, 1983, 199.

50. Modderman, E. S. M., Merkus, F. W. H. M., Zuidema, J., Hilbers, H. W., and Warndorff, T., Dapsone levels after oral therapy and weekly oily injections in Ethiopian leprosy patients, *Int. J. Lepr.,* 51, 191, 1983.

51. Modderman, E. S. M., Merkus, F. W. H. M., Zuidema, J., Hilbers, H. W., and Warndorff, T., Sex differences in the absorption of dapsone after intramuscular injection, *Int. J. Lepr.,* 51, 359, 1983.

52. Modderman, E. S. M., Ph. D. thesis, University of Amsterdam, 1983.

53. Ballard, B. E., Biopharmaceutical considerations in subcutaneous and intramuscular drug administration, *J. Pharm. Sci.,* 57, 357, 1968.

54. Evans, E. F., Proctor, J. D., Fratkin, M. J., Velandia, J., and Wasserman, A. J., Blood flow in muscle groups and drug absorption, *Clin. Pharmacol. Ther.,* 17, 44, 1975.

55. Modderman, E. S. M., Hilbers, H. W., Zuidema, J., Merkus, F. W. H. M., and Warndorff, T., Injection into fat instead of muscle, *N. Engl. J. Med.,* 307, 1581, 1982.

56. Cockshott, W. P., Thompson, G. T., Howlett, L. J., and Seeley, E. T., Intramuscular or intralipomatous injections?, *N. Engl. J. Med.,* 307, 356, 1982.

57. Beck, L. R., Ramos, R. A., Flowers, E., Lopez, G. Z., Lewis, D. H., and Cowsar, D. R., Clinical evaluation of injectable biodegradable contraceptive system, *Am. J. Obstet. Gynecol.,* 140, 799, 1981.

58. Shaw, J. E. and Urquhart, J., Programmed systemic drug delivery by the transdermal route, *Trends Pharmacol. Sci.,* 1, 208, 1980.
59. Karim, A., Transdermal absorption of nitroglycerin from microsealed drug delivery (MDD) system, *Angiology,* 34, 11, 1983.
60. Wolff, M., Cordes, G., and Luckow, V., In vitro and in vivo-release of nitroglycerin from a new transdermal therapeutic system, *Pharm. Res.,* 2, 23, 1985.
61. Wester, R. C., Role of skin in nitroglycerin transdermal delivery, 10th International Symposium on Controlled Release of Bioactive Materials, (Abstracts), 329, 1983.
62. Koch-Weser, J. and Schechter, P. J., Slow-release preparations in clinical perspective, in *Drug Absorption,* Prescott, L. F. and Nimmo, W. S., Eds., ADIS, New York, 1981, 217.

Chapter 3

DRUG INPUT FUNCTIONS AND BODY TRANSFER FUNCTIONS IN PHARMACOKINETICS

J. M. van Rossum, H. J. M. Snoeck, O. M. Steijger,
H. W. A. Teeuwen, J. T. W. M. Tissen, and T. J. F. van Uem

TABLE OF CONTENTS

I. INTRODUCTION

The human body may be considered as a dynamical system. It is not only reacting to inputs from the outside world, but it is also a self-organizing system, to some extent controlling its input and even controlling its environment.[1]

Obviously, a large number of linear and nonlinear feedback control systems regulating posture, movements, blood pressure, etc. is involved. To understand such a complicated system, it is logical to apply knowledge gained in systems dynamics and control theory. Recent developments in the applied mathematics of dynamical systems may greatly facilitate the study of the behavior of the body and its responses to the input of drugs.[2,3]

II. DYNAMICAL SYSTEMS THEORY OF BODY FUNCTIONING

In systems dynamics, the body can be characterized by a large number of state variables: the state vector X.[4] Depending on the type of study one does, one may consider various state variables since it is impractical to consider all possible state variables at the same time. State variables may be the blood pressure in the aorta, the core temperature, the autonomic drive to the intestine, the tension in the sensors of a muscle, the degree of muscle contraction, the hypothalamic drive on the growth hormone of the hypophysis, etc. See Figure 1.

The future state of the system depends on the present state, the memory of the system, the input, and the time. The change in the state variables is therefore a function of the state X, the time T, the memory M, and the input I:

$$\dot{X} = F(X, M, I, T)$$

This relationship may be highly nonlinear so that the differential equation cannot be solved by classic methods, but new ways of analysis have been developed.[2,3,5]

Although the system is of an extremely high dimension, it behaves as a relatively low dimensional control system. This implies that attractors are involved. In the course of time, the systems settle down to point attractors, periodic attractors (oscillation), or so-called strange attractors.[3]

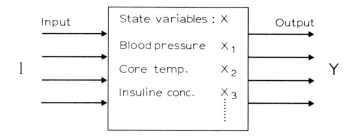

FIGURE 1.   Schematic presentation of the body as a dynamical system. Many thousands of state variables together may fully characterize the entire body behavior. Such a multidimensional dynamical system would be impossible to study were it not that attractors are involved by which the actual behavior is of a much lower dimension.

III. THE BEHAVIOR OF PHYSIOLOGICAL SYSTEMS IS DOMINATED BY ATTRACTORS

The multidimensional state space of a living system is dominated by asymptotic behavior of much lower dimension. Attractors may be considered as low dimensional subsets of the state space to which its behavior quickly settles down.[3]

In this way, the dynamical system can be visualized by its phase portrait; that is, the state space of the systems can be divided in basins, which are areas of influence of its attractors separated by lines of bifurcations or separatrices.[3,5]

The best known attractor is the point attractor. It is the steady state of a system. Garfinkel[3] recently pointed out that thinking in physiology has been dominated by point attractors; so students are still taught in medical schools the importance of homeostasis, whereas reality is much more complicated.

Periodic attractors are the basis of oscillation, which is abundant in biology (ECG, EEG, etc.). The cyclic behavior of dynamical systems on basis of periodic attractors is reasonably well understood.

The interest now is on aperiodic, chaotic, or strange attractors. A nice clarification has been given by Hofstadter.[6] Details can be found in an article by Abraham and Shaw[5] and by Ott.[7]

IV. DYNAMICAL SYSTEMS THEORY IN PHARMACOKINETICS

In pharmacokinetics one may often disregard a large number of the state variables of the system, since they are irrelevant for the understanding of the disposition of drugs in the body. The relevant state variables in pharmacokinetics are the concentration of drugs in the aorta, the central venous pool, the liver sinusoids, etc. The differential equation may even be a linear one:[8]

$$\dot{X}(t) = A \cdot X(t) + B \cdot I(t)$$

where $X(t)$ is the state vector, $I(t)$ the input vector, and A and B matrices.

If there is linearity, the differential equation can be solved:[8]

$$X(t) = \phi(t) \cdot X(o) + \phi(t) * B \cdot I(t)$$

The further behavior is completely determined by the state transition matrix $\phi(t)$, the initial state, and the input. Also the output of the system is uniquely described. The attractor of the system is a point attractor so that a constant input always leads to a steady state situation.

For a better understanding of the systems dynamics approach in pharmacokinetics and the implications of various input functions, we will first consider the subsystems of the body, which are the individual organs and tissues.

V. DYNAMICS OF SUBSYSTEMS

In contrast to the total body system, the subsystems are relatively homogeneous; therefore, only a few state variables fully characterize those systems.

A. Drug Transport in Tissues and Organs

When a drug is injected into the blood supply of a tissue or organ, the individual drug molecules may pass the tissue via quite different routes. The transit time, that is, the time from entry to exit for the individual molecules depends on the length of the pathway and whether or not the molecules enter cells surrounding the blood vessels and remain there for some time. Some molecules may leave the tissue already after a few seconds whereas others may have a much longer transit time.

Figure 2A is an illustration of a two-dimensional network of part of the wing of a bat.[9] It may be seen from this two-dimensional network that even drug molecules that do not leave the lumen of the blood vessels may have quite different transit times as some molecules may even temporarily proceed in the wrong direction. Obviously, a much larger variation may occur in all mammalian organs and tissues as the capillary network is three-dimensional and the bloodflow is not the same all the time.

B. The Density Function of Transit Times

With regard to drug transport, a tissue or organ may be characterized by a density function of transit times. This will be a continuous distribution function, since even the slightest amount of drug (say 1 μg) consists of a huge number of molecules (more than 10^{15}). For each subsystem, therefore, a density function of transit times is the characteristic transport function which dictates what occurs on the venous site when drug is offered to the arterial site. See Figure 2B.

Figure 3 is an illustration of the output concentration of brom fluorescein when given by a pulse injection to a lung lobus of a dog. The input pulse is dispersed by the subsystem analogous to the dispersion in a liquid chromatograph. In general, there is a delay or lag-time, a steep rise, a peak, and a decline. See Figures 2A and 3.[10]

Obviously, when the drug is given as a very small pulse, all drug molecules enter the tissue at the same time and the output curve is *directly* proportional to the density function of transit times. The transport function of a subsystem may therefore be regarded as the unit impulse response of that subsystem.

As an abstraction of its shape, the density function of transit times of a subsystem can be characterized by the modal transit time (the time when the peak occurs), the median transit time (the time when half the molecules have passed), and the mean transit time (MTT). See Figure 4. In addition, the volume of the subsystem (V), the bloodflow through it ($\dot{V}_B$), and, in case of elimination, the extraction ratio (E) are of importance.

In a subsystem, the central volume principle requires that the volume equals the product of the flow and the mean transit time. This principle is generally applied in circulation research.[11]

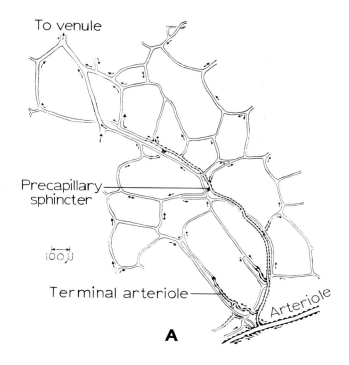

To venule

Precapillary
sphincter

100 μ

Terminal arteriole

Arteriole

A

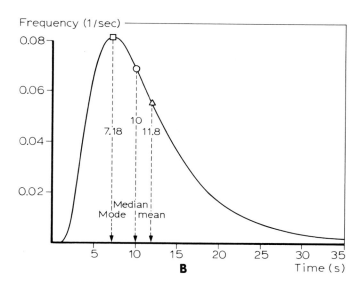

Frequency (1/sec)

0.08

0.06

0.04

0.02

7.18   10   11.8

Median
Mode   mean

5   10   15   20   25   30   35

B   Time (s)

FIGURE 2.   (A) Two dimensional capillary network of part of the
wing of a bat.[9] Molecules entering at the arterial site may pass the
network via different pathways. In addition, they may leave the capillary and remain in the cells surrounding the capillaries. Consequently
the transit time of the molecules will be distributed according to a
certain density function. (From Nicoll, P. A. and Webb, R. L., *Ann.
N. Y. Acad. Sci.,* **46,** 697, 1946. With permission.) (B) Example of a
log normal density function of transit times showing that most molecules have a transit time of about 7 sec, while some molecules may
have a very large transit time.

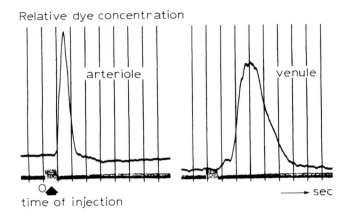

FIGURE 3.   Arterial concentration input function and the venous concentration output function of a fluorescent dye in a part of the lung. The mean transit time is ± 3 sec. (Reproduced from **Wagner, W. W.** et al., *Science,* 218, 379, 1982. With permission.)

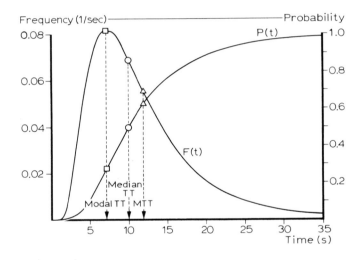

FIGURE 4.   Density function of transit times and its integral, the probability function. In this case the modal transit time is 7.2 sec, the median transit time is 10 sec, and the mean transit time is 11.8 sec. The large transit times have a considerable influence on the mean transit time.

C. Flow Vessel Analog of a Tissue

A flow vessel is a reasonably good analog of a tissue or organ. See Figure 5A. If the content of the vessel is thoroughly mixed, the drug concentration is the same in all parts of the vessel. As a result, the decrease in the concentration following a pulse input at the entrance is proportional to the concentration in the vessel. This implies that the transfer function is exponential. See Figure 5B.

$$F(t) = \frac{e^{-(t-T)/\tau}}{\tau} \quad \text{and} \quad F(s) = \frac{1}{s\tau + 1} \cdot e^{-Ts}$$

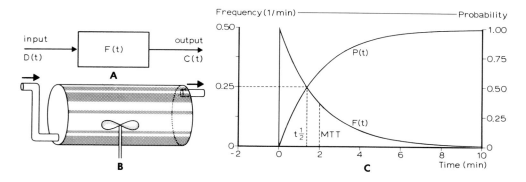

FIGURE 5. (A) Block diagram of a subsystem with simple input, simple output. (B) A good example is a flow vessel. The volume and the flow, provided that mixing is efficient, fully determine the subsystem behavior. (C) Density function of transit times of an ideal flow vessel. This function is monoexponential, so its median transit time equals the half-life time while the mean transit time is 1.44 times the half-lives. In this example the MTT = TF = 2 sec.

where τ is the time constant and T is the delay. The mean transit time of the flow vessel equals the time constant. It is interesting to note that the median transit time equals the half-life $t_{1/2}$, while the modal transit time equals the delay.

In the actual situation, the rise will be less steep and the decline not exactly exponential. The flow vessel is, however, a good model of a tissue or organ.

VI. CONTROL SYSTEM DYNAMICS OF A SUBSYSTEM

A subsystem is fully described by its transport function (F(t)), which is in fact a density function of transit times. Control systems theory can be used to understand the input-output relations. See Figures 2 and 5 and Table 1. According to conventions in systems dynamics, the input/output can be considered in the time domain as well as in the Laplace s-domain. The transport function F(t) in the time domain corresponds to the transfer function F(s) in the Laplace s-domain. See Table 1.

The relationship between the input function D(t), which is a dosage flow of drug (e.g., in μg/min), and the output function C(t), which is the concentration in the venous blood leaving the subsystem (e.g., in μg/mℓ), is governed by the transport function and the bloodflow:

$$C(t) = \frac{D(t)}{\dot{V}} * F(t) \quad \text{and} \quad F(s) = \frac{D(s)}{\dot{V}} \cdot F(s)$$

where * is the symbol of the convolution integral. See Table 1.[8,12]

If elimination in the subsystem occurs, e.g., as in the liver and the kidneys, the extraction ratio is also involved. See Table 1. In general, the output concentration is the convolution of input function and transport function in the time domain and merely the product of input and transfer function in the Laplace domain.

The transport function (that is, the density function of transit times) may resemble a log normal distribution, a gamma function, a Poisson distribution, or a sum of exponentials. The analysis is obviously best if one needs not to take into account what kind of function is involved. This implies that integral analysis, using the entire curve, is of advantage.

Table 1
SYSTEMS DYNAMICS IN A SUBSYSTEM[a]

The systems equation
  Laplace domain   Without extraction   With extraction

$$C(s) = \frac{D(s)}{\dot{V}_B} \cdot F(s) \qquad C(s) = \frac{D(s)}{\dot{V}_B} \cdot (1 - E) \cdot F(s)$$

Time domain

$$C(t) = \frac{D(t)}{\dot{V}_B} \cdot (1 - E) * F(t) = \frac{(1 - E)}{\dot{V}_B} \int_0^t D(t - \lambda) \cdot F(\lambda) \cdot dt$$

where * is the operator symbol of the convolution integral

Analysis
  Areas

$$AC = \frac{AD}{\dot{V}_B} \cdot AF \qquad AC = \frac{AD}{\dot{V}_B} \cdot (1 - E) \cdot AF$$

$$AUC = \frac{dose}{\dot{V}_B} \qquad AUC = \frac{dose}{\dot{V}_B} \cdot (1 - E)$$

  Mean times

$$TC = TD + TF \quad \text{where } TF = MTT$$

  Variance

$$VC = VD + VF$$

  Volume of distribution

$$V = \dot{V}_B \cdot MTT$$

Note: D(t) is the dosage input function (e.g., in mg/hr), F(t) is the subsystem transport function which is the density function of transit times, $\dot{V}_B$ is the bloodflow, E the extraction ratio. For the explanation of the other symbols, see Table 2. The symbol A in AC, AD, and AF stands for area under the C(t), D(t), and F(t) curve. The symbol T in TC, TD, and TF stands for the mean time of the functions C(t), D(t), and F(t). The symbol V in VC, VD, and VF stands for the variance in the functions C(t), D(t), and F(t).

[a]   Input: dosage flow in the subsystem (e.g., mg/min). Output: concentration in the blood leaving the subsystem (mg/l).

A. Analysis Of Input-Output Relations

In systems analysis, we use the statistical moments as a useful type of integral analysis, disregarding the shape of the functions involved.[13,14] See Table 1. We then obtain directly the area under the curve of the functions, the mean times, and their variance. There is a simple relationship between the moments and the so-called final value theorema of the Laplace transforms.[13,15] See Tables 1 and 2.

Whatever the input function D(t) may be, its area equals the total dose administered.

Table 2
ANALYSIS OF TRANSPORT AND TRANSFER FUNCTIONS BY STATISTICAL MOMENTS

Function

In time domain F(t)   In Laplace domain F(s)

Definition of the kth general moment:

$$m_k = \int_0^\infty t^k \cdot F(t) \cdot dt$$

For a density function of transit times

$$m_o = 1 \text{ (the area)} \qquad m_1 = TF = MTT \text{ (mean transit time)}$$

$$\text{or the expected value } E(F(t))$$

Definition of the kth central moment:

$$\mu_k = \int_0^\infty (t - m_1)^k \, C(t) \cdot dt$$

For a density function of transit times

$$\mu_0 = 1 \qquad \mu_1 = 0 \qquad \mu_2 = VF = \text{the variance}$$

Symbols used in the text

Areas

$$AF = \lim_{s \downarrow 0} F(s) = \int_0^\infty F(t) \cdot dt$$

Mean time

$$TF = -\lim_{s \downarrow 0} \frac{d \cdot \ln F(s)}{ds} = \int_0^\infty t \cdot F(t) \cdot dt/AF$$

Variance

$$VF = \lim_{s \downarrow 0} \frac{d^2 \cdot \ln F(s)}{ds^2} = \int_0^\infty t^2 \cdot F(t) \cdot dt/AF - TF^2$$

The area under the transport function is obviously equal to unity as is the case in a density function, because the integral is the probability function.

The mean time of the transport function is the mean transit time of the subsystem. The mean time of the input is the mean time for the dose to enter the subsystem. Obviously, the mean input time is zero if the dose is given as a short lasting pulse. The variance is the variance of the respective mean times.

B. Special Input Functions to a Subsystem

The Dirac δ pulse — A pulse injection is a special input, since in that case all the molecules enter the subsystem at the same moment. The output is then directly proportional to the transport function. This implies that the convolution operator then reduces to a *proportionality*. See Figure 6 and Table 3. The proportionality factor is the area under the output concentration curve. This implies that the transport function F(t) can be calculated simply by dividing the output concentration by its area under the curve following a pulse injection.

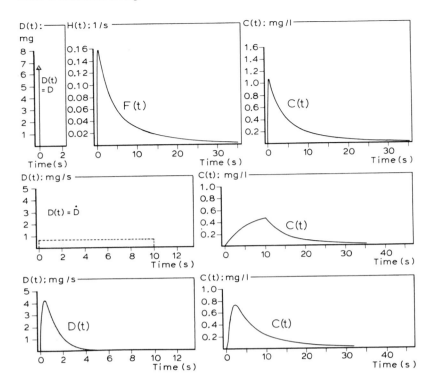

FIGURE 6.   The influence of various types of input functions on the output of a subsystem. (A) The input is a pulse or Dirac Delta function. This implies that all the molecules enter at the same time so that the output is *directly proportional* to the transport function so convolution reduces to multiplication. (B) The input is a step function or constant infusion. The output is *the integral* of the input function, so the convolution integral reduces to a simple interval. (C) Any input function. As a result the output is the convolution integral of the transport function.

Table 3
SPECIAL INPUT FUNCTIONS INTO A SUBSYSTEM

General equation

$$C(s) = \frac{D(s)}{\dot{V}_B} \cdot (1 - E) \cdot F(s) \quad \text{and} \quad C(t) = \frac{D(t)}{\dot{V}_B} \cdot (1 - E) * F(t)$$

Pulse input, Dirac delta pulse: $D(t) \rightarrow D \cdot \delta(t)$

$$C(s) = \frac{D}{\dot{V}_B} \cdot (1 - E) \cdot F(s) \qquad\qquad C(t) = \frac{D}{\dot{V}_B} \cdot (1 - E) \cdot F(t)$$

Step function input: $D(t) \rightarrow \dot{D} \cdot U(t)$

$$C(s) = \frac{\dot{D}}{s} \cdot \frac{(1 - E)}{\dot{V}_B} \cdot F(s) \qquad\qquad C(t) = \frac{\dot{D}}{\dot{V}_B} \cdot (1 - E) \int_0^t F(\lambda) \cdot d\lambda$$

Steady state situation: $t \rightarrow \infty$

Table 3 (continued)
SPECIAL INPUT FUNCTIONS INTO A SUBSYSTEM

$$C(\infty) = \frac{\dot{D}}{V_B} \cdot (1 - E)$$

Note: $\delta(t)$ = the unit impulse function. $U(t)$ = the unit step function. $C(\infty)$ = the concentration at steady state.

The step function input — A constant infusion or step function is also a special input. It may be regarded as a sequence of pulse injections of equal size applied after progressively longer periods. The convolution operator then reduces to a *normal integration*. See Figure 6 and Table 3. If the constant infusion is continued over a sufficiently long period of time, that is, long with respect to the mean transit time, the output concentration is also constant and equal to the quotient of constant dosage flow and bloodflow. See Table 3. Obviously, if extraction occurs, the output would be lowered by a factor equal to $(1 - E)$ since only that fraction passes the subsystem intact. Since the central volume principle holds, the *amount* of drug in the tissue during steady state is also constant and is equal to the product of the dosage flow and the mean transit time. See Table 3.

C. The Output in the Steady State

Depending on the dynamics of the transport function, the steady state will be reached rapidly or more slowly. The dynamics of small, highly vascularized tissues are fast as reflected by a small MTT of seconds so that the output of such a tissue practically follows the input and steady state is reached very rapidly. The dynamics of poorly vascularized tissues are much slower, in the order of several minutes, and its output will not readily follow input variation.

The dynamics of the individual tissues may vary greatly, but their dynamics are, in general, much faster than the kinetics of drugs in the entire system. The mean transit time of drugs in tissues and organs is from several seconds to several minutes, whereas the mean residence time of drugs in the total body is in the order of hours to many hours. Obviously, for the total system it is of great importance how the various subsystems as the organs and tissues are arranged. See handbooks of anatomy, e.g., Gray's.[49]

VII. THE ARRANGEMENT OF SUBSYSTEMS

In principle, the subsystems may be arranged in series or in parallel. For reasons of simplicity, we will restrict ourselves here to two subsystems with transport functions $F_1(t)$ and $F_2(t)$. For more complicated arrangements, see handbooks such as DiStefano et al.[12]

A. Subsystems in Series

If two subsystems are connected in series, the output of the first is input to the second. See Figure 7A. Consequently, the overall transport function is the convolution of the two transfer functions of the subsystems:

$$F(t) = F_1(t) * F_2(t)$$

The flow to the two subsystems is equal, so that the overall system equation can easily be written down. See Table 4.

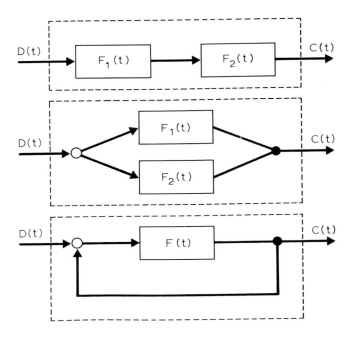

FIGURE 7.   Arrangement of subsystems. **(A)** Two subsystems in series. The overall transport function is the product of the two transfer functions. **(B)** Two subsystems in parallel. The overall transfer function is the weighted sum of the two transfer functions. **(C)** A subsystem with feedback arrangement. The output is feedback to the input site. The overall transfer function is typical for a positive feedback control system.

Table 4
ARRANGEMENT OF SUBSYSTEMS

General systems equation

$$C(s) = \frac{D(s)}{\dot{V}} \cdot F(s) \qquad C(t) = \frac{D(t)}{\dot{V}} * F(t)$$

Two subsystems in series

$$F(s) = F_1(s) \cdot F_2(s) \qquad F(t) = F_1(t) * F_2(t)$$

Analysis
Areas

$$AC = \frac{AD}{\dot{V}} \cdot AF_1 \cdot AF_2 = \frac{dose}{\dot{V}}$$

Mean times

$$TC = TD + TF_1 + TF_2 \qquad MTT = TF_1 + TF_2$$

Two subsystems in parallel

Table 4 (continued)
ARRANGEMENT OF SUBSYSTEMS

$$F(s) = f_1F_1(s) + f_2F_2(s) \qquad\qquad F(t) = f_1F_1(t) + f_2F_2(t)$$

$$(f_1 + f_2) = 1$$

Analysis
Areas

$$AC = \frac{AD}{\dot{V}} \cdot (f_1AF_1 + f_2AF_2) = \frac{dose}{\dot{V}}$$

Mean times

$$TC = TD + \frac{f_1TF_1 \cdot AF_1 + f_2TF_2 \cdot AF_2}{f_1AF_1 + f_2AF_2} = TD + f_1TF_1 + f_2TF_2$$

Note: A in AF, etc. is the symbol for area. T in TF, etc. is the symbol for mean time.

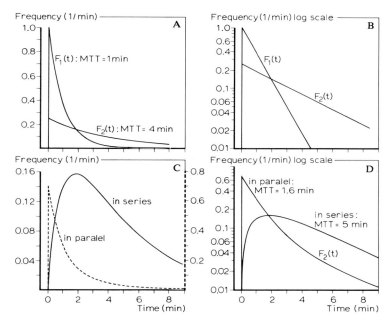

FIGURE 8. (A) Individual monoexponential transfer functions $F_1(t)$ and $F_2(t)$ with time constants of 1 and 4 min, respectively. (B) The same function on a log scale. (C) The result of the arrangement of $F_1(t)$ and $F_2(t)$ in series and in parallel. Note the great difference in the two curves. (D) The same functions on a log scale showing that the two time constants of 1 and 4 min still dominate the overall curves.

If a pulse injection is given to the first system, there is dispersion in the first, while the second system causes a further dispersion. See Figure 8. Obviously, the mean transit time of the total system equals the sum of the mean transit times of the two subsystems, and the delays in the subsystems add to a total delay.

B. Subsystems in Parallel
The input is divided over the two subsystems simultaneously dependent on their

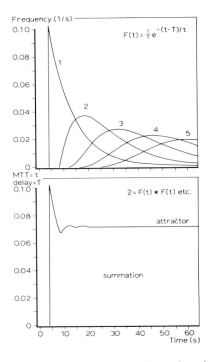

FIGURE 9. (Top) The forward path and the first nine recirculations of the feedback arrangement. The curves become flatter and the delays are added. (Bottom) The overall output is the summation of all the individual curves. Note that after a slight oscillation the curve attracts to a fixed point simply because recirculation mixing occurs very rapidly.

relative flows. The total transfer function is the weighted sum of the transfer functions of the subsystems:

$$F(t) = f_1 F_1(t) + f_2 F_2(t)$$

where f_1 and f_2 are the fractions of the flow for the two subsystems. The overall systems equation is given in Table 3. The mean transit time is also the weighted sum of the transit times of the two subsystems.

An example is given in Figure 8. For instance, if both $F_1(t)$ and $F_2(t)$ are exponential transfer functions, the overall transfer function is biexponential.

C. Subsystems in Feedback Arrangement

If the output of a subsystem is fed back to the system again, the next output is again the result of a convolution operation. Repetitive passage through the subsystem causes progressive dispersion. See Figure 9. In this figure, a pulse is given to the subsystem showing an exponential dispersion during the first pass. It is like feeding back the output of a gas chromatograph to the input. The progressive dispersion results in a constant concentration after many recirculations. See bottom of Figure 9. This is the attractor of the recirculation system following a single input. See Table 5.

It is obvious that if, during a single pass, some degree of extraction occurs, the point attractor will be zero as finally the drug leaves the system.

Table 5

A SUBSYSTEM IN FEEDBACK ARRANGEMENT

Laplace domain   Time domain

First pass

$$C_1(s) = \frac{D(s)}{\dot{V}_B} \cdot F(s) \qquad C_1(t) = \frac{D(t)}{\dot{V}_B} * F(t)$$

Second pass

$$C_2(s) = \frac{D(s)}{\dot{V}_B} \cdot F(s) \cdot F(s) \quad C_2(t) = \frac{D(t)}{\dot{V}_B} * F(t) * F_{(2x)}(t)$$

n^{th} pass

$$C_n(s) = \frac{D(s)}{\dot{V}_B} \cdot F(s)^n \qquad C_n(t) = \frac{D(t)}{\dot{V}_B} * F(t) * F(t) * \ldots$$

Summation

$$C(s) = \frac{D(s)}{\dot{V}_B} \cdot \frac{F(s)}{1 - F(s)} \qquad C(t) = C_1(t) + C_2(t) + \ldots\ldots$$

Attractor following a single dose D

$$C(\infty) = \frac{D}{\dot{V}_B} \cdot \frac{1}{MTT}$$

Note: Here a steady-state level is reached, so the attractor is a point attractor.

VIII. SYSTEMS DYNAMICS OF THE TOTAL BODY

The behavior of the total body system depends on the behavior of the subsystems and anatomical organization of the subsystems. See Figure 10.

A. Anatomical Organization of the Subsystems

The various organs and tissues of the body that receive arterial input are in essence arranged in parallel. The liver is an exception, since it is in series with the small intestines. See Figure 11. According to control systems theory,[8,12] the overall transfer function of a system consisting of subsystems arranged in parallel is an addition of the individual subsystem transfer functions. The transfer function of subsystems in series are to be multiplied.[8,12]

We have grouped together all tissues and organs that receive arterial input, while the gut and liver in series is considered as one subsystem. See Figure 12. The heart-lung system is considered as a separate subsystem that is arranged in series with the rest of the body. See Figure 12. If one injects a drug into the vena cava, molecules first pass the heart-lung system. So, if one observes the concentration in the aorta, one sees the dispersion or distortion through the heart-lung system. The drug molecules then pass on to the rest of the body, again being dispersed. Still observing in the aorta, one sees after some time again the dispersed concentration after the second pass through the heart-lungs. In essence, one sees the result of several recirculations. The concentration, however, finally dies out as during each pass through the body a certain fraction of drug is eliminated. This fraction is called the extraction ratio. In general, extraction occurs not in the heart-lung system, but in the rest of the body in which the liver and the kidneys are included. The observed concentration of drug in the aorta, when a drug

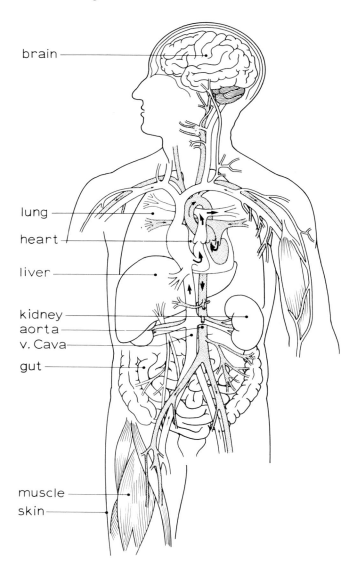

FIGURE 10.   Semischematic anatomical arrangement of organs and
tissues with their blood supply. The system is "viewed" by measuring
the concentration of a drug in the blood of the aorta or some peripheral venous observation sites.

input function is given to the vena cava, is therefore the sum of a series of convolutions
because of the recirculation. The sum of the products reduces to a simple equation
showing a positive feedback system. In fact, conventions of control systems theory
immediately let one write down the total systems equation of the systems of Figure 12.
See Table 6.

It may be emphasized here that the study of pharmacokinetics essentially deals with
the result of the recirculations. Circulation research mainly aims at the study of the
density functions of transit times of individual organs and tissues or the total system.
The circulation times of the tissues and organs is on the order of seconds to minutes,
whereas the time constants of the residence of drugs in the body are in the order of

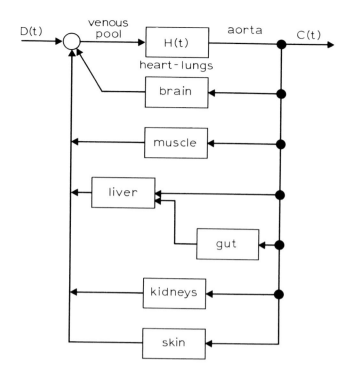

FIGURE 11. Diagram of the arrangement of the most important tissues and organs. Most tissues receive arterial blood and are therefore arranged in parallel. The blood leaving these tissues comes together in the vena cava from which it flows to the heart and the lungs. The lungs are therefore in series with the tissues of the rest of the body. An overall system equation can easily be derived. (From Van Rossum, J. M. et al., *Pharmacol. Ther.*, 21, 77, 1983. With permission.)

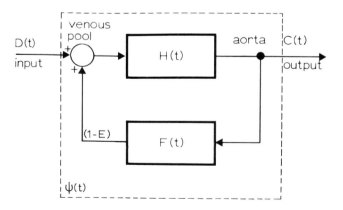

FIGURE 12. Reduced block diagram of the body. All the tissues that are arranged in series have been grouped together. In essence this results in a simple positive feedback arrangement with the lungs (H(t)) in the forward path and the tissues and organs of the rest of the body in the feedback path (F(t)).

Table 6
THE POSITIVE FEEDBACK BODY TRANSFER FUNCTION[a]

Systems equation
  Laplace domain

$$C(s) = \frac{D(s)}{\dot{V}_B} \cdot \frac{H(s)}{1 - (1 - E) \cdot F(s)H(s)} = \frac{D(s)}{\dot{V}_{cl}} \cdot \psi(s)$$

$$\text{where } \psi(s) = \frac{E \cdot H(s)}{1 - (1 - E) \cdot F(s)H(s)}$$

  Time domain

$$C(t) = \frac{D(t)}{\dot{V}_{cl}} * \psi(t)$$

Analysis
  Areas

$$AC = \frac{AD}{\dot{V}_B} \cdot \frac{AH}{1 - (1 - E) \cdot AF \cdot AH} = \frac{dose}{\dot{V}_B \cdot E} = \frac{dose}{\dot{V}_{cl}}$$

  Mean times

$$TC = TD + T\psi = TD + MRT$$

$$\text{where } MRT = TH + MTT \cdot \frac{1 - E}{E} = \frac{MTT}{E} - TF$$

$$\text{and } MTT = TF + TH$$

Note: $\psi(s)$ = the normalized overall positive feedback transfer function. $\Psi(t)$ = the total body transport function, i.e., density function of residence times. MTT = the body mean transit time, i.e., the mean time for a single pass. MRT = the body mean residence time. $\dot{V}_B$ = the cardiac output. E = the extraction ratio. $\dot{V}_{cl}$ = the clearance.

[a]   Input: dosage flow directly into the mixed venous pool. Output: drug concentration in the aorta.

hours or days. In accordance, data sampling in pharmacokinetics is not frequent, in contrast to data sampling in circulation research.

B. The Feedback Control System

The output of the aorta is fed to the rest of the body with transfer function F(t), while its output is again fed back to the mixed venous pool. The result is a positive feedback with a forward transfer function H(t) and a feedback transfer function F(t). The two in succession give the open-loop transfer function governing a single pass through the entire body. See Table 7. In essence, this is a density function of body transit times.

The closed-loop transfer function is the combination of F(t) and H(t) according to a positive feedback control system. See Table 7. From this equation, we derive the overall body transfer function by normalizing so that it, in fact, becomes a density function of residence times. The steady-state error of this positive feedback control system equals 1/E, so that the error is larger when the extraction is smaller. Needless to say, if the error is zero, the positive feedback system blows itself up.

Table 7

THE TOTAL BODY POSITIVE FEEDBACK CONTROL SYSTEM OF DRUG DISPOSITION

$H(s)$	The forward transfer function
$F(s)$	The feedback transfer function
$F(s) \cdot H(s)$	The *open*-loop transfer function
$F(t)*H(t)$	The transport function governing a single transit through the body. It therefore is a density function of the body *transit* times
$\dfrac{H(s)}{1 - (1 - E) \cdot F(s) \cdot H(s)}$	The *closed*-loop transfer function governing the repetitive transit through the body
$1/E$	The steady-state error of the closed-loop feedback system
$\psi(s)$	The normalized closed-loop transfer function obtained by multiplication with E
$\psi(t)$	The transport function governing repetitive transport through the body. It therefore is a density function of body *residence* times
E	The extraction ratio
$\dot{V}_B$	The cardiac output

C. The Total Body Transport Function $\psi(t)$

The total body transfer function is essentially a normalized positive feedback transfer function. We prefer not to include the cardiac output in the overall transfer function. As remarked, it is a normalized function obtained by multiplying the closed-loop transfer function with the extraction ratio E and at the same time multiplying the cardiac output in the numerator with E. The reason for this is that the so-called steady-state error constant of the feedback equation is $1/E$. For definition of error constants in feedback systems, see d'Azzo and Houpis.[8] Using the definition of the clearance $(\dot{V}_{el} = \dot{V}_B \cdot E)$, the overall positive feedback transfer function of Table 7 can be rewritten and transformed back to the time domain. See Tables 6 and 7.

The overall body transport function has the dimensions of a statistical density function and can be defined as a frequency distribution of *residence times*. The concentration in the aorta is the convolution of input function and this body transport function $\psi(t)$. See Table 6.

The body transport function can be calculated by deconvolution of the concentration curve with a known input function. As mentioned before, in case of pulse injection directly into the vena cava, all molecules enter the system at once. Consequently the output concentration is directly proportional to the transport function. The proportionality factor is dose/$\dot{V}_{el}$, which equals the area under the concentration curve. So, from plasma concentration curves following a rapid bolus injection, the body transport function can be obtained by dividing the concentration data by the AUC. See Figure 13.

Often i.v. plasma concentrations can be fitted to a sum of exponentials (1, 2, or 3), so that then also the transport function can be described by a sum of exponentials. It should be realized that the largest errors are made during the first minutes after injection because the first pass through the heart-lungs is very fast, while there is still a delay of some seconds. The plasma concentration curve should start at zero concentration in any case. Extrapolation to zero time therefore has little meaning. The so-called zero time concentration will strongly depend on the number of data points shortly after injection. In fact, it is the concentration at the modal transit time of the pulmonary system. Consequently, the calculation of the so-called central volume of distribution, as usually done in compartmental kinetics, is of little meaning.

D. Dependence of the Body Transport Function on Forward and Feedback Transfer Functions

If one ''observes'' the output by looking at the concentration in the aorta, the first

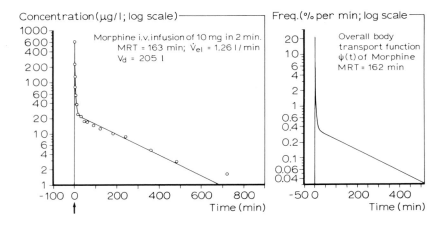

FIGURE 13.   The i.v. concentration of a short infusion of morphine in a human subject and the overall body transport function derived from the concentration curve. Calculated from data by Stanski. (From Stanski, D. R. et al., *Clin. Pharmacol. Ther.*, 24, 52, 1978. With permission.)

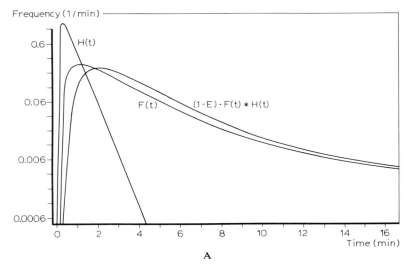

A

FIGURE 14.   (A) Theoretical transport functions of the heart lungs, (feedforward H(t)) and the rest of the body (feedback, F(t)) as well as the open loop feedback transfer function. (B) The forward path (t) and a number of recirculations which show an increasing degree of dispersion. Finally the curves reduce to zero. (C) The actual curve is the summation of the forward and all the recirculations. It is a highly damped oscillation. Irrespective of the type of H(t) and F(t) functions, the result is largely a biexponential decay curve except for the first minute or so.

pass is due to dispersion in the heart-lung system. See Figure 14A. The second pass includes convolution of H(t)*F(t)*H(t), while only a fraction (1 − E) will be seen the second time. The following passes show progressive dispersion and progressive reduction due to repetitive extraction. See Figure 14B. The observer in the aorta sees a cumulation of the first and next passes through the body. This cumulative curve relates to a overdamped oscillation. It approaches zero, because there is diminution. Compare Figure 14 with Figure 9.

Except for the initial oscillations, the curve very much resembles a biexponential

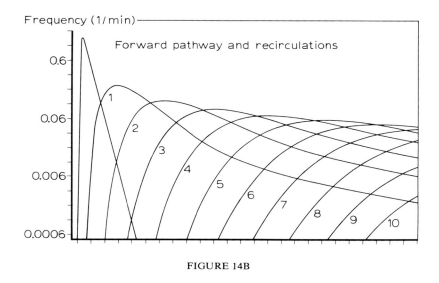

FIGURE 14B

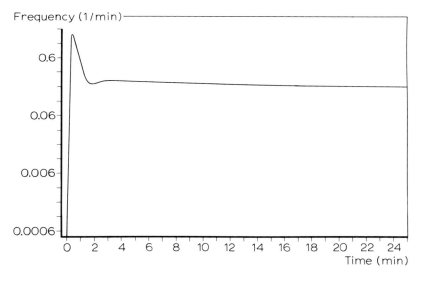

FIGURE 14C

curve. In fact, the shape of the forward and feedback transfer functions is not critical with respect to the shape of the entire output curve except during the first minutes after i.v. injection. Consequently, pharmacokinetic experiments provide little information on the forward and feedback transfer function. The importance of recirculation in pharmacokinetics has been emphasized by Vaughan[18] and Cutler.[19,20]

E. Dependence of the Body Transport Function on the Extraction Ratio

It is obvious that if the extraction were complete, no recirculation would occur, and the output would be equal to the first pass through the heart-lung subsystem. If, on the other hand, the extraction were zero, the drug would recirculate the whole life span of the body. It is evident that the extraction ratio strongly influences the profile of the body transport function. This influence is shown in Figure 15. The extraction ratio has a greater influence than the profile of the forward and feedback transfer functions because the extraction ratio determines the average number of recirculations.

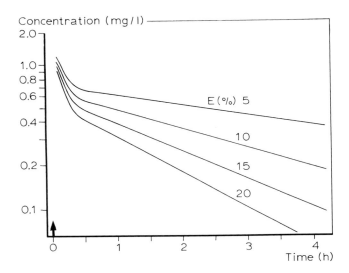

FIGURE 15. Output concentration curves of drugs with the same feedforward and feedback transfer functions as those of Figure 14, but with varying extraction rates, E. The initial concentration has been left out. The decay of the curves strongly depend on the extraction ratio.

F. Analysis of the Body Transport Function

As for the analysis of subsystems, statistical moments are the methods of choice for the analysis of the system's transport function since they are integral methods using the entire plasma concentration curve. The analysis is therefore independent of fitting data to a sum of exponentials or other polynomials.

1. Areas

The area under the plasma curve (AC = AUC) equals the areas under the input and transport functions according to the system equations (see Table 6). Realizing that the area under a density function equals 1, the AUC equals the dose divided by the clearance. It is also evident that if one estimates the AUC of the first pass through the pulmonary system, the AUC then equals the dose divided by cardiac output.

2. Mean Times

The mean times are calculated from the concentration curve and equal the sum of the mean time of the dose to enter the system and the mean residence time of the drug molecules in the system.

The mean residence time is composed of the mean times to pass the pulmonary system and the mean number of recirculations through the entire body. The mean number of recirculations depends merely on the extraction ratio ($N_{rc} = (1 - E)/E$). A mean number of recirculations of 25 means that on the average, the molecules pass the system 25 times, but some molecules may be eliminated already at the first pass while others may make more than 100 transits through the body. The mean residence time is therefore largely dependent on the mean transit time through the body and the average number of recirculations. See Tables 6 and 8A.

Approximately, the MRT equals the MTT divided by the extraction ratio. This approximation is correct if the extraction ratio is small, as is the case for most drugs. See Table 8B. The mean transit time of fenazon is in the order of 10 min, the extraction

Table 8A
PHARMACOKINETIC SYSTEM PARAMETERS

V_B = cardiac output

V_{el} = clearance

MRT = mean body residence time

MIT = mean input time

MAT = mean absorption time

E = extraction ratio

MTT = mean body transit time

V_{dss} = volume of distribution

h_a = bioavailability (fraction of dose absorbed)

N_{rc} = average number of recirculations

Relationship between system parameters
  By definition

$$\dot{V}_{el} = E \cdot \dot{V}_B \qquad V_{dss} = MTT \cdot \dot{V}_B \qquad N_{rc} = \frac{1 - E}{E}$$

Approximately, if E is less than 10%

$$MRT = MTT/E \qquad V_{dss} = \dot{V}_{el} \cdot MRT \qquad N_{rc} = 1/E$$

System parameters derived from concentration data following an i.v. pulse injection
  In general

$$AUC = \int_0^\infty C(t) \cdot dt \qquad TAUC = \int_0^\infty t \cdot C(t) \cdot dt$$

If C(t) can be fitted to a sum of exponentials

$$C(t) = \Sigma A_i \cdot e^{-t/\tau_i} \qquad AUC = \Sigma A_i \tau_i \qquad TAUC = \Sigma A_i \tau_i^2$$

Always

$$MRT = TAUC/AUC \qquad \dot{V}_{el} = D/AUC \qquad V_{dss} = \dot{V}_{el} \cdot MRT$$

and provided that the cardiac output is known:

$$E = \dot{V}_{el}/\dot{V}_B \qquad MTT = E \cdot MRT \qquad \psi(t) = C(t)/AUC$$

Table 8B
PHARMACOKINETIC SYSTEMS PARAMETERS OF SOME DRUGS

Drug	V_{el} (hr⁻¹)	MRT (hr)	V_f (ℓ)	E (%)	MTT (min)	N_{rc}	Ref.
Fluorouracil	65	0.15	9.8	22	1.8	3.5	25
Warfarin	0.32	40	12.8	0.16	2.6	624	26
Sulfinpyrazone	1.17	6.5	7.62	0.39	1.5	255	27
Thiamphenicol	9.42	2.6	24.5	3.14	4.9	31	28
Theophylline	3.54	7.85	28	1.16	5.56	84	29
Prazosin	10.4	2.8	29	3.47	5.8	28	30
Phenazon	2.17	14.5	32	0.7	6.3	142	31
Aminophenazon	22.7	1.94	44	7.6	8.8	12	32
Proquazon	43	1.9	82	14	16	6	33
Paracetamol	19.3	3.24	63	6.4	12	15	34
Phenacetin	66	1.36	89	22	15	3.5	35
Terbutaline	14	5.35	75	4.7	25	20	36
Nicotine	77	2.37	183	2.5	36	3	37

Table 8B (continued)
PHARMACOKINETIC SYSTEMS PARAMETERS OF SOME DRUGS

Drug	V_{el} (hr^{-1})	MRT (hr)	V_f (l)	E (%)	MTT (min)	N_{rc}	Ref.
Pindolol	18.8	2.94	55	6.3	11	15	38
Butobarbital	1.08	54	58	0.36	12	275	39
Lormetazepam	11.4	10.5	120	3.5	24	28	40
Caffeine	6	8	48	2	7	46	41
Dexamphetamine	21	9.8	210	7	42	13	42
Morphine	76	2.7	205	25	41	3	17
Codeine	45	4	182	15	36	6	43
Meperidine	57	3.7	209	19	42	4	44
Methadon	8	30	240	2.5	48	39	45
Fentanyl	37	3.8	141	12	28	7	46
Buprenorphine	54	2	90	15	18	5	47
Pentazocine	82	1.2	96	27	20	3	48

Note: The cardiac output $\dot{V}_B$ was assumed to be $5l \cdot min^{-1}$. V_f is the volume of distribution $\dot{V}_{el}$ the clearance, MRT the mean residence time, E the extraction, MTT the mean transit time and N_{rc} the mean number of recirculations.

ratio about 0.7%, and the mean residence time about 15 hrs. The MTT of aminophenazon is also in the order of 10 min, but its extraction ratio is about 7% and therefore its MRT is about 1.5 hr.

IX. PHARMACOKINETIC SYSTEMS PARAMETERS

Irrespective of the fitting procedures used on the plasma concentration curve, the area under the curve (AUC) and the area under the time-concentration curve (TAUC) can be obtained either by applying numerical integration methods or by analytical integrations of equations to which the data have been fitted. In fact, the AUC and TAUC are analogous to the statistical moments used to characterize statistical distribution functions.

When the drug is given by i.v. bolus or pulse injection, the plasma concentration is directly proportional to the body transport function or density function of residence times. The moment calculations applied to the plasma concentration curve is therefore a logical way of calculating kinetic systems parameters. See Tables 6 and 8. The total body clearance is directly related to the dose and to AUC. The mean residence time is by reasonable approximation equal to the quotient of TAUC and AUC.

The cardiac output in general cannot be obtained simultaneously, but could be obtained with conventional methods such as thermodilution or i.v. indicator dilution methods. The recently developed noninvasive laser Doppler methods and NMR techniques allow cardiac output determination on a larger scale. This will be very important for a better understanding of pharmacokinetics. For the moment, simultaneous cardiac output and pharmacokinetic measurements are lacking. The combined methods would also deepen the insight into the pathology of the circulation for which the MTT is a good indicator.

If the cardiac output is known, the extraction ratio and the body mean transit time can be found. The steady-state volume of distribution is approximately the product of clearance and mean residence time.

The system parameters of a number of drugs have been given in Table 8. The shortest mean body transit time is found to be in the order of 1 min. The MTT correlates

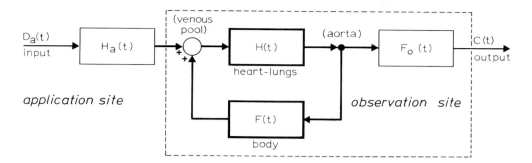

FIGURE 16. Realistic block diagram of the body transport function with input not into the venous pool, but at an application site and observation not in the aorta, but some peripheral observation site. Two additional transfer functions are involved. See Table 9.

with the volume of distribution. Drugs having a large volume, as many psychopharmacological agents, also have a relatively long MTT of 0.5 hr. For most drugs, the mean residence time is many hours because of a considerable number of recirculations.

X. CALCULATION OF THE BODY TRANSPORT FUNCTION

The profile of the body transport function $\psi(t)$ can be calculated from the plasma concentration, provided that the input function is known by the inverse operation of deconvolution:

$$\psi(t) = \dot{V}_{el} \cdot C(t) * D(t)^{-1} \quad \text{or} \quad \psi(s) = \dot{V}_{el} \cdot C(s)/D(s)$$

Several numerical methods have been developed to carry out deconvolution.[21,22]

If the input function is the Dirac delta pulse, the output is directly proportional to the transport function. Consequently, the inverse operation deconvolution is equal to division. This implies that in case of i.v. pulse injection, the transport function can be calculated by dividing the concentration curve by the area under the concentration curve. An example is given in Figure 13.

XI. INPUT FUNCTIONS OF THE BODY

As the overall body transport function is the characteristic function, fully dominating what the output will be for a given input, knowledge about the transport function is important in order to calculate what the output will be when various inputs are offered (convolution), or it can be used to calculate which input function ought to be offered when a certain output is required.

A. Input Functions at the Application Site

In general, the input function is not offered directly to the venous pool, but at some application site which may be the skin, the GI tract, a muscle, or any other location. This implies that a transport function $H_a(t)$ has to be included in the systems equation which determines the transport from application site to the venous pool. See Figure 16.

The area under this function AH_a may be less than one if some drug is lost during this transport. In fact, the $AH_a = h_a$ is the biological availability. It will also take some time to pass the $H_a(t)$ function as indicated by a mean absorption time MAT.

The output is, in general, not measured in the aorta but in a peripheral vein or at some other observation site. See Figure 16. Therefore, again a transport function $F_o(t)$ has to be included describing the transport from aorta to observation site. Often this function is very fast with respect to the total body transport function $\psi(t)$, so that it may be neglected.

The general systems equation, then, has to be extended, but the principles as discussed before remain valid. See Table 9.

B. The Intravenous Input Function

If drugs are not injected directly into the vena cava, but into a vein of the arm, the application transport function is short. A pulse input function is, however, already dispersed or distorted to some extent when the drug reaches the vena cava or mixed venous pool. The additional transfer function governing transport from injection site to mixed venous pool has no influence on the positive feedback body transfer function, except that when very fast processes are observed, as in the first passage through lungs, these may cause great errors in the output.

During passage from injection site to mixed venous pool, in general no drug is lost so that from the analysis by statistical moments, the clearance still can be calculated. The mean time from injection site to venous pool is in the order of seconds so that this transport function often may be neglected. Consequently, the overall body transport function can be obtained most easily from i.v. drug application.

The input functions usually applied by the i.v. route are the pulse or bolus injection and the step function or constant i.v. infusion.

Pulse injection — The output concentration is directly proportional to the convolution of $H_a(t)$, $\psi(t)$, and $F_o(t)$, or approximately to $\psi(t)$ alone, neglecting $H_a(t)$ and $F_o(t)$. This approximation is certainly allowed for the plasma concentration with a large mean residence time, but large errors may occur for the fast time constants of the curve, that is, just after injection.

Step function — The output concentration is the integral of the convolution of $H_a(t)$, $\psi(t)$, and $F_o(t)$. Since $H_a(t)$ and $F_o(t)$ may be neglected, in fact, the output is simply the integral of the transport function $\psi(t)$. If the infusion is continued long enough, a steady-state output concentration is obtained since the area under $\psi(t)$ is one. See Table 10.

From concentration curves during and after infusion, it is relatively easy to calculate the body transport function. See Figures 17 and 18.

XII. ANALYSIS OF INPUT FUNCTIONS AND APPLICATION SITE TRANSPORT FUNCTIONS

Once the body transport function is known by calculation from a measured output following a known i.v. input function, unknown input functions can also be calculated as well as the transport function from application site to venous pool. The general equation is (see Table 9):

$$C(t) = D(t) * \frac{H_a(t)}{\dot{V}_{el}} * \psi(t) * F_0(t)$$

So, if $\psi(t)$ is known, $D(t) * H_a(t)$ can also be obtained. An example is given for the oral intake of a capsule of quinine in Figure 17.

A. Analysis of the Application Function $H_a(t)$

From input-output studies with known $\psi(t)$, one still does not have $D(t)$ or $H_a(t)$

Table 9
SYSTEMS DYNAMICS OF DRUG APPLICATION IN GENERAL[a]

Systems equation
  Laplace s-domain

$$C(s) = \frac{D_a(s)}{\dot{V}_B} \cdot H_a(s) \cdot \frac{H(s)}{1 - (1 - E) \cdot F(s)H(s)} \cdot F_0(s)$$

$$= \frac{D_a(s)}{\dot{V}_{el}} \cdot H_a(s) \cdot \psi(s) \cdot F_0(s)$$

  Time domain

$$C(t) = \frac{D_a(t)}{\dot{V}_{el}} * H_a(t) * \psi(t) * F_0(t)$$

Analysis
  Areas

$$AC = \frac{AD_a}{\dot{V}_{el}} \cdot AH_a \cdot A\psi \cdot AF_0 = \frac{dose \cdot h_a}{\dot{V}_{el}}$$

  Mean times

$$TC = TD + TH_a + MRT + TF_0$$

$$or \quad TC = MIT + MRT$$

Special input functions
  i.v. Application

$$H_a(t) \rightarrow H_i(t) \quad and \quad h_a = 1$$

  Pulse or bolus $D(t) \rightarrow D$

$$C(t) = \frac{D}{\dot{V}_{el}} \cdot H_i(t) * \psi(t) = \frac{D}{\dot{V}_{el}} \cdot \psi(t)$$

  Step function or constant infusion $D(t) \rightarrow \dot{D}$

$$C(t) = \frac{\dot{D}}{\dot{V}_{el}} \int_0^t \psi(\lambda) \cdot d\lambda$$

  Steady state

$$C_{ss} = \frac{\dot{D}}{\dot{V}_{el}}$$

Note: h_a = the bioavailability (fraction of the dose taken up). MIT = the mean input time. $\dot{D}$ = the constant step function input, e.g., in mg/h.

[a] Input: drug dosage flow at application site.
   Output: drug concentration at observation site.

Table 10

ANALYSIS OF INPUT FUNCTIONS AND APPLICATION TRANSPORT FUNCTIONS

General systems equation (Laplace domain)

$$C(s) = D(s) \cdot \frac{H_a(s)}{\dot{V}_{el}} \cdot \psi(s) \cdot F_o(s)$$

Analysis of $H_a(s)$ from i.v. input ($D(t) = D_i$ and $H_a(s) = 1$) and pulse input ($D(t) = D_a{}^*$) at application site

$$H_a(s) = \frac{C^*(s)}{C(s)} \cdot \frac{D_i}{D_a^*}$$

when $C^*(s)$ is the concentration function of the D_a dose

$$h_a = \frac{AUC^*}{AUC} \cdot \frac{dose\ (iv)}{dose\ (a)}$$

$$TH_a = TC^* - TC$$

mean time of transport from application site to venous pool

Analysis of $D^*(s)$ from a dose as a solution (D) and a dose as a particular dosage form (D(t))

$$\frac{C^*(s)}{C(s)} = \frac{D^*(s) \cdot H_a(s) \cdot \psi(s) \cdot F_o(s)}{D \cdot H_a(s) \cdot \psi(s) \cdot F_o(s)} \qquad or \qquad D^*(s) = D \cdot \frac{C^*(s)}{C(s)}$$

$$Dose^* = Dose(sol) \cdot \frac{AUC^*}{AUC} \qquad TD^* = TC^* + TC \quad as\ TD_{sol} = 0$$

separately. If, however, D(t) is reduced to a pulse as in, for instance, the intramuscular injection of a small volume solution, the general solution reduces to:

$$C(t) = D \cdot \frac{H_a(t)}{\dot{V}_{el}} * \psi(t)$$

This implies that $H_a(t)$ then can be calculated from the output concentration, provided that $\psi(t)$ has been determined using analytical or numerical deconvolution. The analysis is summarized in Table 10 using Laplace transforms. Figure 17 shows the results of calculating $H_a(t)$ of a quinine solution. The results show that this function is certainly not a monoexponential decay curve. Swallowing a solution of a drug brings the drug practically directly to the application site, so that again $H_a(t)$ can be calculated from output concentration measurements. Figure 17 is an example for the oral intake of a quinine solution in a human subject. There is quite a variation in the transport of quinine from GI tract to the venous pool in different individuals.[23] A similar experiment for cromoglycate via input in the respiratory tract is given in Figure 18.

B. Analysis of the Input Function by Eliminating the Transport Function

The input function of an oral tablet or capsule can be calculated by a deconvolution operation on the output concentration of that tablet and a solution of the drug. This

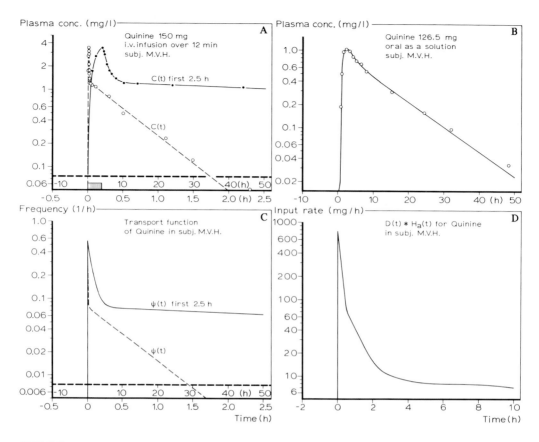

FIGURE 17.   (A) Venous concentration curves of quinine following a known input as a step function in a human subject. (B) Total body transport function of quinine as calculated from (A). (C) Venous concentration curve of a quinine solution in the same individual following an unknown input via the GI tract. (D) Input function in the GI tract calculated from the data of (C) and the transport function of (B). (Reproduced from Teeuwen, H. W. A. and Van Rossum, J. M., in preparation.)

implies that in the two experiments, the $H_a(t)$ is expected to remain the same. In essence, the $H_a(t)$ is not separated from $\psi(t)$. So, by measuring the output of a solution, one calculates $H_a(t) * \psi(t)$. A deconvolution operation on the output following the tablet using the previously found $H_a(t) * \psi(t)$ directly gives $D(t)$.

If one measures the output concentration following oral intake of a tablet and a retard preparation, obviously deconvolution does not give the input of the retard preparation. It does, however, provide a good measure of the relative performance of the two formulations. Again it is not necessary to know the body transport function nor the application site transport function as may easily be concluded from the systems equations in the Laplace domain. See Table 10.

It must be realized that it is not always possible to perform the analysis since it may occur that the application transport function is different for the two pharmaceutical dosage forms that are compared. For instance, a solution may pass immediately from stomach to duodenum, whereas the retard tablet may distribute over a different part of the GI tract.

XIII. METABOLIC INPUT FUNCTION

Most drugs are transformed in the body into metabolites which may have pharma-

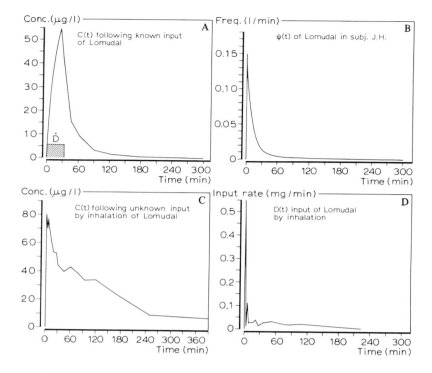

FIGURE 18.   (A) Venous concentration curve of cromoglycate in a human subject following a known input as a step function of 30 min duration. (B) Total body transport function of cromoglycate as calculated from (A). (C) Venous concentration curve following an unknown input in the respiratory tract by inhalation of cromoglycate powder. (D) Input function calculated from the data of (C) and the transport function of (B). Note a very fast and slow component in the input function. (Reproduced from Houben, J. J. G., Festen, J., Meulenberg, E., and Van Rossum, J. M., in preparation.)

cological activity. With regard to a metabolite concentration profile, the parent drug concentration is input to the metabolite transport function. See Figure 19. The system equation for the parent drug and metabolite is given in Table 11. It is evident that the two transport functions are in series. Consequently, the metabolite curve is more dispersed than the concentration curve of the parent drug. An example is given for nicotine input by smoking cigarettes and the output of nicotine and of its metabolite, cotinine. During smoking, there is a rapid uptake of nicotine in the body. Since the body transport function of nicotine is fast, the output follows the input. Consequently there is a rise and fall in the nicotine concentration with every individual cigarette smoked. See Figure 20. The body transport function of cotinine, however, is slower so that the cotinine output concentration cannot follow the input variation of nicotine. Such computational experiments demonstrate that if one desires an estimate of the daily intake of nicotine in tobacco smokers, the cotinine level should be measured instead of the nicotine concentration.

XIV. CONCLUSION

The body is a dynamical system whose future state depends on its present state and inputs to the system. In pharmacokinetics, only a limited number of state variables are sufficient to characterize the system behavior.

The various tissues and organs may be considered as subsystems. Their kinetic be-

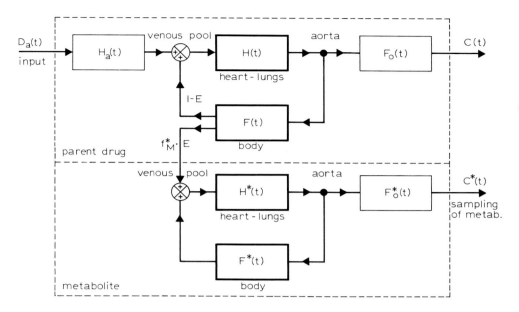

FIGURE 19. Feedback diagram for the parent drug and its major metabolite. If the metabolite concentration is observed, the parent drug concentration is input to the transport function of the metabolite, so we have the two transport functions in series. See Table 11.

Table 11
CONTROL SYSTEMS DYNAMICS OF DRUG METABOLISM[a]

Systems equation
  In Laplace domain

$$C_m(s) = D_a(s) \cdot \frac{H_a(s)}{\dot{V}_B} \cdot \frac{H(s)}{1 - (1 - E) \cdot F(s)H(s)} \cdot E \cdot f_m \cdot F(s) \cdot \frac{H_m(s)}{1 - (1 - E_m) \cdot F_m(s)H_m(s)} \cdot F_{mo}(s)$$

$$C_m(s) = D_a(s) \cdot \frac{H_a(s)}{\dot{V}_{mel}} \cdot \psi(s) \cdot f_m \cdot F(s) \cdot \psi_m(s) \cdot F_{mo}(s)$$

where $\psi(s) = \dfrac{E \cdot H(s)}{1 - (1 - E) \cdot F(s)H(s)}$ and $\psi_m(s) = \dfrac{E_m \cdot H_m(s)}{1 - (1 - E_m) \cdot F_m(s)H_m(s)}$

  In time domain

$$C_m(t) = D_a(t) * \frac{H_a(t)}{\dot{V}_{mel}} * \psi(t) * f_m \cdot F(t) * \psi_m(t) * f_{mo}(t)$$

Analysis
  Areas

$$AC_m = AD_a \cdot \frac{AH_a}{\dot{V}_B} \cdot \frac{AH \cdot AF \cdot E}{1 - (1 - E) \cdot AF \cdot AH} \cdot f_m \cdot \frac{AH_m \cdot AF_{mo}}{1 - (1 - E_m) \cdot AF_m \cdot AH_m}$$

$$AC_m = \frac{dose}{\dot{V}_{mel}} \cdot f_a \cdot f_m$$

Table 11 (continued)
CONTROL SYSTEMS DYNAMICS OF DRUG METABOLISM[a]

Mean times

$$TC_m = TD_a + TH_a + T\psi + TF + T\psi_m + TF_o$$

where $T\psi = MRT = TH + \dfrac{1 - E}{E} \cdot MTT$ and $T\psi_m = MRT_m = TH_m + \dfrac{1 - E_m}{E_m} \cdot MTT_m$

approximately $TC_m = MAT + MRT + MRT_m$

Special input functions
  i.v. pulse injection: $D(t) \rightarrow D\delta(t)$ and $f_a + 1$, $H_a(t)$ is fast

$$C_m(t) = \frac{D}{V_{el}} \cdot \psi(t) * f_m \cdot F(t) * \psi_m(t) * F_{mo}(t)$$

  i.v. constant infusion: $D(t) \rightarrow \dot{D}$ and $f_a = 1$, $H_a(t)$ is fast

$$C_m(t) = \frac{\dot{D}}{V_{mel}} \cdot f_m \int_0^t \psi(t) * F(t) * \psi_m(t) * F_{mo}(t) \cdot dt$$

Steady state $(t \rightarrow \infty)$

$$C_m(pl) = \frac{\dot{D} \cdot f_m}{V_{mel}}$$

[a] Input: parent drug dosage flow at application site.
    Output: metabolite concentration at observation site.

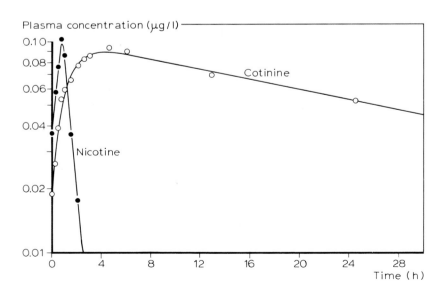

FIGURE 20.   Concentration curves of the parent drug nicotine and its major metabolite cotinine. The transport function of nicotine is fast while that of cotinine is much
slower (unpublished data).

havior is fully characterized by density functions of transit times and their bloodflow. The important subsystem parameters are the mean transit time and the bloodflow.

The total body is an arrangement of the subsystems according to a *positive* feedback control system. The open-loop feedback transfer function is a density function of body transit times, while the closed-loop transfer function is, in essence, a density function of residence times.

The important pharmacokinetic system parameters are the mean body transit time, the mean residence time, the cardiac output, the extraction ratio, the clearance, and the volume of distribution.

The overall body transport function can be found from measuring the output concentration when applying a known input function using deconvolution methods. Dosage input functions to the body, either by oral intake, intramuscular injection, or otherwise, can be found from measuring the output concentration of such an unknown input after first obtaining the body transport function.

Since the body transport function is fixed for a given individual and a given drug, a required output can only be obtained by devising the correct input function. Computational experiments may be helpful to design the adequate dosage form in order to fulfill such requirements.

REFERENCES

1. Yates, E. E., *Self-Organizing Systems,* Plenum Press, New York, 1983.
2. Abraham, R. H., Dynamical models for physiology, *Am. J. Physiol.,* 245, R467, 1983.
3. Garfinkel, A., A mathematics for physiology, *Am. J. Physiol.,* 245, R455, 1983.
4. Rosen, R., *Dynamical System Theory in Biology,* John Wiley & Sons, New York, 1970.
5. Abraham, R. H. and Shaw, C. D., *Dynamics, the Geometry of Behavior,* Vol. I, Aerial, Santa Cruz, 1982.
6. Hofstadter, D. R., Metamagical themas, *Sci. Am.,* 245, 16, 1981.
7. Ott, E., Strange attractors and chaotic motions of dynamical systems, *Rev. Mod. Phys.,* 53, 655, 1979.
8. D'Azzo, J. J. and Houpis, C. H., *Linear Control System Analysis and Design,* McGraw-Hill, New York, 1981.
9. Nicoll, P. A. and Webb, R. L., Blood circulation in the subcutaneous tissue of the living bat's wing, *Ann. N.Y. Acad. Sci.,* 46, 697, 1946.
10. Wagner, W. W., Jr., Latham, L. P., Gillespie, M. N., and Guenther, J. P., Direct measurement of pulmonary capillary transit times, *Science,* 218, 379, 1982.
11. Grodins, S., *Control Theory and Biological Systems,* Columbia University Press, New York, 1963.
12. DiStefano, J. J., Stubberub, A. R., and Williams, I. J., *Feedback and Control Systems,* McGraw-Hill, New York, 1975.
13. Churchill, R. V., *Operational Mathematics,* McGraw-Hill Kogakusha, Tokyo, 1972.
14. Papoulis, A., *Probability, Random Variables and Stochastic Processes,* McGraw-Hill Kogakusha, Tokyo, 1965.
15. Yamaoka, K., Nakagawa, T., and Uno, T., Statistical moments in pharmacokinetics, *J. Pharmacokinet. Biopharm.,* 6, 547, 1978.
16. Van Rossum, J. M., Van Lingen, G., and Burgers, J. P. T., Dose-dependent pharmacokinetics, *Pharmacol. Ther.,* 21, 77, 1983.
17. Stanski, D. R., Greenblatt, D. J., and Lowenstein, E., Kinetics of intravenous and intramuscular morphine, *Clin. Pharmacol. Ther.,* 24, 52, 1978.
18. Vaughan, D. P. and Hope, I., Applications of a recirculatory stochastic pharmacokinetic model: limitations of compartmental models, *J. Pharmacokinet. Biopharm.,* 7, 207, 1979.
19. Cutler, D. J., Properties of the recirculation model: matrix description and conditions for a monotonic decreasing single pass response, *J. Pharmacokinet. Biopharm.,* 9, 217, 1981.
20. Cutler, D. J., Properties of the recirculation model: calculation of the amount of drug in the body from blood concentration data with application to absorption rate calculations, *J. Pharmacokinet. Biopharm.,* 9, 225, 1981.

21. Veng-Pedersen, P., Novel deconvolution method for linear pharmacokinetic systems with polyexponential impulse response, *J. Pharm. Sci.*, 69, 312, 1980.
22. Vaughan, D. P. and Dennis, M., Mathematical basis of point-area deconvolution method for determining in vivo input functions, *J. Pharm. Sci.*, 67, 663, 1978.
23. Teeuwen, H. W. A. and Van Rossum, J. M., Selective high-performance liquid chromatographic method for estimating quinine levels in biological fluids, in preparation.
24. Houben, J. J. G., Festen, J., Meulenberg, E., and Van Rossum, J. M., The transport function of disodiumcromoglycate in healthy volunteers, in preparation.
25. Phillips, T. A., Howell, A., Grieve, R. J., and Welling, P. J., Pharmacokinetics of oral and intravenous fluorouracil in humans, *J. Pharm. Sci.*, 69, 1428, 1980.
26. Breckenridge, A. and Orme, M., Kinetics of warfarin absorption in man, *Clin. Pharmacol. Ther.*, 14, 955, 1973.
27. Lecaillon, J. B., Souppart, C., Schoeller, J. P., Humbert, G., and Massias, P., Sulfinpyrazone kinetics after intravenous and oral administration, *Clin. Pharmacol. Ther.*, 26, 611, 1979.
28. Azzollini, F., Gazzaniga, A., Lodola, E., and Natangelo, R., Elimination of chloramphenicol and thiamphenicol in subjects with cirrhosis of the liver, *Int. J. Clin. Pharmacol.*, 6, 130, 1972.
29. Mitenko, P. A. and Ogilvie, R. I., Pharmacokinetics of intravenous theophylline, *Clin. Pharmacol. Ther.*, 14, 509, 1973.
30. Grahnén, A., Seideman, P., Lindström, B., Haglund, K., and Von Bahr, C., Prazosin kinetics in hypertension, *Clin. Pharmacol. Ther.*, 30, 439, 1981.
31. Van Ginneken, C. A. M., *Pharmacokinetics of Antipyretic and Anti-inflammatory Analgesics: A Fundamental Kinetic Study in Men and its Clinical-Pharmacological Implications*, Ph.D. thesis, Catholic University, Stichting Studentenpress, Nijmegen, 1976.
32. Breyer-Pfaff, U., Harder, M., and Egberts, E.-H., Plasma levels of parent drug and metabolites in the intravenous aminopyrine breath test, *Eur. J. Clin. Pharmacol.*, 21, 521, 1982.
33. Hinderling, P. H. and Roos, A., Pharmacokinetics of the antirheumatic proquazone in healthy humans, *J. Pharm. Sci.*, 73, 332, 1984.
34. Rawlins, M. D. Henderson, D. B., and Hijab, A. R., Pharmacokinetics of paracetamol (acetaminophen) after intravenous and oral administration, *Eur. J. Clin. Pharmacol.*, 11, 283, 1977.
35. Raaflaub, J. and Dubach, U. C., On the pharmacokinetics of phenacetin in man, *Eur. J. Clin. Pharmacol.*, 8, 261, 1975.
36. Leferink, J. G., Lamont, H., Wagemaker-Engels, I., Maes, R. A. A., Pouwels, R., and Van der Straeten, M., Pharmacokinetics of terbutaline after subcutaneous administration, *Int. J. Clin. Pharmacol.*, 17, 181, 1979.
37. Benowitz, N. L., Jacob, P., Jones, R. T., and Rosenberg, J., Interindividual variability in the metabolism and cardiovascular effects of nicotine in man, *J. Pharmacol. Exp. Ther.*, 221, 368, 1982.
38. Gugler, R., Herold, W., and Dengler, H. J., Pharmocokinetics of pindolol in man, *Eur. J. Clin. Pharmacol.*, 7, 17—24, 1977.
39. Breimer, D. D., *Pharmacokinetics of Hypnotic Drugs: Studies on the Pharmacokinetics and Biopharmaceutics of Barbiturates and Chloral Hydrate in Man*, Ph.D. thesis, Catholic University Drukkerij Brakkenstein, Nijmegen, 1974.
40. Hümpel, M., Nieuweboer, B., Milius, W., Hanke, H., and Wendt, H., Kinetics and biotransformation of lormetazepam. II. Radioimmunologic determinations in plasma and urine of young and elderly subjects: first-pass effect, *Clin. Pharmacol. Ther.*, 28, 673, 1980.
41. Bonati, M., Latini, R., Galletti, F., Young, J. F., Tognoni, G., and Garattini, S., Caffeine disposition after oral doses, *Clin. Pharmacol. Ther.*, 32, 98, 1982.
42. Wan, S. H., Matin, S. B., and Azarnoff, D. L., Kinetics, salivary excretion of amphetamine isomers, and effect of urinary pH, *Clin. Pharmacol. Ther.*, 23, 585, 1978.
43. Rogers, J. F., Findlay, J. W. A., Hull, J. H., Butz, R. F., Jones, E. C., Bustrack, J. A., and Welch, R. M., Codeine disposition in smokers and nonsmokers, *Clin. Pharmacol. Ther.*, 32, 218, 1982.
44. Kuhnert, B. R., Kuhnert, P. M., Prochaska, A. L., and Sokol, R. J., Meperidine disposition in mother, neonate and nonpregnant females, *Clin. Pharmacol. Ther.*, 27, 486, 1980.
45. Ånggard, E., Nillson, M.-I., Holmstrand, J., and Gunne, L.-M., Pharmacokinetics of methadone during maintenance therapy: pulse labeling with deuterated methadone in the steady state, *Eur. J. Clin. Pharmacol.*, 16, 53, 1979.
46. Michiels, M., Hendriks, R., and Heykants, J., A sensitive radioimmunoassay for fentanyl, *Eur. J. Clin. Pharmacol.*, 12, 153, 1977.
47. Bullingham, R. E. S., McQuay, H. J., Moore, A., and Bennett, M. R. D., Buprenorphine kinetics, *Clin. Pharmacol. Ther.*, 28, 667, 1980.
48. Ehrnebo, M., Boreus, L. O., and Lönroth, U., Bioavailability and first-pass metabolism of oral pentazocine in man, *Clin. Pharmacol. Ther.*, 22, 888, 1977.
49. Williams, P. L. and Warwick, R., *Gray's Anatomy*, 36th ed., Churchill Livingstone, Edinburgh, 1980.

Chapter 4

SPATIAL CONTROL OF DRUG ACTION: THEORETICAL CONSIDER-ATIONS ON THE PHARMACOKINETICS OF TARGET-AIMED DRUG DELIVERY

J. F. M. Smits and H. H. W. Thijssen

TABLE OF CONTENTS

I. INTRODUCTION: SIDE EFFECTS VS. SITE EFFECTS

The assumption that an effect of a drug is in some way related to its concentration at the site of action (or receptor) forms the basis of all quantitative thinking in pharmacology. It also is the justification for considering controlled drug delivery. Thus, systemic controlled drug delivery is generally aimed at obtaining some programmed pattern of drug concentration in plasma and hence a desired pattern of drug at the receptor sites. The latter, of course, only holds if we assume that plasma levels reflect, in some way, concentrations at the site of drug action. With regard to the patterns one may want to generate, there are several options. Usually, constant controlled drug delivery is used to circumvent the fluctuations in plasma drug levels that normally occur during oral therapy and that result in temporary too high (toxic) or too low (subtherapeutic) levels of the drug.

In other therapies, these time-related inconstancies may be in fact the aim of drug delivery control. Thus, insulin used for diabetes mellitus should not be delivered in such a way that plasma levels are constant; rather, at mealtime, a peak concentration should be reached which should then gradually return to a low steady-state level. Applications of this inconstant delivery can be found in both clinical[1,2] and experimental literature[3] (see also: Struyker-Boudier et al., Chapter 7).

In the above considerations, we have only implicated one aspect of the control of drug delivery, i.e., control in the time domain. Several authors deal with that aspect of drug delivery in this book. However, besides temporal control, there is also the option of spatial control. Thus, it can be imagined that a disease or discomfort is localized at some specific site within an organism. If one would choose for a pharmacotherapeutic approach in such a case, that specific site is the target site for the drug, and drug reaching other sites is, at best, redundant. There are instances where drugs outside of the pathological process are disadvantageous and therefore unwanted. In those cases, the beneficial interaction of a drug with pathological processes may be paralleled by undesired similar interaction with nonpathological processes. If the mechanisms underlying both damaging effects are the same, it would be short-sighted to call the unwanted phenomena side effects, as they are usually referred to. In these instances, the term "site effects" gives a more accurate description of the complications. Temporal control of drug delivery will obviously not offer a solution to the occurrence of "site effects". In such cases, an attempt could and should be made to restrict the presence of the drug, and thereby its action, to the desired sites.

Localized drug delivery has, in some forms, already acquired a place in daily routine. We are all familiar with the existence of, for instance, steroid ointments for treatment of certain topical skin rashes. In this case, systemic corticosteroid therapy would never be considered because the "site effect" would be a generalized immunosuppression. Another example may be found in the use of alpha$_1$-adrenoceptor agonists as nasal decongestants. These drugs cause vasoconstriction and by their application to the nasal mucosa, they shrink that tissue. The "site effect" after systemic administration would be a general vasoconstriction, and before the nasal mucosa would be shrunk, death from severe hypertension probably would occur. As a final example, we could consider the beta$_2$-adrenoceptor agonists that are contained in some aerosols for relieving symptoms in bronchial asthma. These drugs, when inhaled, primarily cause dilation of the bronchi. However, systemic administration would result in serious "site effects" such as tachycardias and palpitations because of the chronotropic and dromotropic properties of beta-adrenoceptor agonists on the myocardium.

The above are all examples where the specific target tissues may be reached with relative ease. Unfortunately, however, this is not a general rule. In cases where the target tissue is not at the body surface, other less obvious routes of administration may be explored to get the drug at the desired site. In fact, in clinical practice numerous attempts have been made, especially in chemotherapy of neoplastic disease, to treat patients by local delivery of the drugs. What is amazing, though, is the often lacking theoretical basis for these interventions.

The present chapter will be aimed at providing a pharmacokinetic framework for thinking about localized drug delivery. It will present a simple model in which the factors contributing to possible successful attempts may be examined. Two different approaches will be discussed: one in which site-specificity may or may not be obtained through administering the drug at or near the target site and another, in which site-specificity relies upon local generation of the active substance, i.e., through the use of prodrugs. Also, theoretical implications for considering local drug therapy will be discussed.

II. SYSTEMIC VS. LOCAL DRUG DELIVERY

A. The Advantage

Before evaluating any advantage of target-directed drug delivery, we should consider how to express selectivity. In fact, there are two approaches, depending on what is aimed by target-directed delivery:

1. If the aim is to achieve higher concentrations at the target site, the advantage may be formulated as the gain in drug concentration at the target site following target-directed over systemic delivery. Such a definition is meaningful only for steady-state conditions. For nonsteady-state conditions (for instance, following a bolus injection at the target site), the advantage can be formulated as the gain in total amount of drug that passed the target organ, integrated over time.
2. If, on the other hand, the aim of target-directed drug delivery is reduction of systemic drug exposure at any given target exposure, the advantage may be formulated as the reduction in the dose that may be achieved or the reduction in the systemic bioavailability of the drug due to a first-pass extraction by the target organ.

Mathematical descriptions for the advantages formulated above have been derived from classical pharmacokinetics[4] and from physiologically based pharmacokinetics.[5,6] Both approaches lead to the same conditions for successful target-directed (i.e., intra-arterial) drug delivery. The physiological model which conceptually describes flow-related processes of drug transport and drug elimination in physiologically defined compartments[7-9] will be discussed briefly here. The base of a physiological model is a flow scheme that interconnects anatomically described organs (Figure 1). One main (nonphysiological) assumption is made: the organ is described as a well-mixed phase (or as well-mixed subphases) in which the drug concentration is proportional to the drug concentration in the efferent blood (plasma). In its simplest form, the mass balance of a drug in organ i is written as:

$$V_i \cdot \frac{dC_i}{dt} = Q_i \cdot \left(C_p - \frac{C_i}{R_i} \right) - K_i \cdot C_i \tag{1}$$

where V_i is the volume of organ i, C_i and C_p the organ and the afferent blood (plasma) concentration, respectively; Q_i is the blood flow through the organ, R_i is the drug's distribution coefficient between organ tissue and plasma at equilibrium; K_i is the clearance constant for drug elimination in the organ. A similar relationship can be given for the drug in the blood (plasma) compartment:

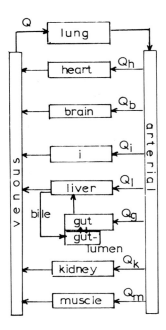

FIGURE 1.   The physiologically based pharmacokinetic model. Blood flow Q is represented by arrows and the organs or volume compartments are represented by blocks.

$$V_p \cdot \frac{dC_p}{dt} = \sum_{i=1}^{n} Q_i \cdot \frac{C_i}{R_i} - Q \cdot C_p - K_p \cdot C_p \qquad (2)$$

where Q represents total blood flow, i.e., cardiac output. Depending on the site of drug administration, the right hand terms of Equation 1 or Equation 2 have to be extended by an input function I(t), the mathematical form of which depends on the form of administration, e.g., bolus injection (pulse), infusion (step input), etc.

B. Intra-Arterial Drug Delivery

To derive mathematical expressions of the formulated advantages for intra-arterial over systemic drug delivery, we use a simplification of the physiological model, viz. the organs — with exception of the target organ (T) — are lumped together to form one compartment (Figure 2). The following expressions for steady-state C_T and C_p for intravenous and intra-arterial infusion from Equations 1 and 2 can be derived, respectively:

$$C_{p,II} = 1/R_{T,II} \times C_{T,II} = 1/R_{NT,II} \times C_{NT,II} = \frac{\text{infusion rate}}{Kp}$$

•i.v. infusion

$$C_T = \frac{Q_T \cdot R_T}{Q_T + K_T} \cdot C_p \qquad (3)$$

$$C_p = k_0 / \left(K_s + \frac{Q_T \cdot K_T}{Q_T + K_T} \right) \qquad (4)$$

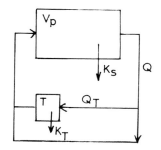

FIGURE 2. A two-compartment physiological pharmacokinetic model. V is a volume compartment, T is a tissue or target compartment. Q is the total blood (plasma) flow, i.e., the cardiac output. Q_T is the flow through the tissue compartment. K_T and K_s are clearance constants operating in T and V, respectively.

where K_s represents total body clearance of the drug outside the target organ and k_o is the constant rate infusion input.

• i.a. Infusion

$$C_T = (k_0 + Q_T \cdot C_p) \cdot R_T/(Q_T + K_T) \qquad (5)$$

$$C_p = \frac{Q_T}{Q_T + K_T} \cdot k_0 / \left(K_s + \frac{Q_T \cdot K_T}{Q_T + K_T} \right) \qquad (6)$$

$$C_{TA} = \frac{k_0}{Q_T} + C_p \qquad (7)$$

where C_{TA} is the concentration in the artery supplying the target organ. The advantage of target-directed delivery R_d at steady state as defined by approach 1 (see above) is given by:

$$R_d = C_{TAia}/C_{TAiv} \qquad (8)$$

which by substitution of Equation 6 into 7 and division by 4 leads to:

$$R_d = 1 + K_s/Q_T \qquad (9)$$

The same relationship is obtained when defining R_d as C_{Tia}/C_{Tiv}. In fact, this relationship has been shown previously by Chen and Gross.[5] An identical relationship is obtained for the ratio between the total amounts of drug delivered to the target organ following an intra-arterial or intravenous bolus injections.[4,6] The advantages according to approach 2 are described by:

$$k_{oia}/k_{oiv} = Q_T/(Q_T + K_s) \qquad (10)$$

where k_{oia} and k_{oiv} are the intra-arterial and intravenous infusion rates, respectively, needed to attain a defined steady-state drug concentration in the arterial bed supplying the target organ, and by:

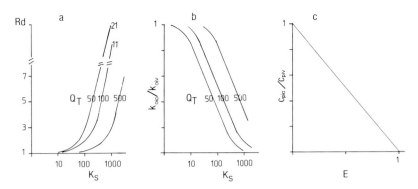

FIGURE 3.   (a) The gain R_d of target directed drug delivery as a function of Q_T (ml/min) and K_s (ml/min) (Equation 9). (b) The gain through dose reduction as a function of Q_T and K_s (Equation 10). (c) The gain as the reduction in systemic exposition, its dependency on E (Equation 11).

$$C_{pia}/C_{piv} = (1 - E) \cdot Q_T/(Q_T + K_s) \qquad (11)$$

where C_{pia} and C_{piv} are the systemic steady-state blood (plasma) concentrations following intra-arterial and intravenous infusion at a rate adjusted according to Equation 10, and E is the extraction ratio, i.e., $(C_{in} - C_{out})/C_{in}$, of the target organ.

The relationships in Equations 9 to 11 show that the only parameter that determines any advantage of target-directed (intra-arterial) drug delivery is the ratio of the blood flow, Q_T, through the target organ and the body clearance K_s of the drug. Equations 9 and 10 approach to 1 when drug clearance outside the target organ is small with respect to Q_T. Hence, under that condition, no advantage from target-directed drug delivery is to be expected at steady-state conditions according to these definitions. Advantage of intra-arterial drug delivery with respect to reduction of systemic exposure is obtained if reduction in dosing can be carried through, e.g., when K_s is high (Equation 10) or if the target organ shows a high extraction ratio. Here, Equation 11 approaches zero (an infinite advantage) when E approaches 1. The above-discussed principles are visualized in Figure 3.

In the discussion of the advantages of intra-arterial drug delivery, it is assumed tacitly that the drug distribution between organ tissue and organ venous blood remains constant (i.e., constant R), and as we have seen, the gain in the effective drug concentration within the target organ can be described by the same relationship describing the gain in arterial concentration supplying the organ, i.e., Equation 9.

However, deflection of linearity in pharmacokinetics may be the rule rather than the exception. For instance, the high drug concentration that may be obtained by intra-arterial infusion into the blood supplying the target organ might surpass the range of linearity in plasma protein binding or saturate (active) carrier systems for transport into the target organ. Second, the high intracellular concentrations that may be reached might saturate drug elimination processes in the target organ.

To evaluate the effect of saturation kinetics on the intracellular concentration, the target compartment can be divided into subcompartments. Such an approach is presented schematically in Figure 4, where, as a simplification, the target compartment is divided into a volume comprising the vascular and the interstitial space, and an intracellular space. Considering that only free drug participates in transport and elimination processes and both the compartments are well-mixed, the follwing mass-balance equations for the intracellular and vascular/interstitial space can be formulated:

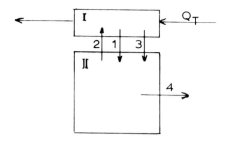

FIGURE 4. A physiological approach of the pharmacokinetics in the tissue compartment. The vascular and interstitial space are treated as one compartment, I. Compartment I is in exchange with the intracellular compartment II
via passive diffusion of free drug in (arrow 1) and out (arrow 2) and carrier-mediated or active transport inwards (arrow 3). Drug elimination occurs intracellularly (arrow 4)
according to Michaelis-Menten kinetics.

$$V_{II} \cdot \frac{dC_{II}}{dt} = K_1 \cdot C_{I,F} + \frac{T \cdot C_{I,F}}{K_T + C_{I,F}} - K_2 \cdot C_{II,F} - \frac{V_M \cdot C_{II,F}}{K_M + C_{II,F}} \tag{12}$$

$$V_I \cdot \frac{dC_I}{dt} = Q_T(C_p - C_I) - K_1 \cdot C_{I,F} - \frac{T \cdot C_{I,F}}{K_T + C_{I,F}} + K_2 \cdot C_{II,F} \tag{13}$$

where the subscripts I, II denote the vascular/interstitial and the intracellular compartment, respectively, and F denotes the free drug concentration. K_1 and K_2 are transfer
constants (vol·time^{-1}) for passive diffusion across the cellular membrane of the target
cell. T is the maximal capacity for carrier-mediated transport of free drug
(mass·time^{-1}), K_T is the free drug concentration for half maximal transport, V_M is the
maximal capacity for (intracellular) drug elimination (metabolism) with K_M as the intracellular free drug concentration for half-maximal elimination. The free drug concentration in each compartment is related to its total drug concentration according to:

$$C_F = C - \sum_{i=1}^{m} \frac{n_i \cdot P_i \cdot C_F}{K_i + C_p} \tag{14}$$

where P_i is the binding protein i, n_i is the number of binding sites on P_i with K_i as its
dissociation constant. It may be obvious that quantitative descriptions of the mass
balances are hard to give, because with the exception of the protein binding constants,
the different constants (diffusion, transport elimination, etc.) are difficult to explore
experimentally. Therefore, only a qualitative discussion of what might occur may be
given. Equations 15 to 17 describe intracellular drug concentrations under conditions
of first-order processes of transport and elimination, saturation of transport, and saturation of elimination, respectively:

$$\beta \cdot C_{II} = C_{I,F} \cdot \left(K_1 + \frac{T}{K_T}\right) \bigg/ \left(K_2 + \frac{V_M}{K_M}\right) \tag{15}$$

$$\beta \cdot C_{II} = (T + K_1 \cdot C_{I,F}) \bigg/ \left(K_2 + \frac{V_M}{K_M} \right) \tag{16}$$

$$\beta \cdot C_{II} = \frac{C_{I,F}}{K_2} \cdot \left(K_1 + \frac{T}{K_T} \right) - V_M \tag{17}$$

where β is the intracellular unbound fraction. To visualize the consequences of deviations from linear pharmacokinetics, computer simulations were performed on a DEC MINC 11 computer using THTSIM as the simulating language (THTSIM is a simulation language developed at the Technical University of Twente, Enschede, the Netherlands.[10]) The physiological model of Figure 2 in combination with the target compartment of Figure 4 was used with the following parameters (per kilogram body weight): $V = 600$ mℓ, $V_{II} = 6$ mℓ, $V_I = 0.6$ mℓ, $Q = 50$ mℓ/min, $Q_T = 0.5$ mℓ/min, $K_s = 10$ mℓ/min. For clarity, plasma protein binding was simulated for one binding site only with $P = 0.5$ mM and $K = 10$ μM (Equation 14). The intracellular protein binding was held linear, i.e., in Equations 15 to 17 β was 0.02. The parameters should be interpreted as follows: the drug distributes over the total body water and the drug's half-life is about 40 min. The volume of the target organ represents 1% of the distribution volume and the target obtains 1% of the cardiac output. Plasma protein binding is restricted to plasma albumin.

The effect of plasma protein binding on the intracellular concentration (C_{II}, Equation 15) is shown in Figures 5A and B. At the end of the 100-min i.v. infusion of 0.1 μM/min, the concentration in the vascular space of the target organ was 7.5 μM. The intracellular peak concentration was 5 μM at 2.25 hr. The unbound drug fraction in the vascular space appeared to be constant during the infusion, i.e., $f = 0.0196$ (Figure 5A). During infusion directly into the artery supplying the target tissue, total drug concentration in the vascular space reached between 140 and 195 (end of infusion) μM. The intracellular peak concentration was 220 μM at the end of the infusion (Figure 5B). The unbound drug fraction in the vascular space during the infusion time appeared to be 0.032. Thus, whereas the concentration in the vascular space increased 25-fold by target-directed delivery, the intracellular concentration rose 44-fold, reflecting the effect of the increase in the free fraction. It may be obvious that nonlinearity of plasma protein binding is of importance only for drugs that are extensively bound to plasma proteins. A decrease of the bound fraction from 0.98 to 0.96 means a doubling of the free fraction, whereas by lowering the protein bound fraction from 0.70 to 0.60, an increase of the unbound fraction of only about 30% will be observed.

The effect of saturation of carrier-mediated transport (Equation 16) is clearly demonstrated in Figure 6A and B. For clarity, the coefficient of transport by diffusion in and out of the intracellular compartment has been taken low (i.e., 0.5 mℓ/min). During intra-arterial infusion, the concentration in the vascular compartment was more than 25-fold the maximal concentration obtained following systemic infusion, i.e., 200 vs. 7.3 μM. The intracellular concentration, however, was 12 times higher only, 80 vs. 6.6 μM (Figure 6A and B).

The effect of saturation of the intracellular elimination mechanism (Equation 17) is depicted in Figures 7A and B. The extraction ratio of the target organ observed following systemic infusion was 0.3, i.e., the steady-state plasma and vascular concentrations were 10 and 7 μM, respectively. The intracellular concentration was less, 0.4 μM (Figure 7A). After intra-arterial infusion of the same amount of drug, the observed systemic concentration at steady state was 9.4 μM and the intracellular concentration was 285 μM (Figure 7B). Thus, the effect of saturation of the intracellular elimination was of two kinds: (1) the extraction of drug by the target organ declined to a minimum,

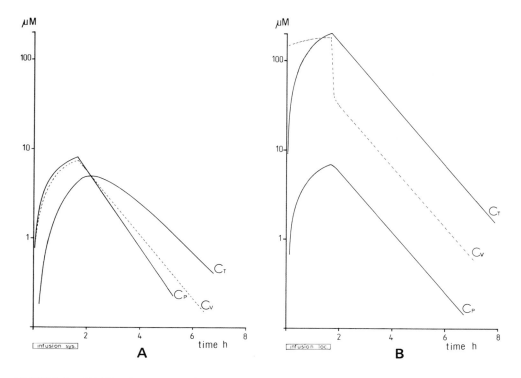

FIGURE 5. (A) The time course of drug concentrations simulated for constant rate i.v. infusion (0.1 $\mu mol \cdot min^{-1} \cdot kg^{-1}$) for 100 min. Exchange between the vascular/interstitial compartment I and the intracellular compartment II (Figure 4) was by diffusion only. Elimination by the tissue compartment was zero. The diffusion transfer constants for free drug K_1 and K_2 were 5 mℓ/min. The parameters for plasma protein binding were n = 1, [P] = 0.5 mM, K = 10 μM (Equation 14). C_p = plasma drug concentration, C_v = drug concentration in the vascular/interstitial space, C_T = intracellular drug concentration (see text for discussion). (B) As for Figure 5A, except that drug delivery was via the artery supplying the target.

i.e., hardly any differences in steady-state systemic concentration were obtained whether systemic or local drug delivery had been applied; (2) the intracellular drug concentration had increased far more than proportionally, in the present case, 700-fold.

These obvious events of saturation kinetics (Figures 5 to 7) have been discussed in some detail to illustrate that, although for particular drugs the conditions for intra-arterial drug delivery appear to be optimal[5] (cf. Equations 9 and 11), the gain of the target-directed drug delivery can be lost due to deviations from linear pharmacokinetics. For the sake of completeness, deviation from linearity may also lead to additional gain in selectivity (see Figures 5 and 7).

Let us turn back to Equation 9. According to this relationship, in steady state, there will be no benefit from intra-arterial delivery when K_s/Q_T is small. However, as long as steady state has not yet been reached, higher concentrations are delivered to the target organ by intra-arterial infusion compared to systemic delivery. For instance, after an infusion period corresponding to the drug's half-life, the concentration that is delivered to the organ at that time by local infusion is still twice the concentration that would be delivered by systemic infusion. For an infusion period of one fourth the half-life of the drug, the arterial concentration perfusing the organ following intra-arterial delivery is six times the concentration following systemic infusion. So for those drugs, the pharmacokinetics of which in terms of Equation 9 are unfavorable for steady-state intra-arterial target-directed drug delivery, intermittent short-lasting intra-arterial infusions might be worth trying (Figure 8).

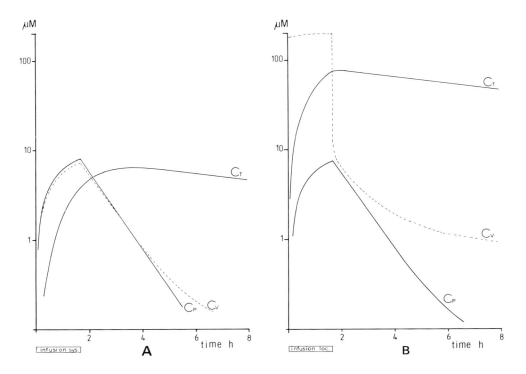

FIGURE 6.   The effect of carrier-mediated cellular drug uptake on the cellular drug concentration C_T following (A) systemic, and (B) intra-arterial infusion. Maximal capacity of transport T was 5 nmol·min⁻¹, K_T was 1 μM. K_1 and K_2 were 0.5 ml·min⁻¹. Other conditions as for Figure 5A.

C. Peritarget Drug Delivery

Another method of target-directed drug delivery is administration of the drug directly in the target or in a space, the peritarget cavity, which surrounds the target. A successful example of this method of local therapy is the well-known delivery system Ocusert® that delivers pilocarpine to the eye in the treatment of glaucoma. Also, the administration of drugs in the cerebrospinal fluid,[11] is an example of intratarget drug delivery. As was done for the intra-arterial administration, the benefit of (peri-)target drug delivery can be formulated as the gain in (peri-)target concentration as compared to systemic administration. For ease of evaluation, a simple compartment model is used, where the target compartment is in exchange with the plasma compartment via diffusion transport functions with the dimension of ml/min (Figure 9). From the mass-balance equations (Figure 9), the following equations for the steady-state concentration in the target or peritarget compartment following systemic or local delivery, respectively, can be derived:

$$C_T = R_{T,P} \cdot \frac{k_0}{K_S} \tag{18}$$

$$C_T = R_{T,P} \cdot \frac{k_0}{K_S} \cdot \left(\frac{K_{T,P} + K_S}{K_{T,P}} \right) \tag{19}$$

Thus, the gain R_d in (peri-)target tissue concentration can be given by:

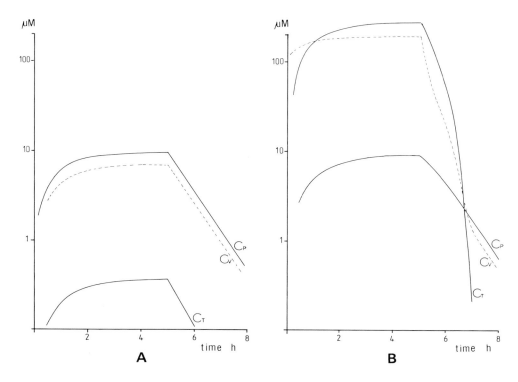

FIGURE 7. The effect of Michaelis-Menten kinetics of intracellular elimination of drug on the cellular C_T and systemic C_P drug concentration following (A) systemic, and (B) intra-arterial infusion. Conditions: exchange between the vascular/interstitial and cellular compartment was by passive diffusion, K_1 and K_2 were set at 10 m$\ell \cdot$min^{-1}. Maximal capacity of elimination V_M was 5 nmol$\cdot$min^{-1}. Constant K_M was 1 μM. Constant rate infusion of 0.1 μmol$\cdot$min^{-1}, was for 300 min.

$$R_d = 1 + \frac{K_S}{K_{T,P}} \tag{20}$$

The equation shows that the advantage of (peri-)target delivery is defined by the body clearance K_S and the transport "clearance" $K_{T,P}$ from the target into the plasma compartment. Either a high body clearance or a low transport "clearance" favors target delivery. As may be clear, Equation 20 has much in common with Equation 9 which describes the conditions for the advantage of intra-arterial over systemic drug delivery.

It may be obvious that the ideal way of target-site drug delivery would be to administer the drug directly into the extracellular space of the target organ. This situation is met by the intrathecal drug administration because of the cerebrospinal fluid and the extracellular brain space are almost a homogenous compartment.[12] Another example is the bladder. The peritoneal cavity and the pleural and pericardial spaces under certain circumstances can be looked at as the extracellular space of the target site too; for instance, when dealing with the free-floating tumor cells or small tumors within the cavity which do not have their own blood supply yet.[13] If these conditions are not met, drug delivery via such anatomical spaces is, in fact, peritarget delivery. However, in contrast to the situation described by Figure 9, the peritarget as well as the target space are in exchange with the plasma compartment by transport functions (Figure 10). The following relationships can be derived for the steady-state target drug concentration following systemic or peritarget drug delivery, respectively (Figure 10):

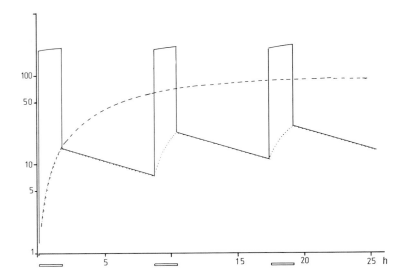

FIGURE 8.   The time course of drug concentration delivered to the target organ
(——) by intermittent intra-arterial infusion. Conditions: $Q_T = 0.5$ and $K_s =$
1 mℓ/min, t½ of drug = 7 hr, infusion period = 100 min, interval time = t½. The
dashed line (---) represents the drug concentration following continuous systemic infusion. The dotted line (...) represents drug concentration that would be delivered if intermittent infusion was performed systemically.

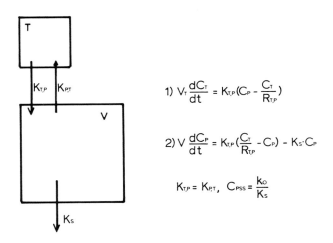

1) $V_T \dfrac{dC_T}{dt} = K_{T,P}\left(C_P - \dfrac{C_T}{R_{T,P}}\right)$

2) $V \dfrac{dC_P}{dt} = K_{T,P}\left(\dfrac{C_T}{R_{T,P}} - C_P\right) - K_s \cdot C_P$

$K_{T,P} = K_{P,T}, \quad C_{PSS} = \dfrac{k_0}{K_s}$

FIGURE 9.   A diagrammatical presentation of the interchange between the target (T) and plasma (P) compartment together with the
mass-balance equations. The subscripts T, P, SS stand for target,
plasma and steady state, respectively.

$$C_T = \frac{k_0}{K_S} \cdot \frac{K_{T,p} + K_{PT,T} \cdot R_{PT,p}}{(K_{T,p} + K_{PT,T} \cdot R_{PT,p})/R_{T,p}} = R_{T,p} \cdot C_p \qquad (21)$$

$$C_T = \frac{k_0}{K_S} \frac{K_{T,p} + K_{PT,T} \cdot R_{PT,p}\left(1 + \dfrac{K_S}{K_{PT,p}}\right)}{(K_{T,p} + K_{PT,T} \cdot R_{PT,p})/R_{T,p}} \qquad (22)$$

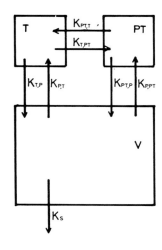

1) $V_T \dfrac{dC_T}{dt} = K_{T,P}(C_P - \dfrac{C_T}{R_{T,P}}) + K_{PT,T}(C_P - \dfrac{C_T}{R_{T,PT}})$

2) $V_{PT} \dfrac{dC_{PT}}{dt} = K_{PT,T}(C_T - \dfrac{C_{PT}}{R_{PT,T}}) + K_{PT,P}(C_P - \dfrac{C_{PT}}{R_{PT,P}})$

3) $V \dfrac{dC_P}{dt} = K_{T,P}(\dfrac{C_T}{R_{TP}} - C_P) + K_{PT,P}(\dfrac{C_{PT}}{R_{PT,P}} - C_P) - K_S \cdot C_P$

$R_{PTP} \cdot R_{T,PT} = R_{T,P}, \quad C_{PSS} = \dfrac{k_O}{K_S}, \quad C_{PTSS}/C_{PSS} = R_{PT,P}(1 + \dfrac{K_S}{K_{PT,P}})$

FIGURE 10. A schematic presentation of the interchange between the peritarget (PT), the target (T) and the plasma (P) compartment together with the relevant mass-balance equations.

The advantage R_d of peritarget drug delivery is given by:

$$R_d = \frac{K_{T,p} + K_{PT,T} \cdot R_{PT,p}\left(1 + \dfrac{K_S}{K_{PT,p}}\right)}{K_{T,p} + K_{PT,T} \cdot R_{PT,p}} \tag{23}$$

Although R_d in Equation 23 is always greater than 1, $(1 + KS/K_{PT,p} > 1)$, hardly any advantage from peritarget drug delivery is obtained if the transport from the target into the plasma compartment, $K_{T,P}$, is high with respect to the transport $K_{PT,T}$ from the peritarget space into the target.

As was discussed for the intra-arterial drug delivery, reduction in systemic exposure to a drug is achieved if by peritarget drug delivery dose reduction can be achieved or if the target organ eliminates the drug. In the latter case, the gain is proportional to $1 - E$ (Equation 11).

In general, considering the conditions for peritarget delivery being of advantage over systemic delivery, it is questionable whether this way of target-directed delivery will ever have a future. For instance, the prime condition is a low "clearance" from the peritarget space into the plasma. This condition is met for highly polar substances, e.g., methotrexate,[14] but not for lipophilic substances that easily pass membrane barriers. However, unless there are carrier-mediated or active transport systems for such a polar substance, the restricted diffusion also holds for the transport from the peritarget space into the target.

III. PRODRUGS FOR SITE-SPECIFIC DRUG DELIVERY

A. The Prodrug Concept

The term "prodrug" is used in reference to a group of substances that by themselves are inactive. Within the organism, however, they undergo a change into an active drug. This conversion may or may not be an enzymatic reaction.

Prodrugs have been recognized as such since the 1950s.[15] However, examples date back to the 19th century. Methenamine, for instance, is probably one of the oldest

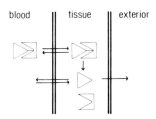

FIGURE 11. Schematic description for the generation of an active drug (D) from a prodrug. Following diffusion of the prodrug into tissue, the active drug D is generated. From there, it behaves as any drug diffusing freely over membranes. For further explanation, see text.

prodrugs. It is used as a urinary tract antiseptic agent and its action depends on the formation of formaldehyde from methenamine under acidic conditions. Another example of an old prodrug may be aspirin, which really is a prodrug for salicylic acid. However, it is still not clear whether aspirin by itself has analgesic and antipyretic properties too.

Prodrugs may be developed for a number of different purposes as diverse as improving the taste of a drug, increasing its bioavailability, extending the duration of action (or rather smoothing its release inside the organism), or obtaining a site-specific action. The general considerations in designing prodrugs for different reasons have recently been reviewed extensively.[16] In the present context, we will only deal with the possibility of obtaining some degree of site-specificity for a drug by conversion into a prodrug.

The principles governing the formation of an active drug from its prodrug are depicted in Figure 11. The prodrug as such diffuses from the bloodstream into tissues. There it undergoes the crucial change, resulting in the active drug D and, if the reaction is a cleavage reaction, the "pro"-moiety P. In the further reasoning, we will consider P to be inactive and therefore not take its pharmacokinetics into account. After formation of P and D, they may both diffuse out of the tissue, resulting in spillover into the circulation. Thereafter, they will behave like any other drug, meaning that they will distribute and eventually be eliminated from the body.

From the simple picture in Figure 11, it may be concluded that, basically, the concentration of a drug that is generated from a prodrug is going to depend on four processes:

1. Partitioning of the prodrug between blood and tissue
2. The rate of formation of the active drug from the prodrug
3. Partitioning of the active drug between tissue and blood
4. Possible elimination of the active drug directly from the target tissue, i.e., not in remote tissue

With regard to the latter process, one may think of metabolic inactivation as well as extrusion from the tissue into a space that that does not readily take part in the process of drug partitioning, e.g., into urine, for a drug which is not reabsorbed in the renal tubules, or into bile. The other three factors will be discussed in more detail below.

To examine the relative relevance of the different processes for the pharmacokinetic behavior of a prodrug with regard to its site-specificity, a model may be developed, which is a physiologically based/classical model for pharmacokinetics.[17] Although it is possible, as before, to include a large diversity of tissue compartments in the model,

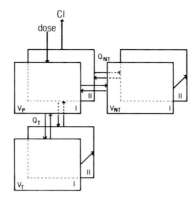

FIGURE 12. Layout of the simulation model for a prodrug behavior. The foreground describes compartments of
the prodrug in a physiological model. In the background,
the same parameters are used to simulate behavior of the
active drug. The only elimination from the foreground
model takes place in target (V_T) and nontarget compartments (V_{NT}) through first-order enzymatic reactions.

we chose here for a simpler approach to illustrate our points. The layout of the model
is shown in Figure 12. In fact, it consists of two parallel physiological models, that we
have depicted as a foreground and a background model. Each of these, in turn, consists of a blood or plasma compartment (V_P), a target tissue (V_T) and the lump sum of
nontarget tissues (V_{NT}). Both models, since they are physiological models, use the same
parameters for compartment volumes and flows Q_T and Q_{NT}. In our simulations, the
prodrug P is restricted to the foreground model. Concatenation of the two models is
accomplished by assuming that the active drug D is generated by an enzymatic reaction
in both target tissue and nontarget tissue. The rates of formation are described by the
classical Michaelis-Menten equations. After its formation, the drug D is restricted
to the background model where it behaves as any drug, being distributed and eventually eliminated. In order not to complicate the basic mathematics, we have made the
following assumptions that may be derived from Figure 12:

•   Clearance of the prodrug from the body depends entirely upon metabolic trans-
    formation, resulting in the active drug
•   Metabolism takes place only in tissue, leaving plasma as an inert means of trans-
    portation of the active drug
•   Partitioning of both the prodrug and the active drug depends on passive diffusion
    only

In this model, we did not take plasma protein binding as such into account, but rather
we used the tissue distribution coefficient R which comprises both plasma protein binding and tissue binding and which is specified for target and nontarget tissue. In the
present simulations, we assumed R to be constant.

All compartments may now be described by the mass-balance equations:

$$V_T \cdot \frac{dC_{T,I}}{dt} = Q_T \cdot \left(C_{p,I} - \frac{C_{T,I}}{R_{T,I}} \right) - \frac{V_{M,T} \cdot C_{T,I}}{K_M + C_{T,I}} \quad (24)$$

$$V_{NT} \cdot \frac{dC_{NT,I}}{dt} = Q_{NT} \cdot \left(C_{p,I} - \frac{C_{NT,I}}{R_{NT,I}} \right) - \frac{V_{M,NT} \cdot C_{NT,I}}{K_M + C_{NT,I}} \tag{25}$$

$$V_p \cdot \frac{dC_{p,I}}{dt} = Q_T \cdot \left(\frac{C_{T,I}}{R_{T,I}} - C_{p,I} \right) + Q_{NT} \cdot \left(\frac{C_{NT,I}}{R_{NT,I}} - C_{p,I} \right) \tag{26}$$

The above equations all apply to the prodrug which is nominated as I in the subscript. A similar set of equations applies to the active drug, which will be identified by the subscript II:

$$V_T \cdot \frac{dC_{T,II}}{dt} = \frac{V_{M,T} \cdot C_{T,I}}{K_M + C_{T,I}} + Q_T \cdot \left(C_{p,II} - \frac{C_{T,II}}{R_{T,II}} \right) - K_T \cdot C_{T,II} \tag{27}$$

$$V_{NT} \cdot \frac{dC_{NT,II}}{dt} = \frac{V_{M,NT} \cdot C_{NT,I}}{K_M + C_{NT,I}} + Q_T \cdot \left(\frac{C_{p,II}}{R_{NT,II}} - C_{NT,II} \right) - K_{NT} \cdot C_{NT,II} \tag{28}$$

$$V_p \cdot \frac{dC_{p,II}}{dt} = Q_T \cdot \left(\frac{C_{T,II}}{R_{T,II}} - C_{p,II} \right) + Q_{NT} \cdot \left(\frac{C_{NT,II}}{R_{NT,II}} - C_{p,II} \right) - K_p \cdot C_{p,II} \tag{29}$$

Abbreviations in the above equations are: V = volume, C = concentration, R = partitioning coefficient during steady state, Q = flow, K = clearance, V_M = maximal velocity, K_M = Michaelis-Menten constant. Subscripts: I = prodrug, II = active drug, T = target tissue, NT = nontarget tissue, P = plasma.

The above equations, although they resemble the normally used equations, are complicated in the sense that Equations 27 to 29 do not only contain terms related to the behavior of the active drug, but also to the behavior of the prodrug, in the widest pharmacokinetic sense. Therefore, only extremes resulting in approximations and simplifications can be solved by analytical mathematics. Rather, we simulated the concentration profiles on a DEC MINC 11 minicomputer, using THTSIM[10] as the simulating language (see before). Furthermore, we not only simulated steady-state infusions, but also the results of bolus injections of the prodrug into the plasma compartment. Under those conditions, we obviously cannot express selectivity in simple figures, as will also follow from simulations. Finally, it should be noted that in the following, only concentrations of the active drug were calculated because, ultimately, these are the ones that count.

As parameters in our model we used as standards:

- V_P = 2500 ml
- V_T = 500 ml
- V_{NT} = 50,000 ml
- Q_T = 50 ml/min
- Q_{NT} = 5000 ml/min
- $V_{M,NT} = V_{M,T}$ = 0.1 mmol/min
- K_M = 0.001 mM.

This means that we simulate a target tissue comprising 1% of the total body mass. It is not overperfused nor underperfused. Total enzyme activity in the target tissue equals activity in the total nontarget tissue. Note here that normally enzyme activity is expressed per tissue weight, which means here that enzyme activity is 100 × higher in target tissue than in nontarget tissue. K_M was taken arbitrarily to be 1 μM. Clearances from tissues were all taken to be 0 in the simulations in order not to complicate them. Their influences will be discussed separately.

In the following, parameters were varied systematically to study their influence on drug behavior. A division was made between infusions and injections of the prodrug, because in the former case, analytical solution of the Equations 27 to 29 is sometimes possible. For that reason, let us first compare infusion of the active drug to infusion of a very high dose and infusion of a very low dose of the prodrug.

B. Infusions of a Prodrug
1. Infusion of the Active Drug
Under this condition, one always reaches tissue levels that relate to plasma levels as:

$$C_{p,II} = 1/R_{T,II} \times C_{T,II} = 1/R_{NT,II} = \frac{\text{infusion rate}}{K_P}$$

Thus

$$\frac{C_{T,II}}{C_{p,II}} = R_{T,II} \text{ and } \frac{C_{T,II}}{C_{NT,II}} = \frac{R_{T,II}}{R_{NT,II}} \tag{30}$$

This situation was not simulated.

2. Infusion of a High Dose of a Prodrug
Infusion of a prodrug at a rate of 20 mmol/min is simulated in Figure 13. Total duration of the simulation was 10 hr. As can be seen from the figure, steady state of active drug in the target tissue is reached in approximately 2 hr, whereas both plasma and nontarget tissue reach a steady state around 6 hr after the start of the infusion. During steady state, $C_{T,II}$ is approximately 10 $\times$ $C_{p,II}$, whereas $C_{NT,II} \sim C_{p,II}$. In this situation, where the infusion rate is very high, the Equations 27 to 29 may be solved. The only condition is, in fact:

$$C_{T,I} \text{ and } C_{NT,I} >> K_M$$

If this holds, then the enzymatic reaction is saturated and Equations 27 to 29 derive to:

$$V_T \cdot \frac{dC_{T,II}}{dt} = Q_T \cdot \left(C_{p,II} - \frac{C_{T,II}}{R_{T,II}} \right) + V_{M,T} \tag{31}$$

$$V_{NT} \cdot \frac{dC_{NT,II}}{dt} = Q_{NT} \cdot \left(C_{p,II} - \frac{C_{NT,II}}{R_{T,II}} \right) + V_{M,NT} \tag{32}$$

and

$$V_P \cdot \frac{dC_{p,II}}{dt} = Q_T \cdot \left(\frac{C_{T,II}}{R_{T,II}} - C_{p,II} \right) + Q_{NT} \cdot \left(\frac{C_{NT,II}}{R_{NT,II}} - C_{p,II} \right) - K_p \cdot C_{p,II} \tag{33}$$

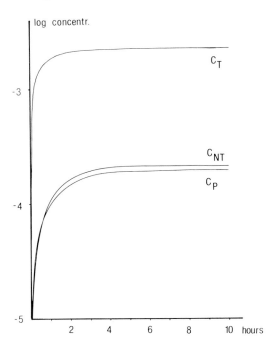

FIGURE 13.   Concentrations of active drug in plasma (C_p), nontarget (C_{NT}) and target tissue (C_T) during infusion of prodrug at a rate of 20 mmol/min. All other parameters were set at basal levels (see text). In this situation, $K_M \ll C_T$ and $K_M \ll C_{NT}$.

Under steady-state conditions, all differentials equal zero and furthermore:

$$K_p \cdot C_{p,II} = (V_{M,T} + V_{M,NT}) \tag{34}$$

Rearrangement of 31 and 32 yields:

$$Q_T \cdot \left(1 - 1/R_{T,II} \cdot \frac{C_{T,II}}{C_{p,II}} \right) + \frac{V_{M,T}}{C_{p,II}} = 0 \tag{35}$$

$$Q_{NT} \cdot \left(1 - 1/R_{NT,II} \cdot \frac{C_{NT,II}}{C_{p,II}} \right) + \frac{V_{M,NT}}{C_{p,II}} = 0 \tag{36}$$

Substitution of 34 into 35 and 36 allows calculation of

$$\frac{C_{T,II}}{C_{p,II}} = (Q_T + \overline{V}) \cdot \frac{R_{T,II}}{Q_T} \tag{37}$$

and

$$\frac{C_{T,II}}{C_{NT,II}} = \frac{Q_{NT}}{Q_T} \times \frac{R_{T,II}}{R_{NT,II}} \left(\frac{Q_T + \overline{V}}{Q_{NT} + \overline{V}}\right) \tag{38}$$

where

$$\overline{V} = \frac{V_{M,T} \cdot K_p}{V_{M,T} + V_{M,NT}}$$

Substitution of the parameters used in the simulation in Figure 13 yields:

$$\frac{C_{T,II}}{C_{p,II}} = \left(50 + \frac{0.1 \times 1000}{0.1 + 0.1}\right) \times \frac{1}{50} = 11.0$$

and

$$\frac{C_{T,II}}{C_{NT,II}} = 10.0$$

which is in accordance with results from the simulation in Figure 13.

Figure 14 shows the effect of an increase of flow through the target organ in this situation. In a physiological sense, the target organ would be a tissue receiving a high percentage of the cardiac output, e.g., brain, kidneys, or lungs. Increasing Q_T by a factor of 10, both increases $C_{p,II}$ and $C_{NT,II}$, whereas it decreases $C_{T,II}$. This results in a ratio:

$$\frac{C_{T,II}}{C_{p,II}} = 1.82$$

which corresponds to the outcome of Equation 37 after substitution of the new values. The reduced ratio seems to be logical, because input into the target tissue has remained constant ($V_{M,T}$) but the active drug is simply washed out at a higher rate.

Figure 15 shows the effect of a tenfold increase in K_p. Thus, clearance of the active drug is increased drastically. The increase in K_p leads to an increase of $\overline{V}$, thus increasing $C_{T,II}/C_{p,II}$. The increase is tenfold. Because in Equation 37 the influence of an increase of V is greater in the numerator than in the denominator (because $Q_T < Q_{NT}$), the ratio $C_{T,II}/C_{NT,II}$ also increases as again evidenced in the figure. The effect of a change of K_p will, however, diminish with decreasing ratio between Q_{NT} and Q_T.

Finally, in Figure 16 we simulated a 100-fold reduction of $V_{M,NT}$. This would mean, in our model, that the measured enzymatic activity in the target tissue would be $10^4 \times$ the activity in nontarget tissue. Both ratios do now increase, although $C_{T,II}$ remains almost constant. If we would assume $V_{M,NT} = 0$, i.e., enzymatic activity would be confined to the target organ only, then Equation 37 would derive to:

$$\frac{C_{T,II}}{C_{p,II}} = (Q_T + K_p) \cdot \frac{R_{T,II}}{Q_T} = R_{T,II} \cdot \left(1 + \frac{K_p}{Q_T}\right) \tag{39}$$

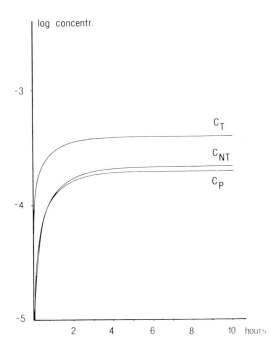

FIGURE 14.   Concentrations of active drug in plasma (C_P), nontarget (C_{NT}) and target tissue (C_T) during infusion of prodrug at a rate of 20 mmol/min. The flow through the target tissue (Q_T) was increased tenfold as compared to Figure 13. All other parameters were set at basal levels (see text).

and

$$\frac{C_{T,II}}{C_{NT,II}} = \frac{R_{T,II}}{R_{NT,II}} \tag{40}$$

In other words, as before with intra-arterial infusion, in this situation the ratio between target tissue and plasma concentration is dependent on the ratio between plasma clearance and organ blood flow (cf. Equation 9).

3. Infusion of a Low Dose of a Prodrug

If $C_{T,I}$ and $C_{NT,I}$ are not high as compared to K_M, analytical solution of Equations 24 to 29 is no longer possible. Figures 17 and 18 show simulations of infusions of doses that are 0.01 and 0.0001 times smaller, respectively, than the one in Figure 13, whereas all other parameters were identical. During the simulated 10-hr infusion period steady state is not reached. In Figure 17, $C_{T,I}$ at 10 hr was $0.7 \times K_M$, whereas in Figure 18, $C_{T,I}$ at this time was approximately $0.004 \times K_M$. Thus, in the latter situation delivery of active drug was almost purely first-order ($V_{M,T}/K_M \times C_{T,I}$, if $C_{T,I} \ll K_M$) whereas in the situation in Figure 17, the delivery was neither zero- nor first-order

$$\frac{V_{M,T} \cdot C_{T,I}}{K_M + C_{T,I}}$$

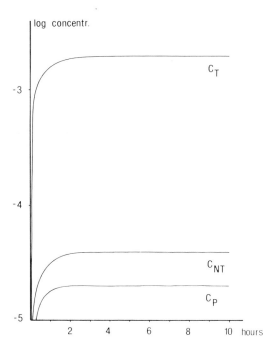

FIGURE 15. Concentrations of active drug in plasma (C_p), nontarget (C_{NT}), and target tissue (C_T) during infusion of prodrug at a rate of 20 mmol/min. Clearance of the active drug (K_p) was increased tenfold as compared to Figure 13. All other parameters were set at basal levels (see text).

Extension of the simulation period by 90 hr resulted in ratios

$$\frac{C_{T,II}}{C_{p,II}} = 10.7 \text{ for infusion of 0.2 mmol/min and}$$

$$\frac{C_{T,II}}{C_{p,II}} = 6.4 \text{ during the infusion of 0.002 mmol/min.}$$

In the latter case, an almost perfect steady state was reached by this time. However, during infusion of the intermediate dose, steady state was not achieved in the first 100 hr. The reason for this is that during low-dose infusion, generation of the active drug follows first-order kinetics, as long as $C_{T,I} \ll K_M$. During high-dose infusion, zero-order formation of the active drug is to be expected. Thus, in the intermediate range where $C_{T,I} \sim K_M$, saturation of formation starts to occur and, with it, saturation of elimination of the prodrug. Hence, $C_{T,I}$ will increase and a situation where $C_{T,I} \gg K_M$ is inevitable.

C. Bolus Injections of a Prodrug

At first sight, site-specific drug delivery should also be possible, using bolus administration of a prodrug. This would, in fact, be the most charming aspect of the concept, meaning that during everyday therapy, patients would be able to accomplish site-specific therapy by simply taking a prodrug pill. An analysis of the principles governing drug distribution after bolus injection of a prodrug has been presented before.[17] However, these authors only compared calculated areas under the concentration-time curves to evaluate specificity. As stated before, in our view, this is not a generally ade-

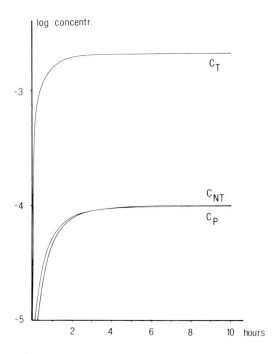

FIGURE 16.   Concentrations of active drug in plasma (C_p), nontarget (C_{NT}) and target tissue (C_T) during infusion of prodrug at a rate of 20 mmol/min. $V_{M,T}$ was kept constant, whereas $V_{M,NT}$ was reduced tenfold as compared to Figure 13. All other parameters were set at basal levels (see text).

quate approach to express selectivity or specificity. Therefore, we carried out a number of simulations in our model for pharmacokinetics of prodrugs. We did not consider oral administration of the prodrug, but rather we simulated the kinetics of intravenously given bolus injections.

1. Effects of Varying the Dose of the Prodrug

Figures 19A to D illustrate the behavior of the active drug after administration of, respectively, 500, 50, 5, and 0.5 mmol of the prodrug. All parameters in the model were set at their "normal" values. When comparing Figures 19A to D, a number of things may be noted. First of all, peak levels reached in plasma and tissues do not relate linearly to the doses. Although increasing the dose from 0.5 to 5 mmol increases peak levels tenfold, further increases in the dose increase peak levels much less. Second, half-lives of the active drug diminish with increasing dose. Finally, at the end of the simulations, the ratios between $C_{T,II}$ and $C_{p,II}$ also increase with dose from 5.4 after injection of 0.5 mmol, to 10.8 after 500 mmol.

The explanation for the above phenomena depends, again, on the rate of the enzymatic conversion. Thus, after a high dose, the level of prodrug in tissue becomes so high that throughout the 10-hr period, the condition $C_{NT,I}$ and $C_{T,I} \gg K_m$ holds. Comparing Figures 19A and 13 confirms this idea, and really we obtain a zero-order release of active drug after a very high dose of prodrug. Following the lowest dose, the condition for zero-order conversion does no longer hold and we see a semi first-order delivery of the active substance.

After the 5 mmol dose, first-order release still occurs, as evidenced from the fact

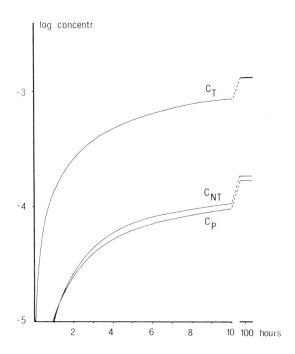

FIGURE 17. Concentrations of active drug in plasma (C_p), nontarget (C_{NT}) and target tissue (C_T) during infusion of prodrug at a rate of 0.2 mmol/min. All parameters were set at basal levels (see text); cf. also Figure 13.

that peak levels increase almost tenfold and half-life in the late phase hardly changes. A further tenfold increase of the dose to 50 mmol finally brings concentrations of the prodrug into the intermediary range, where release of active drug, immediately after injection, is neither first nor zero-order. In the late phase, obviously first-order release is going to occur.

Because of the intermediary behavior, for later simulations the 50 mmol dose was used.

2. Influence of K_M on Prodrug Behavior

The effect of changing K_M is predictable and may, in fact, be derived from earlier reasonings. Increasing K_M will tend to push the release of active drug in the direction of a first-order process. At the same time, the release rate will slow down. The net result will be a constant slow release of active drug. The opposite manipulation, i.e., decreasing K_M, will result in an initially high, zero-order generation of active drug. Both effects are simulated in Figure 20. Simulations in Figure 20 may be compared to Figure 19B, where the same parameters were used except for K_M, which was 0.001 mM.

3. Effect of Changing $V_{M,T}$ and $V_{M,NT}$

Changing $V_{M,T}$ and $V_{M,NT}$ to an equal degree will also shift release towards first-order and zero-order release, respectively. Increasing V_M will exhaust $C_{T,I}$ and $C_{NT,I}$ at a higher rate. Therefore, the ratios $C_{T,I}/K_M$ and $C_{NT,I}/K_M$ will more rapidly decrease and thus result in a faster occurrence of the first-order release. Decreasing V_M will have the opposite result. These phenomena are illustrated in Figure 21. Again, simulations may be compared to Figure 19B, where V_M was 0.1 mmol/min.

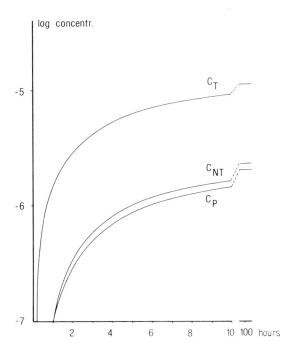

FIGURE 18.   Concentrations of active drug in plasma
(C_p), nontarget (C_{NT}), and target tissue (C_T) during infusion
of prodrug at a rate of 0.002 mmol/min. All other parameters were set at basal levels (see text); cf. also Figure 13.

4. Effect of Increasing $V_{M.T}/V_{M.NT}$

In simulations of acute dosing of the prodrug so far, we have assumed $V_{M.T} = V_{M.NT}$.
As stated before, this would mean that measured enzyme activity in the target tissue
would be 100-fold higher than in the average nontarget tissue. Increasing the ratio by
decreasing $V_{M.NT}$ results in the profiles depicted in Figure 22. Obviously, because the
total amount of prodrug is going to decrease at a lower rate, the release of active drug
is going to be semizero-order for a prolonged time. Also, the ratios $C_{T.II}/C_{p.II}$ and $C_{T.II}/$
$C_{NT.II}$ are going to increase. However, as evidenced from Figure 22, a 10- and 100-fold
increase , respectively, in the ratio $V_{M.T}/V_{M.NT}$ is only going to result in marginal decrease of $C_{p.II}$ and $C_{NT.II}$, whereas $C_{T.II}$ increases only slightly. This illustrates the dominance of the generation of the active drug in the target tissue over nontarget tissue.

5. Contribution of Q_T to Prodrug Behavior

Changing Q_T has a dual effect. First of all, it influences the rate at which the prodrug
concentration in the target tissue $C_{T.I}$ is going to increase after injection. Thus, lowering Q_T will result in initially lower $C_{T.I}$, and therefore a lower rate of formation of
active drug in the target tissue. Eventually, equilibrium for the prodrug is reached and
the other effect, i.e., an effect on kinetics of the active drug, becomes dominant. Because of the lower Q_T, active drug is going to be transported from the target tissue to
the rest of the system at a lower rate. The latter phenomenon, i.e., the effect of flow
on transport of the active drug to the rest of the system, is the only quantitatively
observable change when increasing flow, as illustrated in Figure 23. Thus, relative
overperfusion of the target tissue will result in a lowering of $C_{T.II}$, whereas at the same
time $C_{p.II}$ and $C_{NT.II}$ increase.

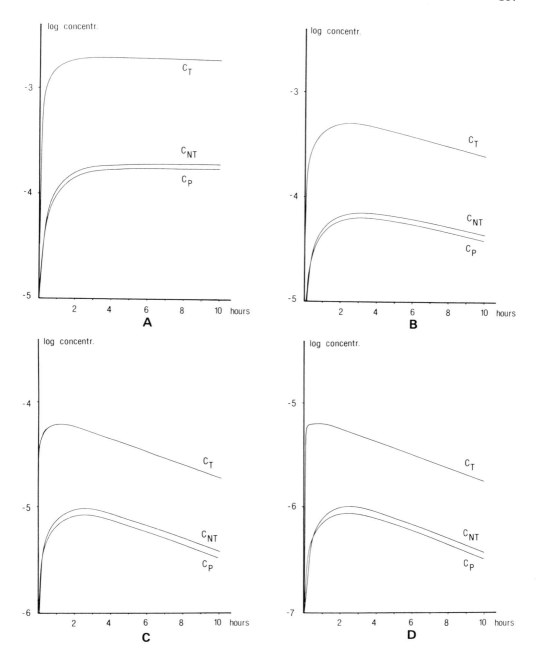

FIGURE 19.   Concentrations of active drug in plasma (C_p), target tissue and nontarget tissue (C_T) following bolus injections of prodrug at doses of 5000 (A), 50 (B), 5 (C), and 0.5 mmol (D). All parameters were set at basal levels (see text).

6. Influences Not Simulated

In the above simulations, the effects of changing a number of parameters were not considered. The only reason for not simulating them was the obvious outcome. For instance, partitioning coefficients were held at unity. This is certainly not a general fact for drugs. However, changing the partitioning coefficient for the active drug will not be very helpful in increasing tissue selectivity, simply because any gain obtained through this factor will also be obtained after direct administration of the active drug.

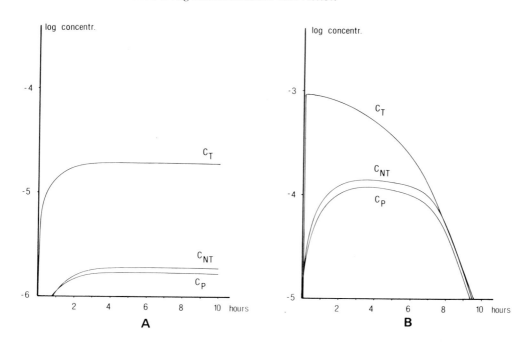

FIGURE 20.   Concentrations of active drug in plasma (C_p), nontarget (C_{NT}), and target tissue (C_T) following bolus injection of 50 mmol of prodrug. K_M for the enzymatic conversion was set at 0.1 mM(A) and 0.00001 mM(B), respectively. Compare to Figure 19B where K_M was 0.001 mM.

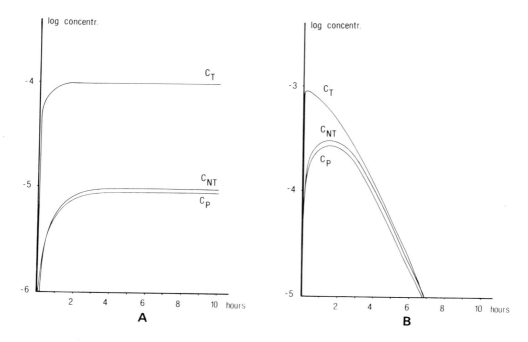

FIGURE 21.   Concentrations of active drug in plasma (C_p), nontarget (C_{NT}), and target tissue (C_T) following bolus injection of 50 mmol of prodrug. V_M for the enzymatic conversion was set at 0.01 (A) and 1 mmol/min (B), respectively, in both target and nontarget tissue. Compare to Figure 19B, where V_M = 0.1 mmol/min.

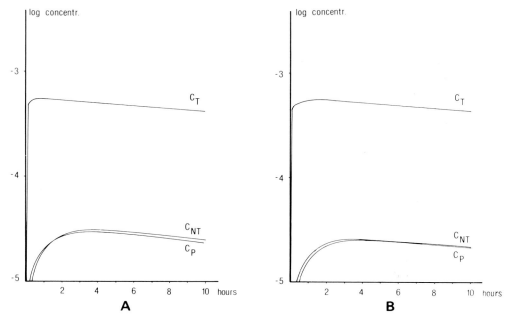

FIGURE 22. Concentrations of active drug in plasma (C_p), nontarget (C_{NT}), and target tissue (C_T) following bolus injection of 50 mmol of prodrug. The ratio $V_{M,T}/-V_{M,NT}$ was set at 10 in (A) and 100 in (B), representing, respectively, a 10^3 and 10^4 higher enzymatic activity in target tissue as compared to nontarget tissue. $V_{M,T}$ was kept constant. Compare to Figure 19B where $V_{M,T}/V_{M,NT} = 1$.

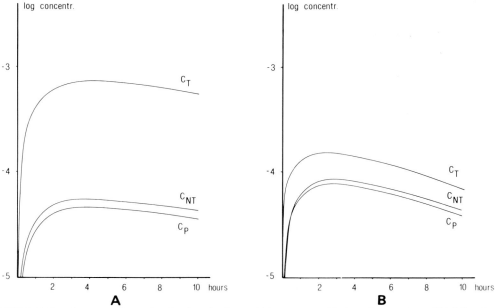

FIGURE 23. Concentrations of active drug in plasma (C_p), nontarget (C_{NT}), and target tissue (C_T) following bolus injection of 50 mmol of prodrug. Flow through the target tissue (Q_T) was set at 5 (A) and 500 ml/min (B), respectively, representing relative tenfold underperfusion and tenfold overperfusion. Compare to Figure 19B where $Q_T = 50$ ml/min.

Furthermore, increasing the partitioning coefficient for the prodrug will only be helpful in these cases where the enzymatic conversion has not been saturated and will result in a shift towards saturation.

Another parameter which we did not vary in our simulations is target organ clearance. This will again result in predictable changes. In Figure 22 where we increased the ratio $V_{M,T}/V_{M,NT}$ by lowering $V_{M,NT}$, it may be seen that plasma concentrations (and nontarget tissue concentrations) are hardly affected by this maneuver, indicating that these concentrations depend largely on leakage of the active drug from the target tissue. Therefore, introducing a clearance term in the target tissue will decrease plasma and nontarget tissue concentrations in a way comparable to what was shown for intra-arterial infusions of drugs earlier (cf. Equation 11).

D. Where and How May Prodrugs Be Used for Site-Specific Drug Delivery?

From the above simulations, we may try to conclude where the prodrug approach to site-specific drug delivery makes sense. First of all, however, we should wonder whether the parameters used in the model influence the outcomes of simulations in any way. Therefore, let us consider the most important parameters separately, being volume of the target tissue, flow through the target tissue, enzyme activities, and total body clearance.

The volume for the target tissue was taken to be 1% of the total volume. In man, most "vital" organs like lungs, liver, brain, and kidneys are in this order of magnitude. Others, like the adrenals and thyroid, are substantially smaller. For these latter tissues, if we would not change $V_{M,T}$, this would mean that our model underestimates selectivity gain, but only because of the "artificial" increase in enzyme activity.

Assuming a volume of 1% of total body weight for the target tissue, a flow of 1% of total cardiac output ($Q_T + Q_{NT}$) is in most cases an underestimation. Tissues like kidneys, brain, heart, and lungs receive a substantially greater amount of flow. From Figures 14 and 23, it may be seen that increasing the flow will tend to decrease the gain in specificity. Thus, with regard to the outcome of the simulations, we may conclude that they will, in most cases, flatter the situation.

$V_{M,T}$ was taken equal to $V_{M,NT}$. As already pointed out, this means that enzyme activity (per unit weight) is 100-fold higher in V_T than in V_{NT}. Increasing this ratio (cf. Figure 22) hardly affects the levels reached, which only illustrates the dependency of plasma and nontarget tissue levels on formation of active drug in the target tissue as was already pointed out. In other words, changing the ratio $V_{M,T}/V_{M,NT}$ is going to have only minor effects on selectivity. Finally, the clearance of the active drug was taken to be 1000 mℓ/min. Since total cardiac output was 5050 mℓ/min, this represents a clearance value of 20% of cardiac output, which is a high clearance. Normally, this value will be lower. The result will be that plasma and nontarget tissue levels increase, leaving target tissue relatively unaffected (cf. Figures 13 and 15).

The above considerations indicate that care must be taken in the interpretation of the simulations in a sense that all parameters that might increase the gain in selectivity are optimal. In other words, in practice, selectivity is going to be less in almost all cases.

Taking the simulations together, the potential of the prodrug approach towards obtaining tissue specificity should not be overestimated, especially if one would want to predict such specificity. In the latter case, one would have to give the prodrug by infusion or some other zero-order way of administration in order to avoid shifts of active drug delivery from zero-order to first-order, resulting in bizarre concentration profiles. If one would choose to deliver prodrugs by infusion, the problem that will be encountered next is the nonlinearity of drug levels and infusion rates. From mathematical considerations (cf. Equations 37 and 38), drug levels and gains in selectivity are going to be determined predominantly by tissue flows, total body clearance of the active drug, and V_M for enzymatic conversion, i.e., the rate of administration is going to play only a minor role. This then implies that the levels that one obtains are going to depend primarily on parameters that are "dictated" by other factors than infusion rates. In synthesizing a specific prodrug, in fact, one would already have to consider these parameters together with the desired levels (see also below).

Of course, there are exceptions to the generally negative remarks above. However, as said before, they did not need to be simulated because of the obvious outcome. In general, one may say that if a prodrug is formed within a tissue that has a physical barrier to the active drug but not to the prodrug, this will greatly enhance selectivity. Examples for this may be found, for instance, in the use of L-dopa for increasing the brain content of dopamine or in the use of methenamine as a urinary tract disinfectant. In both cases, there are biological barriers (the blood-brain barrier and the renal filtration process, respectively) that will prevent most of the active drug formed from entering into the circulation. Of course, these barriers are not necessarily organ boundaries. As discussed earlier, cell membranes and transport processes across these membranes may also pose a barrier to a drug for entering to its site of action. If, for instance, the prodrug would be substituted with a group that would make it liable to be transported over membranes by active processes and the parent compound would not contain this group, then the same considerations that apply to for instance L-dopa and the brain will be applicable to that hypothetical prodrug and the intracellular space. Such considerations might explain the success that seems to have been attained in synthesizing renal prodrugs by introduction of two groups, i.e., an L-α-glutamyl group as well as an acetyl group. α-Glutamyl transpeptidase does occur in a high concentration in the kidney. However, mere introduction of this group into sulfomethoxazole does not improve delivery to the kidney substantially,[18] which may be explained by the fact that flow through this tissue is very high. However, after introduction of an acetyl moiety into the molecule, renal delivery increases drastically. On the basis of enzyme kinetics, one would not expect such an increase, because one of the two enzymatic conversions will probably be rate-limiting and therefore determines the rate for the sequential cleavage reactions. If, however, one would assume that the acetyl group makes active transport of the prodrug into the cell possible, then the success of this intervention might be explicable on this basis. Such an effect of acetyl groups has been shown to exist for renal proximal tubular transport mechanisms.[29]

IV. SITE-SPECIFIC EFFECTS THROUGH SITE-SPECIFIC DRUG DELIVERY?

Although drug concentration-time profiles undoubtedly provide interesting information on the behavior of that drug within the body, the ultimate concern is going to be the effect that is elicited. In contrast to the mathematical approaches that may be used in the description of pharmacokinetics, pharmacodynamics still has to work with "black-box" functions. Even though molecular pharmacologists may describe receptor occupancy by a drug on the basis of several models, receptor-effector coupling is not necessarily a linear process. Therefore, this aspect may be only approached roughly.

It will be obvious that if desired and undesired effects of a drug occur at different concentrations, this concentration difference is going to limit the possibilities for site-specificity to a large degree.

If, for instance, an undesired effect in one tissue occurs at tenfold lower concentrations than the wanted effect in the target tissue, our aim will have to be to keep non-target tissue levels at least a factor of 10 lower than target tissue levels, whereas at the same time target tissue levels have to be in a certain effective range. Thus, the rates of administration or release rates will have to be selected while keeping that in mind. In the case that undesired effects occur at higher concentrations than desired effects, one will hardly ever consider site-specific delivery because the organism already provides site-specificity in the effect.

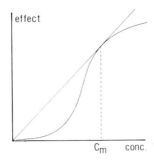

FIGURE 24.   Graph representing a composite concentration-effect relationship, consisting of a convex part, a linear
part, and a concave part. The tangent through the origin to
the convex part of the curve intercepts the curve at a concentration C_m. See further in text.

Now, let us assume that the side effects on a drug are really "site effects", i.e., the
same effect that we want to occur in our target tissue is considered to be an undesired
effect in nontarget tissue. Furthermore, for the sake of reasoning, let us assume that
receptor-effector coupling is the same in target and nontarget tissues. The relationship
between concentration and effect may then be either a linear relationship between concentration and effect, or a convex or concave relationship. In the former case, obviously, any gain in concentration is translated directly to a gain in effect. In the other
two cases, where the concentration-effect relationship is nonlinear, the matter is more
complicated.

Eckman and co-workers[4] defined H(C) as the effect per unit concentration:

$$H(C) = E(C)/C \tag{41}$$

where E(C) is the effect elicited by the concentration C of the drug. They showed that
both concave and convex concentration-effect curves may be analyzed in a similar way.
Therefore, let us consider the composite curve in Figure 24. If one draws a tangent to
the curve through the origin, this line intersects the curve at a point C_m, which in Figure
24 is in the concave region of the curve. Eckman et al.[4] showed that in this case, the
point C_m represents a maximum for H(C) whereas if the intercept is in the convex
region of the curve, C_m is the concentration of minimal H(C). Thus, for a concave
relationship between concentration and effect, the increase in effect is greater than the
increase in concentration for $C < C_m$, whereas if $C > C_m$, the effect increases less with
increasing concentration. If the relationship is convex, this is just the other way
around. The implications for site-specificity with regard to the effects of a drug may
be obvious. In the case of a concave concentration-effect relationship, the gain in effect
will keep increasing up to $C = C_m$. Thereafter, it will diminish again. This means that
the greatest specificity is going to be obtained for target concentrations up to $C_T = C_m$.
Thereafter, assuming that $C_{NT} < C_T$, the effect in the nontarget tissue will increase more
rapidly than the effect in the target tissue and will thus attenuate the gain in specificity.
Ideally, C_T should equal C_m. In case of a convex relationship, again assuming that $C_{NT}
< C_T$, C_T should be greater than C_m, whereas at the same time, C_{NT} should not exceed
C_m. Here, ideally C_{NT} should equal C_m to obtain a maximal gain in specificity with
regard to the effect.

From the above, it should be concluded that it is not only the pharmacokinetic gain
that is going to determine site-specificity, but also the absolute values of the concentrations (C_T and C_{NT}) are going to be crucial for site-specificity of the effects. Therefore,

both the shape of the concentration-effect relationship as well as the exact position of that curve (C_m) have to be considered together with the pharmacokinetics in order to perform an optimal localized therapy.

V. CONCLUSIONS

In the preceding sections, we have discussed two approaches of target-directed drug delivery: (1) local delivery, via intra-arterial delivery or (peri-)target delivery, and (2) the prodrug concept. Although the former approach at first sight seems to be the straightforward one, theoretical evaluation of the principle has shown that only under strict pharmacokinetic and pharmacodynamic conditions, target-directed selectivity can be achieved by local drug delivery. In order to have any reasonable gain in local drug concentration by local drug delivery as compared to systemic delivery, the body clearance of the drug should be much higher than the target blood flow, in the case of intra-arterial delivery, or higher than the efflux from the (peri-)target space, in the case of (peri-)target delivery. Reduction in systemic exposition by local delivery is only obtained if the target organ efficiently extracts the drug.

Nowadays, local drug delivery has become common practice in cancer chemotherapy, e.g., hepatic arterial infusion and intrathecal instillation of chemotherapeutics for hepatic and CNS tumors, respectively. Also the intrathecal administration of aminoglycosides is being used in case of Gram-negative bacillary meningitis.[20] The rationale for local delivery under these circumstances is obvious; to obtain higher, thus more effective, local concentrations and/or less systemic toxicity. It is amazing though understandable, however, that hepatic arterial infusion in particular has been performed with (anticancer) drugs the pharmacokinetics of which are poorly understood yet,[5,21] much less their concentration-effect dynamics. Because of the high hepatic arterial blood flow (300 ml/min), it is hardly to be expected that appreciable gain will be obtained in the amount of drug delivered to the liver via continuous hepatic arterial infusion, unless the flow is reduced, for instance by clamping. However, reduction in systemic exposition should be observed for high hepatic clearance drugs, provided that the elimination process remains first-order over the dosage range. Besides well-designed clinical trials, knowledge about the clinical pharmacokinetics of drugs which might be appropriate for local delivery is a prerequisite. Above all, however, experimental models to evaluate the merits of local delivery are needed.

With respect to the prodrug approach, our simulations have shown that under extreme conditions only (i.e., with the formation of the active compound in the target organ exclusively, preferably in zero-order process, the target blood flow low and the body clearance of the active species high), benefit regarding target selectivity can be expected. In accordance with these findings are the failures of earlier efforts to enhance target selectivity by molecular modification of cytostatic drugs. This modification was expected to be undone by target-specific enzymatic reactions. The classical example is the use of diethylstilbestroldiphosphate in the therapy of prostate cancer. In the prostate tissue, which is rich in the enzyme acid phosphatase, the active drug diethylstilbestrol should be generated from its prodrug. However, the enzyme acid phosphatase is also present in other tissues such as liver, hence selectivity is not obtained.

REFERENCES

1. Schade, D. S., Eaton, R. P., Friedman, N. M., and Spencer, W. J., Intraperitoneal delivery of insulin by a portable microinfusion pump, *Metabolism,* 29, 699, 1980.
2. Eaton, R. P., Portable insulin infusion pumps: what is their role in therapy, *Drugs,* 23, 245, 1982.
3. Lynch, H. J., Rivest, R. W., and Wurtman, R. J., Artificial induction of melatonin rhythms by programmed microinfusion, *Neuroendocrinology,* 31, 106, 1980.
4. Eckman, W. W., Patlak, C. S., and Fenstermacher, J. D., A critical evaluation of the principles governing the advantages of intraarterial infusions, *J. Pharmacokinet. Biopharm.,* 2, 257, 1974.
5. Chen, H. S. G. and Gross, J. F., Intraarterial infusions of anticancer drugs: theoretic aspects of drug delivery and review of responses, *Cancer Treat. Rep.,* 64, 31, 1980.
6. Øie, S. and Huang, J. D., Influence of administration route on drug delivery to a target organ, *J. Pharm. Sci.,* 12, 1344, 1981.
7. Himmelstein, K. J. and Lutz, R. J., A review of the applications of physiologically based pharmacokinetic modeling, *J. Pharmacokinet. Biopharm.,* 7, 127, 1979.
8. Bischoff, K. B., Current applications of physiological pharmacokinetics, *Fed. Proc. Fed. Am. Soc. Exp. Biol.,* 39, 2456, 1980.
9. Gerlowski, L. E. and Jain, R. K., Physiologically based pharmacokinetic modeling: principles and applications, *J. Pharm. Sci.,* 72, 1103, 1983.
10. Van Dixhoorn, J. J., Simulation of bondgraphs on minicomputers, *J. Dyn. Syst. Meas. Control,* 99, 9, 1977.
11. Shapiro, W. R., Young, D. F., and Metha, B. M., Methotrexate: distribution in cerebrospinal fluid after intravenous, ventricular and lumbar injections, *N. Engl. J. Med.,* 293, 161, 1975.
12. Spector, R., Spector, A. Z., and Snodgrass, S. R., Model for transport in the central nervous system, *Am. J. Physiol.,* 232, R73, 1977.
13. Ensminger, W. D. and Gyves, J. W., Regional chemotherapy of neoplastic disease, *Pharmacol. Ther.,* 21, 277, 1983.
14. Dedrick, R. L., Myers, C. E., Buorgay, P. M., and DeVita, V. T., Pharmacokinetic rationale for peritoneal drug administration in the treatment of ovarian cancer, *Cancer Treat. Rep.,* 62, 1, 1978.
15. Albert. A., Chemical aspects of selective toxicity, *Nature,* 182, 421, 1958.
16. Notari, R. E., Prodrug design, *Pharmacol. Ther.,* 14, 25, 1981.
17. Stella, V. J. and Himmelstein, K. J., Prodrugs and site-specific drug delivery, *J. Med. Chem.,* 23, 1275, 1980.
18. Orlowski, M., Mizoguchi, H., and Wilk, S., N-Acyl-γ-glutamyl derivatives of sulfamethoxazole as models of kidney-selective prodrugs, *J. Pharmacol. Exp. Ther.,* 212, 167, 1979.
19. Møller, J. V. and Sheikh, M. I., Renal organic anion transport system: pharmacological, physiological, and biochemical aspects, *Pharmacol. Rev.,* 34, 315, 1983.
20. Overturf, G. D. and Wehrle, P. F., Bacterial meningitis: which regimen? *Drugs,* 18, 65, 1979.
21. Balis, F. M., Holcenbeg, J. S., and Gleyer, W. A., Clinical pharmacokinetics of commonly used anticancer drugs, *Clin. Pharmacokinet.,* 8, 202, 1983.

Chapter 5

OSMOTIC SYSTEMS FOR RATE-CONTROLLED DRUG DELIVERY IN PRECLINICAL AND CLINICAL RESEARCH: THERAPEUTIC IMPLICATIONS

John Fara and Constance Mitchell

TABLE OF CONTENTS

I. INTRODUCTION

Drug delivery systems for pharmacologic research now provide the means for controlled delivery of most drugs, locally or systemically, at rates and for durations chosen by the investigator. This chapter will focus on two of these devices: the implantable osmotic pump (ALZET®) for studies in animals,[1-3] and the OSMET™ module for oral, vaginal, or rectal administration of drugs in clinical research.[2,3] Both of these research tools allow adjustment of drug delivery rate by adjusting the concentration of the drug solution used. The potential impact of their use on basic pharmacologic research, on drug development, and on therapeutics will be discussed.

Researchers are now using these drug delivery devices routinely in the early stages of drug research, such as drug screening, animal toxicology and pharmacology, and also in initial clinical testing.[4-8] Additionally, applications in these areas are creating new therapeutic opportunities. For example, studies to define drug dosage regimens — to minimize side effects, maximize therapeutic effect, and optimize dosing frequency — can now be done early in the development of a new drug. Such investigations provide the logic for selecting the appropriate drug delivery pattern for treatment and eliminate the need for painstaking empirical investigations. The same types of studies are also appropriate for the restudy of older drugs with troublesome side actions or inconvenient dosing schedules.

II. IMPLANTABLE GENERIC RATE-CONTROLLED DELIVERY SYSTEMS

In preclinical studies, the use of implantable osmotic pumps has virtually replaced the clumsy alternative of connecting small animals to heavy infusion pumps.[9,10] Previously, long-duration delivery devices for implantation have proven useful in endocrinology, but outside that field have found limited usefulness. Essentially, these are silastic tubes filled with a drug solution — generally a steroid because of the permeability characteristics of such agents. The properties of the silastic are such that it provides prolonged but continuously declining delivery rates. Moreover, the systems require adjustment of membrane thickness and area for every specific compound studied. Osmotic pumps, on the other hand (Figure 1), provide rate-controlled, unattended administration of a wide range of drug solutions and other bioactive agents for 1 to 4 weeks.

The pumps currently available have delivery rates and durations of 1 or 10 $\mu\ell$/hr for 7 days, 0.5 or 5 $\mu\ell$/hr for 14 days, or 2.5 $\mu\ell$/hr for 28 days. These osmotic pumps consist of the following components (Figure 2): an inert, impermeable, flexible drug reservoir open to the exterior via a single portal; a thin sleeve of osmotic agent surrounding the reservoir; and a semipermeable membrane surrounding the sleeve of the osmotic agent. The researcher fills the reservoir through the portal with the solution or suspension of interest and then inserts a flow moderator to prevent diffusion of solution from the portal. This ensures that the osmotic process will control the delivery rate. After implantation of the filled pump, water from the surrounding tissue moves osmotically through the membrane at a rate controlled by the permeability of the membrane. The rigidity of the membrane causes the swelling osmotic sleeve to displace the liquid drug formulation within the reservoir out through the portal in a continuous, controlled manner. The performance characteristics of one model of the osmotic pump are shown in Figure 3.

III. RESEARCH APPLICATIONS OF IMPLANTABLE PUMPS

Review of nearly 700 publications in endocrinology and drug research in which os-

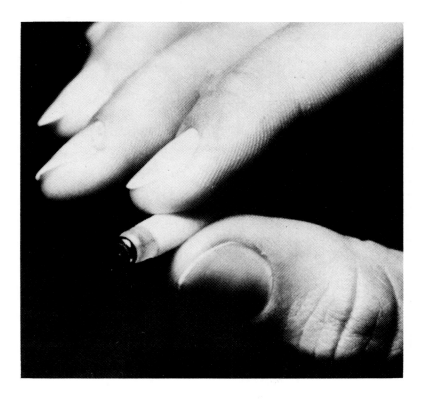

FIGURE 1.   The ALZET® osmotic pump.

motic pumps have been used reveals several general areas of application. More than 150 agents (Table 1) reportedly have been delivered in various animals, including mice, rabbits, rats, dogs, baboons, and sheep. Moreover, several novel approaches have been reported in cold-blooded animals, including fish.[11,12]

A. Delivery of Short-Half-Life Agents

The osmotic pumps have allowed the development of new approaches to the evaluation of potent hormones, peptides, and other short-half-life agents. They have been extensively used in research on peptides, for most of these compounds have a half-life of minutes, and their bolus delivery produces only brief tissue exposure to them. Thus, one must make observations at precisely the right moment to recognize certain of their actions. For such compounds, rate-specified administration is the proper delivery mode.

That mode does not necessarily mean constant-rate administration. Sometimes peptide action persists after delivery has ceased; on the other hand, effects of some agents may fade during constant-rate administration because receptors become refractory to the stimulus. In such cases, the logical step is not to revert to single-dose, bolus administration, but rather to advance to preprogrammed rate-varying patterns of administration. A number of investigators have devised techniques for accomplishing this, which will be discussed in a later section.

B. Minimizing Stress

Handling of animals, subjecting them to frequent injections, or confining them during infusions can all introduce stress into experimental protocols. The biochemical and/or physiological changes that result can be severe. For example, Riley[13] has shown

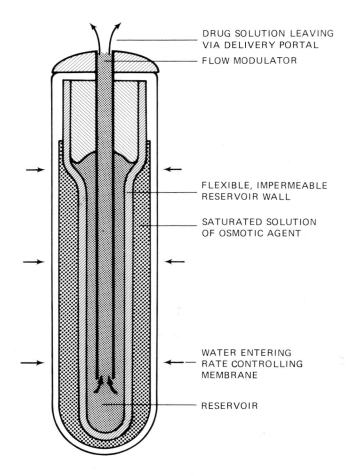

FIGURE 2.   Cross-section of the osmotic pump.

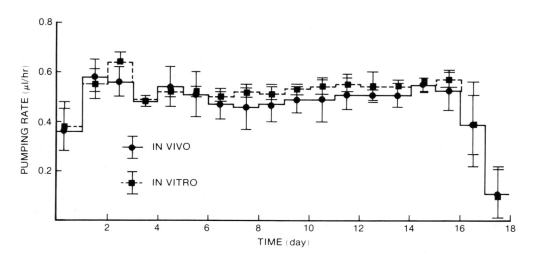

FIGURE 3.   In vivo and in vitro pumping rates of an osmotic pump designed to deliver 0.5 $\mu\ell$/hr of agent for 14 days.

Table 1
AGENTS DELIVERED BY OSMOTIC PUMPS IN RECENTLY REPORTED EXPERIMENTS

Peptides

ACTH	Insulin
Angiotensin	LH
Bombesin	LHRH
Bungarotoxin snake venom	LHRH analogs, agon/antag
Calcitonin	α-MSH
Cholecystokinin	Muramyl dipeptide
Dermorphin	Neurotensin
Endorphins	Parathyroid hormone
Enkephalins	Pentagastrin
Erythropoietin	Pituitary extract
FSH	Prolactin
Gastrin	Somatomedins
Glucagon	Teprotide
Growth hormones	Tetragastrin
IGF	Vasopressin

Steroids

Aldosterone	Estriol
Catecholestrogens	Estrone
Corticosterone	Methoxyesterone
Dexamethasone	Progesterone
DOCA	Spironolactone
Estradiol	Testosterone

Other substances

Anesthetics	G.I. motility modulators
Antibacterials	Heavy metals
Anticancer agents	Immunologic agents
Anticoagulants	Indicator substances
Antiepileptics	Metabolites
Antihypertensives	Neurotransmitters
Anti-Parkinson agents	Nerve growth factors
Antivirals	Nucleosides and nucleotides
Carbonic anhydrase inhibitors	Prostaglandins
Carcinoma antibodies	Radioisotopes
Catecholamines	Renin-angiotensin and inhibitors
Chelators	Thyroid/thyroid-related hormones
Cholinergics	Vitamins and minerals
CNS-acting agents	Miscellaneous test vehicles and solvents
Enzymes	

that the appearance of mammary tumors in female mice of the C3H/He strain carrying an oncogenic virus can be dramatically increased or accelerated by stressful factors, including handling. Less obvious manifestations of stress in small laboratory animals may be the hypersecretion of adrenal steroids, giving rise to interactions with the test agent in undesired and undetected ways. The usual means of differentiating the effects of stress from the agent under study is to administer only vehicle to a control group of animals, according to the same regimen and procedures used to administer drug to treated animals. This procedure simply reveals the effects of drugs in stressed animals rather than eliminating it. Therefore, stress is often an unintended variable in a large proportion of physiological, pharmacological, and toxicological studies. Infusions from implanted pumps offer a means for reducing this variable in many experimental situations.

1. Evidence of Reduced Stress with Implanted Pumps

Delivery systems can replace injections and at the same time reduce handling to once every 1, 2, or 4 weeks. Their implantation, however, adds the need for anesthesia and surgery. Implantation is a minor procedure in an animal that is large relative to the implant, but is more significant when the subcutaneous pocket required involves a tenth or more of the animal's surface area. Yet, in either large or small animals, it can be rapidly accomplished subcutaneously within a minute or so. Intraperitoneal implantation can be done through a "keyhole" incision, avoiding handling of the viscera; otherwise the procedure may be stressful enough to cause one or more postoperative days of diminished food intake and deviation from the normal growth curve (two integrated measures of surgical stress). Additional procedures, such as leading catheters from the implant to veins, arteries, cerebral ventricles, or the gut lumen may accentuate or prolong these manifestations.

A number of investigators have explored possible stress effects of pump implantation. DeLuca et al.[14] compared the effects of 20-week continuous infusions of vitamin D metabolites in vitamin-D-deficient female rats (from weaning through a complete reproductive cycle and lactation) to the effects of oral doses given thrice weekly. The animals were ether-anesthetized every 2 weeks for osmotic pump replacement. The only observed difference between the groups was that half the infused animals receiving 25-hydroxyvitamin D_3 by implant had irregular estrous cycles vs. one fourth of those receiving that agent orally. On the other hand, only one fourth the group receiving 1,25-dihydroxyvitamin D_3 by implant had irregular estrous cycles. Thus, it is not evident that repetitive implantation alone had an adverse effect on estrous cycling. The groups were comparable in maternal growth rates, pregnancy rates, birth rates, litter sizes, litter weights, pup survivorships, and pup weight gains during lactation. These similarities and the favorable comparisons with normal rats led the investigators to conclude that the removal and reimplantation of osmotic pumps every other week "did not place a significant stress on the animals".[14]

Numerous other investigators have reported that neither implantation of the pump nor other procedures accompanying its uninterrupted use over multimonth durations are stressful.[14-22] For example, de la Torre and Gonzalez-Carvajal[17] administered several experimental compounds to the spinal cord of rats using osmotic pumps for as long as 16 weeks. They observed no adverse effects. In monkeys, Akhtar et al.[21] reported normal body weights and no adverse effects during 20 weeks, with weekly replacement of osmotic pumps. Jarnagin et al.[14] concluded in their studies in rats that the removal and reimplantation of the osmotic pumps every other week over a similar time period did not significantly stress the animals.

In general, data on the action of the agent being infused with osmotic pumps can be obtained in the unstressed physiological state after the first day of the experiment. That change could presumably lead to very different results from those seen when stress is present.

2. Advantages of Freedom from Restraint

A related advantage of utilizing implantable delivery devices is the freedom from restraint that they permit. That freedom is especially important in behavioral studies. Animals receiving continuous infusions can, for example, cross grids, interrelate with cage mates, and, in fact, engage in all useful activities.[23-32] Formerly, the animals were tethered to infusion devices, greatly inhibiting their normal activities and responses to stimuli. Clearly, the more normalized situation offers a much better experimental milieu for studying behavior.

For example, until recently, the well-documented dipsogenic action of angiotensin II infusion into the hypothalamus has been observed only briefly.[33,34] This is because of the previous difficulties of continuously infusing peptide into animals whose behavior is unrestrained and the rapid turnover of cerebral spinal fluid. Now, however, week-long duration of dipsogenic action has been described in a study utilizing an osmotic pump/cannula system for angiotensin infusion into the third cerebral ventricle of rats. The animals were offered saline to drink to accentuate the dipsogenic effect.[35,36] One group of rats received no treatment; a second group received infusions of angiotensin II (1 μg/min) for 1 week and then isotonic saline (0.1 mℓ/hr) for week two at the same flow rate; a third group received the same two infusions in reverse order. During the third week neither of these two groups received any treatment. Cross-over design was made possible by changing the osmotic pump. The untreated and saline-infused rats had the same spontaneous intakes of isotonic saline — about 40 to 50 mℓ/day — while rats receiving angiotensin II had an average intake tenfold greater (over 400 mℓ/day). This dipsogenic effect increased steadily as long as the angiotensin II infusion continued. The rats returned to normal fluid intake when the peptide infusions stopped.

C. Delivery Systems as Artificial Organs

Two uses of implantable delivery systems as organs are of special interest: to replace substances secreted by organs removed by surgery or other means; and to study the actions of biological substances on the fetus or on fetal-maternal interactions.

1. Replacement of Endocrine Gland Secretions

One experimental method employed in endocrinology is to remove an organ or part of an organ and then to observe the resulting effect on a single body system or on the whole animal. Replacement of substances normally produced by that organ or tissue is then used to explore the mechanisms of hormone release and hormone action. This approach has been applied to the adrenals, pancreas, pituitary, and, in fact, to virtually all endocrine structures.

Now the capability for uninterrupted multiday infusions without handling of the animals has introduced a type of bioassay. It permits hormonal actions to be assessed in a broader context and over a longer period than in the conventional single-dose hormone bioassay. For example, as an artificial pancreas, delivery systems have been implanted to infuse insulin for 6 days to rats with experimentally (streptozotocin) induced diabetes.[37] Large pulses of insulin release — typical of meal-eaters — do not ordinarily occur in this species because the rat does not eat meals, but instead nibbles day and night. Thus, continuous infusion provides a means for assaying the total daily need for insulin. Osmotic pumps were filled with different concentrations of unmodified crystalline bovine insulin in isotonic saline and implanted subcutaneously to infuse doses of 2, 4, and 10 U per 200-g rat per day. Isotonic-saline-filled pumps were implanted subcutaneously in other (control) rats with induced diabetes. The temporal dose-response curve (Figure 4) showed that a dose of 2 U/day was sufficient to return the streptozotocin-diabetic rat to normoglycemic levels of 90 to 120 mg%.

Patel's[38] study of insulin replacement regimens in streptozotocin-diabetic rats spanned 60 to 80 days, with repeated replacement of 2-week-duration osmotic pumps. Such experiments call for careful attention to detail, as illustrated by contrasting the design of Patel's study with that of Lopaschuk and colleagues.[39] Work of the latter virtually catalogs the technical problems that can confuse the assessment of continuous administration of a peptide hormone for even as short a time as 7 days.

In other studies, the osmotic pump has supplied replacement therapy or drugs in

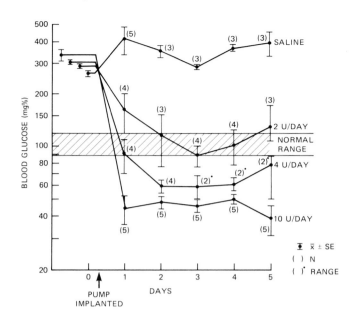

FIGURE 4. Dose-response curves of insulin in the streptozotocin-diabetic rat.[2]

animals who have undergone surgical removal of single or multiple endocrine glands (thyroid,[40,41] pineal,[42,43] adrenal,[44,45] parathyroid,[46,47] hypophysis,[48,49] kidney(s),[50,51] gonads,[52-54] or nervous system structures (ganglionectomy, laminectomy, denervation).[17,55,56] It has also been utilized for replacement therapy in vitamin-deficient animals.

2. Uterine/Fetal Delivery

Investigators have also used this implantable system to deliver agents directly into the uterus or fetus. These infusions permit investigators to regulate events of the estrus cycle and to study maternal-fetal relationships. Pratt et al.[57] positioned pumps in the uterine horn of nonpregnant ewes and administered prostaglandin E_2 in attempts to regulate the life span of the corpus luteum. They were able to sort out whether luteal function could be maintained locally, without influencing the circulatory concentrations of other agents that also regulate corpus luteal events.

Formerly, studying fetal-maternal interactions required the surgical implantation of catheters, with the assorted technical problems inherent in their use. Susa and colleagues[58,59] delivered insulin through implanted osmotic pumps directly into the upper hind leg of the fetus of the rhesus monkey to achieve chronic hyperinsulinemia *in utero* during the 19 days prior to delivery. Fetal plasma insulin concentrations nearly 100 times normal were attained; maternal plasma glucose and insulin concentrations were unaffected. At birth, the neonate was symptomatically hypoglycemic.

Spencer et al. used a similar approach in the fetal pig to achieve chronic hyperinsulinemia and determine the influence of insulin and somatomedin on fetal growth.[60] In this study, pumps containing porcine insulin were implanted in the forearm of the 90-day fetus. Over the next 14 days, each fetus received 3 U of insulin per day. Cesarean section on day 104 revealed that, despite higher levels of somatomedin activity in insulin-treated fetuses, there was no significant difference in fetal growth from control, saline-infused fetuses.

In another application, ALZET® osmotic pumps delivering triiodothyronine were implanted subcutaneously in fetal lambs. The effects of this hormone on placental gas exchange, the fetal cardiovascular system, and on fetal metabolism were then examined.[61,62]

Such procedures for continuous drug administration not only allow experimental manipulation of the fetus, but can, of course, be extended to study the same animal into adulthood by sequentially replacing the pumps.

D. Targeted, Organ- or Tissue-Specific Delivery

S.c., i.v., and i.p. routes of infusion do not provide organ- or tissue-specific delivery and thus hamper the design of experiments to identify the site of action of a drug. Use of implantable pumps has permitted localized delivery, not only to specific organs over prolonged periods, but also microperfusion of specific sites on those organs. The osmotic pump has now been used for chronic delivery of drugs to the surface of the eye, into the uterus and vagina, into the cerebral ventricles and brain tissue, and into the kidney via the renal artery. It has also permitted microperfusion of selected areas of the visual cortex.

Such infusions can produce relatively high concentration in only one organ — or in only one area of an organ — with low systemic levels. For example, after 6 days of continuous infusion of propranolol intracerebroventrically (i.c.v.) or s.c., the ratio of concentrations by the two routes, respectively, were close to 1 in plasma, heart, lungs, and liver, compared with 50 to 600 in different regions of the brain.[63] On pharmacokinetic grounds, it can be shown that the gain in selectivity of tissue concentration obtained by long-term perfusion into tissues depends primarily on tissue blood flow, the blood:tissue partition coefficient of the drug, and the clearance of the drug.[64]

Constant-rate targeted infusions — by eliminating time-dependent, regimen-induced fluctuations in drug levels and actions — can provide a high degree of ability to discriminate between a drug's central and peripheral modes of action. Smits et al.[65] used a unique approach to sort out central from peripheral actions of beta-blockers. They developed a hypertensive rat model in which propranolol could be infused intracerebroventrically or subcutaneously in conscious, unrestrained, spontaneously hypertensive rats (SHR). Over a 5-day infusion, they achieved brain concentrations of propranolol that were approximately 100-fold higher than those prevailing after subcutaneous infusion of equal doses; plasma levels, however, were comparable. In spite of this 100-fold higher brain level, the i.c.v. infusion dose needed for the blood pressure lowering effect was found to be the same as that needed for a subcutaneous infusion. The investigators thus were able to conclude that the antihypertensive effect of propranolol in spontaneously hypertensive rats is due to its peripheral effects. (As discussed elsewhere in this review, these authors have also investigated the effects of propranolol given in the injection mode as opposed to a continuous infusion.) A similar infusion technique[66] also demonstrated the CNS locus of clonidine's antihypertensive effect in the SHR. With continuous s.c. injections of the drug, a tenfold shift of dose-response curve to the right occurred vs. its continuous i.c.v. infusion.

Struyker-Boudier[67] also devised a technique for single-organ (right kidney) infusion via the cardiovascular system by implanting a catheter attached to an osmotic pump into the right suprarenal artery of conscious, unrestrained, uninephrectomized rats. Investigation of various indicators of kidney function showed no changes induced by the catheter itself. The technique was subsequently employed for the intrarenal administration of vasoactive drugs and represents a means of achieving in vivo pharmacologic manipulation of intrarenal processes.[68]

Kasamatsu et al.[26] used continuous microperfusion to demonstrate the effect of neocortical catecholamines (CAs), specifically norepinephrine, on cortical plasticity. As an indicator, they used the marked visual cortical changes in ocular dominance that follow monocular deprivation in kittens. Two separate osmotic pump/cannula systems delivered norepinephrine and control solutions, respectively, to corresponding sites in the left and right visual cortex of kittens who had lost their susceptibility to the effects of monocular lid suture because of prior treatment of the visual cortex with 6-hydroxydopamine. In these animals, norepinephrine restored plasticity, as shown by a shift in ocular dominance. Older animals who had outgrown susceptibility to the effects of monocular deprivation also showed a decrease in binocularity with norepinephrine treatment. The authors cited the following advantages for the microperfusion technique over the intraventricular infusion approach used previously:

- Ability to localize drug effects to a specific brain region and thus to pinpoint more precisely the anatomical locus of drug effect
- Ability to utilize a corresponding site in the opposite hemisphere or a distant site of the same hemisphere as a control in the same animal
- Elimination of side effects that often occur with repeated intraventricular injections (also reported by a number of additional investigators)

E. Models to Study Drugs and Disease

One limitation often encountered by investigators in early pharmacotherapeutic studies is that of the unavailability of suitable animal models of a disease for which a particular class of drugs is being screened. Chronic duodenal ulcers, for example, do not naturally occur in species traditionally used for testing of antiulcer drugs. Histamine injected subcutaneously in bolus doses has long been used to produce hypersecretion of gastric acid, but it is not highly effective in ulcerogenesis. Recently, however, Hosada et al.[69] demonstrated that a continuous subcutaneous infusion of histamine — at doses up to 15 mg/kg/day — produced multiple ulcers in the African rodent, *Praomys (Mastomys) natalensis*. Responses were dose-related, and at higher delivery rates, some perforations occurred. In contrast, histamine given as a single subcutaneous injection of 50 mg/kg/day was not ulcerogenic. These authors believe that this model may well serve for the study of the etiology and treatment of duodenal ulcer disease in humans.

Szabo[70] developed another ulcerogenic model in which cysteamine is delivered by osmotic pumps also implanted subcutaneously, but in Sprague-Dawley-derived Charles River CD female rats. This method is reportedly easily reproducible and economic for producing acute and chronic duodenal ulcer disease.

In both of these models, infusion of saline or water in control animals demonstrated that neither the pump implantation procedure nor the pump's presence changed gastric or duodenal mucosa. Development of these ulcerogenic models has furthermore permitted comparisons of agents that stimulate gastric acid secretion and evaluation of antagonists.

These and other needs in basic research have sparked the development of additional models in a variety of fields. For example, Tze et al.,[71] in a study in diabetic rats, needed to maintain circulation through an implanted artificial capillary unit containing allogeneic islet cells; they infused heparin continuously, 25 U/hr, into the deep circumflex iliac vein via a catheter leading from a heparin-filled osmotic pump implanted intraperitoneally.

Use of implantable continuous-delivery systems has also enabled investigators to evaluate long-term effects of drugs in models that closely resemble chronic therapy. Greenberg and Wilborn, for example, adapted an SHR model to compare effects of the antihypertensive agents clonidine and propranolol on venous and pulmonary arterial smooth muscle function and structure[72] and on biochemical indices of myocardial hypertrophy. Over the 3-week infusion period, both drugs reduced systolic arterial pressure, but only clonidine reversed myocardial hypertrophy. Additionally, chronic administration of propranolol resulted in myocardial necrosis in each SHR tested.[73]

In yet another hypertensive model, continuous delivery of converting enzyme inhibitor SQ14,225 was used to delineate the role of angiotensin II as a renal component in the maintenance of pressure volume relationships in sodium-depleted rats.[27] At the other extreme of manipulating the normotensive rat, investigators have chronically infused catecholamines to raise blood pressure.[74] These investigators achieved labile hypertension after 5 days of administering 40 μg/kg/hr of noradrenaline in unrestrained rats.

In endocrinology, many models have become available with use of preprogrammed, implantable delivery systems. For example, Mills et al.[75] developed a hypoprolactinemic rat model by continuous i.p. infusion of lergotrile mesylate, 0.69 mg/kg/day, for 7 days to suppress prolactin secretion in adult male rats. This suppression allowed the investigators to study spontaneous fluctuations in basal prolactin levels and ether-stimulated prolactin secretion over prolonged periods.

Gruppuso et al.[76] developed a model for fetal growth retardation in the pregnant rat by subcutaneously implanting osmotic pumps that continuously infused exogenous insulin; the resulting chronic maternal hyperinsulinemia significantly decreased the supply of glucose to the fetus. Previously, models for manipulating fetal growth have relied on either uterine vessel ligation, maternal dietary restriction, or other surgical interventions.

Finally, as pointed out in other sections of this review, the use of preprogrammed implanted delivery systems has had an immense impact in developing models for studying agents in the central nervous system. By introducing substances directly into cerebral-spinal fluid, the implanted systems avoid the blood-brain barrier and eliminate important experimental difficulties that have hampered studies with agents having primary or secondary central nervous system effects.

F. Continuous Drug Presence to Study Tolerance and Dependence

It is well known that the continuous presence or the repeated presentation of many agents can produce physical dependence and tolerance to the test agent after a period of exposure. Furthermore, after the agent is withheld, or following the administration of an antagonist, withdrawal syndromes ensue that may persist for some time. Because of the need to maintain the presence of test agents for these events to occur, investigators have utilized implantable drug delivery systems to administer a host of agents in studies on the initiation, prevention, or modulation of tolerance and dependence.

Of particular interest has been the delivery of barbiturates for 3 to 5 days or longer to establish tolerance in physical dependency models. For example, Siew and Goldstein[24] implanted two of the small osmotic pumps subcutaneously in 25 to 30 g mice, each pump delivering approximately 0.25 mg/hr sodium barbital for up to 7 days. Tolerance subsequently developed, as shown by a significant decrease in sleep time after a challenge dose of barbital administered 24 hr after withdrawal. Physical dependence was likewise demonstrated in the model by the withdrawal hypersensitivity measured by convulsions induced either with pentylenetetrazol or by handling.

To study the role of noradrenergic systems in barbiturate tolerance, Tabakoff et al.[77] infused phenobarbital into the CNS of rats for 72 hr and then, under light anesthesia, removed the pumps. A challenge dose of pentobarbital (40 mg/hr) was given 24 hr later to demonstrate tolerance. Selective destruction of noradrenergic neurons by intraventricular administration of 6-hydroxydopamine or by specific lesions of the dorsal or ventral noradrenergic bundles prevented the development of barbiturate tolerance without altering the animal's response to acute administration of barbiturate. Similarly, Wei[78,79] established an animal model of physical dependence and analgesia to enkephalin analogs. Using osmotic pumps, he infused seven enkephalin analogs continuously into the periaqueductal grey 4th-ventricular space of the rat brain; after administering naloxone HCl, 4 mg/kg intraperitoneally, to precipitate the withdrawal syndrome, its intensity was subsequently evaluated.

Interest in ethanol dependency has also sparked the search for new models. Investigators have utilized long-term delivery systems either to establish an animal model or to examine factors that might enhance or lessen the events associated with dependency. For example, Volicer et al.[80] studied the role of chronic intraventricular calcium perfusion, while Rigter et al.[29] looked at the role of vasopressin during ethanol withdrawal. In other models also, calcium infusion studies have identified this ion as playing a role in the development of tolerance to morphine.[81] Similarly, an ACTH-related peptide is also implicated.[82]

In endocrinology, agents are being chronically administered to explore long-term events in reproductive cell function. For example, Akhtar et al.[21] subcutaneously infused the GnRH agonist buserelin by osmotic pumps to rhesus monkeys over 20 weeks. This resulted in an initial rise in serum LH, followed by a decline to undetectable levels, reportedly indicating "pituitary desensitization".

Other studies utilizing delivery systems have explored tolerance and dependence in the fetus following chronic drug delivery to the mother. Hetta and Terenius[83] treated pregnant rats for 7 days with naloxone or saline infusion. Naloxone, administered from day 17 of pregnancy, significantly increased neonatal mortality; by the age of 40 days, the young exposed to naloxone showed a significant analgesic response to morphine (5 mg/kg), in contrast to the saline controls, when tested with the hot plate technique.

Also, the apparent rapid development of behavioral tolerance to chronic administration of the peptide cholecystokinin is reported in a recent study in rats.[84] However, there is some question in this study about the amount of bioactive peptide remaining in the delivery system after several days and also at the conclusion of the experiment. This emphasizes the need to test or verify the in vitro stability and delivery of the test agent over the expected experimental period, before beginning the study.

Another use of implantable delivery systems is the chronic exposure of animals to a test agent and the subsequent removal of their organs to study mechanisms of tolerance and dependence. In two studies,[85,86] guinea pigs were continuously infused with specific opiates by 7-day delivery from implanted osmotic pumps. Subsequently, the animals were sacrificed, the ilea removed, and in vitro tissue studies done in an organ bath. A similar method was employed by Schulz et al.[87] to study the development of opiate tolerance in mouse vas deferens.

Finally, the development of tolerance to chronic treatment with many other agents has been studied. These include dermorphins,[88] de-amphetamine,[89] phencyclidine,[90] and alpha- and beta-agonists.[91]

Closely tied to studies of this nature has been the recent interest in receptor sensitivity and regulation. Delivery systems have been employed to ensure the continuous presence of various agents, often at different, preselected levels. This approach has been used particularly to study angiotensin II and GnRH receptors, as well as other agents (Table 2).

Using the osmotic pump, investigators have been able to deliver agents at preselected, highly dependable rates, and also later to adjust the rate to compare effects at different local tissue concentrations. For example, Clayton[96] demonstrated biphasic autoregulation of pituitary GnRH receptors: up-regulation was consistently observed with low dose continuous infusion; down-regulation or desensitization was produced by continuous exposure to high concentrations.

Table 2
RECEPTOR REGULATION STUDIES DONE BY CHRONICALLY
EXPOSING ANIMALS AND TISSUES TO TEST AGENTS DELIVERED
VIA OSMOTIC PUMPS

	Receptors	Agents delivered	Ref.
Response is to increase receptor population (up-regulation)	Adrenal angiotensin II	Angiotensin II	92—94
	Uterine myometrium Angiotensin II receptors	Angiotensin II	95
	Pituitary GnRH receptors	GnRH (low dose)	96
	Brain opiate receptors	Naltrexone	97
	Brain cholecystokinin receptors	Haloperidol	98
	Brain dopamine receptors	Prolactin	99
	Liver estrogen receptors	Growth hormone	100
	Testicular LH receptor	Luteinizing hormone	101
	Testicular prolactin receptor	Luteinizing hormone	101
	Hepatic prolactin receptor	Growth hormone	102
	Lymphocytes β-adrenergic receptor	Propanolol	103
	Cardiac β-adrenergic receptor	Propanolol	103
	Lung μ-adrenergic receptor	Propanolol	103
	Hepatic growth hormone and prolactin receptor	Growth hormone	104
Response is to decrease receptor population (down-regulation)	Pituitary GnRH receptor	GnRH (high dose)	96, 105
	Ovarian GnRH receptor	GnRH	106
	Testicular LH/hCG receptor	GnRH	107
	Cardiac beta adrenoceptors	Isoproterenol and norepinephrine	108
	Cardiac beta adrenoceptors	Isoproterenol	109
	Brain α_2-adrenoceptors	Clorgyline	110, 111

Studies like these should stimulate development of many additional animal models and testing of numerous other substances in efforts to understand tolerance and dependency and related issues of receptor regulation.

G. Schedule Dependency of Drug Actions

The literature provides a growing number of examples of the way that regimen or rate of drug administration can influence the expression of drug actions.[7,8,46,112-117] Not only anticancer drugs, but those used in a variety of other therapeutic situations demonstrate a changing range of actions with dosing schedule.

Basically, regimen dependence or schedule dependence signifies a shift of the dose-response curve to the right or left according to the time-pattern of drug administration. That is, the same total dose of the drug given over the same time period produces different actions when the schedule of its administration changes.

1. Scaling

Understanding the pharmacokinetics that most drugs have in small laboratory animals is basic to understanding regimen-dependent expressions of drug action. In general, small animals metabolize and/or excrete drugs much more rapidly than humans. Thus, the problem in early drug and toxicity screening and testing is one of scaling — that is, designing the study to permit extrapolating its results from animal to man.

Although experimental designs generally take body weight differences fully into account, they tend to ignore the consequences of time differences in drug metabolism and excretion. Yet differences in plasma half-lives produce very different patterns of drug concentration in species that differ as markedly as mouse and man. The most important consequences are that daily injections of a rapidly absorbed and excreted drug will cause its concentrations in blood and tissues of mice to reach very high peaks followed by a rapid decline to very low levels. In fact, drug will be absent for some time in each dosage interval with the usual 4 to 6 times daily regimen.

According to several investigators,[117] scaling in terms of the plasma half-life is on the order of the body weight to the one quarter power. Thus in rats and mice, plasma half-lives would be one tenth or less of those in humans. For example, in a recent study by Nau and his colleagues, the plasma half-life of valproate in the mouse is only 0.8 hr, compared to 8 to 16 hr in humans.

Extrapolating the results of mouse toxicity data to humans can therefore give rise to two types of errors. The higher peak levels in mice may lead to overestimating human toxicity of a drug; conversely, the long periods of no detectable drug in mice may lead to underestimating its human toxicity.

Efficacy studies are subject to the same sources of error. Does the therapeutic action of the test drug (as has been suggested with some antibiotics) depend on sharp peaking concentrations? If so, then the relatively higher peaks obtained in small animals may lead to false expectations of efficacy in humans. On the other hand, it may be that the effectiveness of a drug depends on its maintenance in plasma at certain critical levels that 3 to 4 times-a-day dosage could maintain in humans; in that case the recurrent absence of the drug in plasma in preclinical testing on a similar regimen can lead to underestimating its therapeutic potential.

Recent studies by Nau, Sikic, and others using continuous infusion from implanted osmotic pumps show that by comparing two types of drug regimens — pulsed vs. continuous drug delivery, for example — it is possible to sort out effects associated with peak and trough levels and constant plasma concentrations. Such protocols illustrate an interesting technique for achieving a valid basis for extrapolation of animal data to the human.

2. The Injection-Infusion Comparison Protocol

Nau et al.[7] administered valproic acid (VPA) by two different regimens in the same total dose to pregnant mice from day 7 to 15 of gestation: by injection once daily and by continuous, constant-rate infusion from implanted pumps. The injections caused drug concentrations in plasma to peak and decline quickly (Figure 5); in fact, for long periods between injections, the drug was undetectable. In humans, the peaks with the usual therapeutic regimen are only one tenth as high, but the trough concentrations are many times higher. These differences arise because the half-life of this widely used antiepileptic drug is only 0.8 hr in the mouse but 8 to 16 hr in humans.

The continuous infusion in mice maintained drug and metabolite levels within a narrow range (Figure 6). Moreover, Nau found that, with the infusion mode, a higher total dose was required to produce embryotoxicity (resorptions and exencephaly) than with daily injections (Figures 7 and 8). Thus, the infusion regimen shifted the dose-response curve for embryotoxicity to the right (Figure 9), such that a tenfold higher dose was required with the infusion regimen to yield the same resorption rate observed with the injection regimen.

Sikic et al.[8] had previously observed regimen dependence for both the toxic and therapeutic actions of the anticancer drug bleomycin. These workers administered doses of the drug in three different 5-day regimens: injections twice daily; alternate-day injections; and continuous infusions by implanted osmotic pumps. Results associated with drug infusion differed in two ways from results obtained with either injection

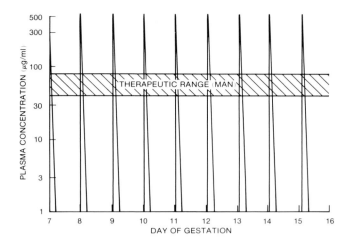

FIGURE 5. Concentrations of valproic acid in mice following once daily s.c. administration of the drug (400 mg/kg) between days 7 and 15 of gestation. The shaded area represents the range of human plasma concentrations during pregnancy and the curves show experimental data.[7]

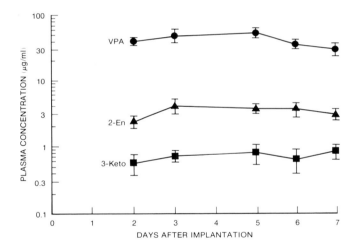

FIGURE 6. Plasma concentrations of valproic acid (VPA) and its metabolites (2-en and 3-keto) in mice after s.c. implantation on day 7 of gestation of two osmotic pumps containing 400 mg/mℓ sodium valproate and delivering 1 μℓ/hr of drug.[7]

regimen: at equal total doses, the infusion reduced the drug's toxicity (Figure 10) but increased its antitumor efficacy (Figure 11). This enhanced efficacy observed with continuous infusion of bleomycin was confirmed by Peng and colleagues.[113] Thus, continuous infusion shifted the dose-response curve for bleomycin toxicity to the right, while shifting the dose-response curve for efficacy to the left. Putting together these two observations leads to the conclusion that the therapeutic index for bleomycin is widened by use of the infusion regimen and narrowed by the injection regimen. Subsequent clinical studies also appear to confirm the prediction that the human use of bleomycin may be made both safer and more efficacious by use of a constant-rate infusion regimen.[118,119]

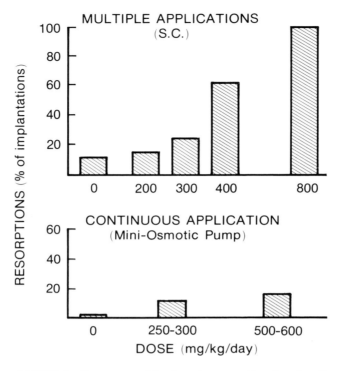

FIGURE 7. Percentage of implantation resorptions in mice after administration of valproic acid between days 7 to 15 of gestation.[7]

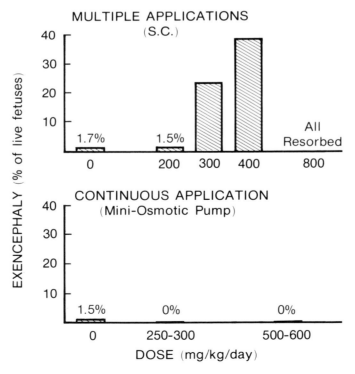

FIGURE 8. Incidence of exencephaly in mice following administration of valproic acid between gestational days 7 to 15.[7]

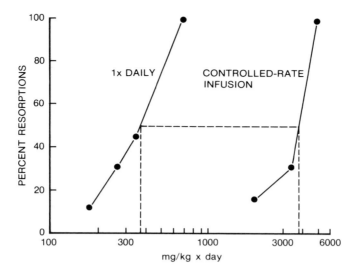

FIGURE 9. Fetal resorption rate observed when valproic acid is administered as a single daily injection or by continuous infusion. (Adapted from Nau, H. et al., *Metabolism of Antiepileptic Drugs*, Levy, R. H. et al., Eds., Raven Press, New York, 1984, 85. With permission.)

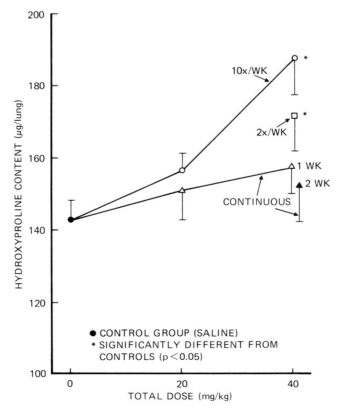

FIGURE 10. Effect of various doses and regimens of bleomycin on pulmonary toxicity in nontumored mice, as measured by the hydroxyproline content of lung after 10 weeks of treatment.[8]

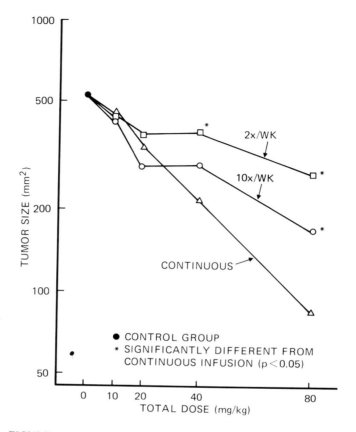

FIGURE 11.   Dose-response curve of bleomycin administered by 3 regimens against Lewis lung carcinoma. Measurements shown in the figure were made on day 15 of treatment but are representative of differences that existed throughout the course of treatment.[8]

Other experimental studies of regimen dependence using continuous infusion have involved exogenous administrations of hormones, whose effects have long been recognized as rate dependent rather than dose dependent. For example, the action of parathormone,[46] human growth hormone,[114] and triiodothyronine[115] have now been studied in comparative injection-infusion protocols.

Two studies using the IIC protocol to explore the action of parathyroid hormone on bone formation and resorption indicated that the net effect on bone mass depended on the regimen used:

Tam et al.[46] compared the effects of parathyroid hormone 6PTH-(1-84) when administered by either daily s.c. injections or by continuous infusion in thyroparathyroidectomized rats. The infusion resulted in increased bone apposition and an increase in both bone formation and resorption surfaces, with a net decrease in trabecular bone. Equal doses in s.c. injection increased bone apposition rate and bone formation surface, but did not increase resorption surfaces; in this case, bone volume increased. The authors conclude that the s.c. injection regimen provides a way of separating the resorptive effects of 6PTH-(1-84) from its effects on apposition rate and that intermittent doses of the hormone would be more effective than continuous infusion in promoting anabolic skeletal effects.

Podbesek et al.[120] obtained similar results in intact greyhounds when they com-

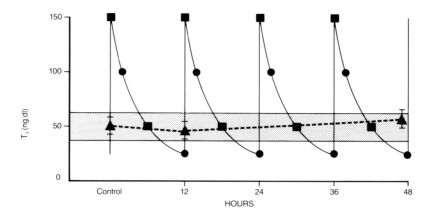

FIGURE 12. Plasma concentrations of T_3 following s.c. injections of 161 mg $T_3/100$ g (■ predicted value, ● measured value) every 12 hr and with continuous infusion (▲ measured value) in thyroidectomized rats. The shaded area is the range of plasma concentrations of T_3 in intact rats.[115]

pared the effects on bone volume of administering human growth hormone (hPTH 1-34) by s.c. injection or continuous infusion. The superior results with injections were in agreement with those in patients similarly treated previously. The authors concluded that an intermittent dosage regimen, though elevating PTH levels only transiently, appears more promising for the treatment of osteoporosis than the infusion regimen. They suggest that the infusion may inhibit the full expression of osteoblastic new bone formation by the "persistently supraphysiologic levels of the peptide" that it maintains.

Connors and Hedge[115] explored quantitative relationships in the control of thyroid hormone secretion in unanesthetized, thyroidectomized rats. Physiologic amounts of T_3 administered by continuous infusion maintained near normal T_3 plasma levels, while TSH levels rose steadily over 144 hr (Figure 12); at higher levels in the physiologic range, T_3 was elevated and TSH was in the normal range. Equivalent amounts of T_3 given twice daily by s.c. injection produced a twice-daily nonphysiologic peak-and-trough pattern of T_3 concentrations and suppressed TSH to below prethyroidectomy levels. The injection regimen also reduced responsiveness to TRH to a greater degree than the infusion. In a second study, the authors administered T_4 in drinking water or by s.c. injection at various doses. At the lower dose, the drinking water regimen produced a rise in plasma T_4 and TSH, and a decrease in T_3; the higher dose produced a greater elevation in T_4, only a transient decrease in T_3 and no change in TSH. Continuous replacement of T_4 caused dose-dependent elevation of T_4, little plasma T_3 generation, and inhibition of the post-thyroidectomy rise in plasma TSH. The authors concluded that T_4 in plasma exerts a negative-feedback effect on TSH secretion in addition to that due to plasma T_3. In the control of pituitary TSH secretion, T_4 acts as both a hormone — conveying feedback information to the pituitary — and as a prohormone, giving rise to a large fraction of plasma T_3. In addition, small amounts of T_4 replacement enhance the TSH responsiveness to exogenous TRH in short-term hypothyroid rats.

Cotes et al.[114] examined the effects in hypophysectomized rats of various dose regimens and vehicles for administering human growth hormone (hGH) to determine the most efficient way to administer the limited amounts available. hGH administered by continuous s.c. infusion induced a greater growth response than hGH administered in higher doses by intermittent daily injection, though it is known that in the rat (and normal child) GH secretion is episodic. The potency of the hormone administered from osmotic pumps was 169% of that administered in intermittent injections of hGH solution.

Obie and Cooper[121] demonstrated that constant exogenous s.c. input of calcitonin or parathormone (CT or PTH) for 1 week in rats produced consistently elevated levels of these agents, but the hypocalcemia produced by CT was transitory, as was the hypercalcemia caused by PTH. Rather than illustrating receptor "down-regulation", this phenomenon was attributed to counter-regulatory action of the other hormone — i.e., the experiment illustrated a double-feedback system. Other investigators have studied regimen-dependent actions of other drugs with the comparative infusion-injection regimen. Smits et al.[122] demonstrated the full range of cardiovascular actions that propranolol evokes in rats over 7 days of subcutaneous infusion.The data are far more conclusive than if injections alone had been the only regimen used for administering this drug. Another interesting demonstration of regimen dependency is found in studies of Prevo et al.[6] and Abood et al.,[123] who explored the effects of nicotine administration on fetal weight gain during pregnancy.

These examples are merely illustrative of the growing number of studies underway to test the advantages or disadvantages of constant-rate infusion vs. intermittent injections in the administration of endogenous substances. The fact that no general or predictable result emerges underlines the importance of using the IIC protocol to assess each agent.

3. Time-Varying Programmed Regimens

Although osmotic systems provide constant-rate delivery, they can be adapted to deliver drugs or hormones at preprogrammed rates that vary over time. That is an important capability, since it is not yet clear which drugs or bioactive agents are best given by a *constant* rate regimen and which might require a *pattern of input* at different rates to obtain an optimal regimen. The true physiological effect of some hormones may be observable only when the agent is given by an on/off or phasic/tonic administration. Various investigators have devised techniques utilizing implanted rate-controlled pumps to achieve these patterns of infusion. The approaches have been either to mimic the circadian rhythm, to infuse agents to alter existing patterns, or to study what the existing pattern does to the test agent.

For example, an adaptation of the osmotic pump has recently permitted mimicking of the circadian rhythm for melatonin. Lynch et al.[42,43] used subcutaneously implanted osmotic pumps to which a coiled polyethylene catheter was attached. By filling the coil with an alternating sequence of vehicle/drug solution/vehicle/drug solution, etc. these investigators infused melatonin slowly and intermittently according to a predetermined temporal test program. To document the 24-hr rhythm in melatonin excretion (which corresponded to the times of infusion by the delivery device) they measured urinary levels of melatonin or of a mixed solution that also contained a dye. They achieved a discrete pattern of 6 hr on and 18 hr off over 6 days. This early use of osmotic pumps to achieve a time-varying pattern of delivery has stimulated other experiments to mimic or uncover temporal patterns of the secretion of physiologic substances.

Knobil's[116] work provides another example of a dynamic mode of rate-controlled administration. Using an on/off pattern of delivery, he demonstrated that the physiologic actions of gonadotropin-releasing hormone — and attempts to mimic those actions in therapy — depend on frequency and amplitude of its administration. Neither dose nor fixed rate provide a rational basis for understanding this hormone's actions. Such results should stimulate explorations of time-varied patterns in the administration of many other biological substances to determine the dependency of their actions on frequency or amplitude of administration.

Other investigators have employed continuous infusion of various agents to influence the characteristics of existing temporal patterns. For example, several studies have used continuously infused antidepressant drugs to study their influence on various cyclic rhythms.[124-126] Wirz-Justice and Campbell[125] found that the circadian rest/activity cycle in female hamsters was lengthened by chronic administration of the monoamine oxidase inhibitor clorgyline. In addition, chronic subcutaneous infusion with clorgyline or imipramine over 2 weeks was found to induce dissociation of many components of the circadian activity rhythm. The authors concluded that chronic use of agents of this nature can modify circadian frequency and/or coupling between circadian rhythms — important considerations in long-term therapy with these drugs. Christensen and Agner[127] studied the effect of lithium on the circadian cycles of food and water intake, urinary concentration and body weight in rats. By then controlling lithium in the diet and at the same time continuously infusing arginine vasopressin at 10 mU/hr i.v. over 1 week, these investigators were able to sort out some of the mediators of diuresis during darkness and antidiuresis during daylight hours in these animals.

Obviously, neither bolus injections nor slow continuous infusions can reproduce normally rhythmic variations in plasma levels of hormones and other cyclic events. Instead, variations of continuous infusion are useful to mimic their precise timing. That approach in animal studies has enabled investigators to explore not only circadian patterns, but also how drugs and other factors affect them. In time, such studies should elucidate the nature of the mechanisms responsible for these time patterns.

IV. OSMET™ DRUG DELIVERY MODULE

The same osmotic technology described for use in preclinical studies has been adapted to clinical studies. The OSMET™ drug delivery module can administer a solution or suspension of an agent of interest either orally or rectally. The capsule-shaped modules transit the human gastrointestinal tract in the same manner as conventional tablets, but are somewhat bulkier in proportion to the amount of drug they can contain. The smaller 0.2-ml capacity modules deliver continuously at a near-constant rate of 8, 15, or 25 μl/hr, respectively, for 24, 12, or 8 hr. The 2-ml capacity modules for rectal or vaginal administration deliver 60 μl/hr for 30 hr or 120 μl/hr for 15 hr.

De Leede and co-workers[4,5] utilized the modules in clinical trials to study rectal administration of antipyrine (Figure 13) and the choline salt of theophylline (Figure 14) over 98 and 72 hr, respectively. For both agents, use by each subject of two modules sequentially resulted in prolonged maintenance of virtually constant plasma levels of drug and good agreement of in vitro and in vivo functionality of the dosage form.

These modules also have been used in clinical investigative studies[127] to deliver anti-inflammatories, antihypertensives, vitamins, and various kinds of receptor-blocking agents.

V. CONCLUSIONS

Until rate-controlled delivery systems became available, drug assessment was severely hampered at both the preclinical and clinical levels by the difficulties of exploring the pharmacodynamics of drug actions. Single-dose pharmacokinetic studies have yielded only limited information in comparison with that now obtainable by studying the agent in a wide array of temporally varied delivery modes. Moreover, the advent of implantable osmotic pumps has greatly facilitated rate-controlled drug administration in preclinical studies by dispensing with the need for animal restraint and special equipment.

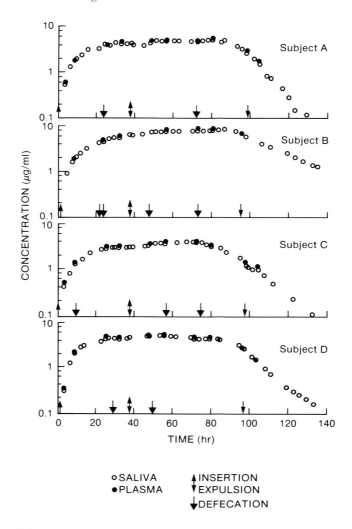

FIGURE 13.   Concentrations of antipyrine in plasma and saliva following administration of an osmotic rectal delivery system (delivering
43 μℓ/hr antipyrine) in four subjects.[5]

For these reasons — and because of the availability of therapeutic rate-controlled
dosage forms — researchers are beginning to view the study of drug actions at steady
state or in programmed, time-varying patterns of delivery as matters of practical importance and not merely of academic interest. Specifically, they are beginning to explore the effects of regimen variation in both pharmacologic and pharmacotherapeutic
research. In the next decade such studies should bring about several developments:

- Testing, registration, and marketing of a growing number of products in which
  innovation is based on rate-controlled release of established agents rather than
  on synthesis of new chemical entities
- Use in routine outpatient therapy of agents with half-lives too short, or therapeutic indexes too narrow, to permit their administration in conventional bolus dosage forms
- Optimization of regimens early in the development phase of new drugs and revi-
  sion of the regimens of many older drugs in the light of data now obtainable
  from rate-controlled preclinical and clinical studies

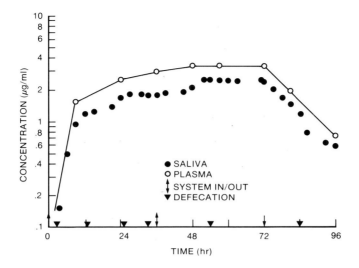

FIGURE 14. Concentrations of theophylline in plasma and saliva after administration of an osmotic rectal delivery system (delivering 11 mg/hr theophylline) in one subject.[4]

ACKNOWLEDGMENT

The authors wish to acknowledge the assistance of James Yuen in the preparation of this manuscript.

REFERENCES

1. Theeuwes, F. and Yum, S. I., Principles of the design and operation of generic osmotic pumps for the delivery of semisolid or liquid drug formulations, *Ann. Biomed. Eng.*, 4, 343, 1976.
2. Eckenhoff, B., Theeuwes, F., and Urquhart, J., Osmotically actuated dosage forms for rate-controlled drug delivery, *Pharm. Technol.*, 5, 35, 1981.
3. Eckenhoff, B. and Yum, S. I., The osmotic pump: novel research tool for optimizing drug regimens, *Biomaterials*, 2, 89, 1981.
4. De Leede, L. G. J., De Boer, A. G., Van Velzen, S. L., and Breimer, D. D., Zero-order rectal delivery of theophylline in man with an osmotic system, *J. Pharmacokinet. Biopharm.*, 10, 525, 1982.
5. De Leede, L. G. J., De Boer, A. G., and Breimer, D. D., Rectal infusion of the model drug antipyrine with an osmotic delivery system, *Biopharm. Drug Dispos.*, 2, 131, 1981.
6. Prevo, M., Amkraut, A., and Fara, J., Regimen-dependent embryotoxicity of nicotine, *Toxicologist*, 3, 156, 1983.
7. Nau, H., Zierer, R., Spielmann, H., Neubert, D., and Gansau, C., A new model for embryotoxicity testing: teratogenicity and pharmacokinetics of valproic acid following constant-rate administration in the mouse using human therapeutic drug and metabolite concentrations, *Life Sci.*, 29, 2803, 1981.
8. Sikic, B. I., Collins, J. M., Mimnaugh, E. G., and Gram, T. E., Improved therapeutic index of bleomycin when administered by continuous infusion in mice, *Cancer Treat. Rep.*, 62, 2011, 1978.
9. Myers, R. D., Ed., *Methods in Psychology: Advanced Laboratory Techniques in Neuropsychology and Neurobiology*, Vol. 3, Academic Press, New York, 1977, 315.
10. Week, J. R., A method for administration of prolonged intravenous infusion of prostacyclin (PGI₂) to unanesthestized rats, *Prostaglandin*, 17, 495, 1979.
11. van Eys, G. J. J. M. and Wendelaar Bonga, S. E., Structural changes in the pars intermedia of the cichlid teleost *Sarotherodon mossambicus* as a result of background adaptation and illumination, *Cell Tissue Res.*, 220, 561, 1981.

12. Martens, G. J. M., Soeterik F., Jenks, B. G., and van Overbeeke, A. P., In vivo biosynthesis of melanotropins and related peptides in the pars intermedia of *Xenopus laevis, Gen. Comp. Endocrinol.,* 49, 73, 1983.

13. Riley, V., Mouse mammary tumors: alteration of incidence as apparent function of stress, *Science,* 189, 465, 1975.

14. Jarnagin, K., Brommage, R., DeLuca, H. F., Yamada, S., and Takayama, H., 1- but not 24-hydroxylation of vitamin D is required for growth and reproduction in rats, *Am. J. Physiol.,* 244, E290, 1983.

15. Cheng, S. W. T., North, W. G., and Gellai, M., Replacement therapy with arginine vasopressin in homozygous Brattleboro rats, *Ann. N. Y. Acad. Sci.,* 394, 473, 1982.

16. Beyler, S. A. and Zaneveld, L. J. D., Antifertility activity of systemically administered proteinase (acrosin) inhibitors, *Contraception,* 26, 137, 1982.

17. de la Torre, J. C. and Gonzalez-Carvajal, M., Steady state drug or fluid delivery to injured or transected spinal cord of rats, *Lab. Anim. Sci.,* 31, 701, 1981.

18. Kroin, J. S. and Penn, R. D., Intracerebral chemotherapy: chronic microinfusion of cisplatin, *Neurosurgery,* 10, 349, 1982.

19. Krause, J. E., Advis, J. P., and McKelvey, J. F., *In vivo* biosynthesis of hypothalamic luteinizing hormone releasing hormone in individual free-running female rats, *Endocrinology,* 111, 344, 1982.

20. Gould, T. R. L., Brunette, D. M., and Dorey, J., Cell turnover in the periodontal ligament determined by continuous infusion of H^3-thymidine using osmotic minipumps, *J. Peridontal Res.,* 17, 662, 1982.

21. Akhtar, F. B., Marshall, G. R., Wickings, E. J., and Nieschlag, E., Reversible induction of azoospermia in rhesus monkeys by constant infusion of a gonadotropin-releasing hormone agonist using osmotic minipumps, *J. Clin. Endocrinol. Metab.,* 56, 534, 1983.

22. Struyker Boudier, H. A. J., Smits, J. F. M., and Kasbergen, C., A new method for long-term continuous drug infusion into the renal artery of the conscious, unrestrained rat, *Naunyn-Schmiedebergs Arch. Pharmakol.,* 319 (Suppl.), R50, 1982.

23. Arimura, A., Predroza, E., Vilchez-Martinez, J., and Schally, A. V., Prevention of implantation of D-Trp6-LH-RH in the rat: comparative study with the effects of large doses of HCG on pregnancy, *Endocr. Res. Commun.,* 4, 357, 1977.

24. Siew, C. and Goldstein, D. B., Osmotic minipumps for administration of barbital to mice: demonstration of functional tolerance and physical dependence, *J. Pharmacol. Exp. Ther.,* 204, 541, 1978.

25. Butcher, R. L., Inskeep, E. K., and Pope, R. S., Plasma concentrations of estradiol produced with two delivery systems in ovariectomized rats, *Proc. Soc. Exp. Biol. Med.,* 158, 475, 1978.

26. Kasamatsu, T., Pettigrew, J. D., and Ary, M., Restoration of visual cortical plasticity by local microperfusion of norepinephrine, *J. Comp. Neurol.,* 185, 163, 1979.

27. Seymour, A. A., Davis, J. O., Freeman, R. H., DeForrest, J. M., Rowe, B. P., Stephens, G. A., and Williams, G. M., Hypertension produced by sodium depletion and unilateral nephrectomy: a new experimental model, *Hypertension,* 2, 125, 1980.

28. Clot, J. P., Bouhnik, J., Baudry, M., and Michel, R., Rat thyroxine metabolism studied by osmotic minipump infusion, *C. R. Acad. Sci.,* 290, 235, 1980.

29. Rigter, H., Rijk, H., and Crabbe, J. C., Tolerance to ethanol and severity of withdrawal in mice are enhanced by a vasopressin fragment, *Eur. J. Pharmacol.,* 64, 53, 1980.

30. Grinker, J., Strohmayer, A. J., Baukal, A., and Catt, K. J., Circulating angiotensin II and adrenal receptors after nephrectomy, *Nature,* 289, 507, 1981.

31. Ogashiwa, M., Hosino, T., Muraoka, I., and Hervatin, S., Variability of radioactive thymidine labeling in the rat brain tumor model, *Neurol. Med. Chir.,* 20, 395, 1980.

32. Yamori, Y., Tarazi, R. C., and Ooshima, A., Effect of B-receptor-blocking agents on cardiovascular structural changes in spontaneous and noradrenaline-induced hypertension in rats, *Clin. Sci.,* 59, 457s, 1980.

33. Severs, W. B. and Daniel-Severs, A. E., Effects of angiotensin on the central nervous system, *Pharm. Rev.,* 25, 415, 1973.

34. Fitzsimons, J. T., Thirst, *Physiol. Rev.,* 52, 468, 1972.

35. Yates, F. E., Saucerman, J., Casper, A., and Urquhart, J., Sustained polydipsia in rats receiving continuous intraventricular infusion of angiotensin II for one to three weeks, presented at 60th Ann. Mtg. Endocrine Society, Miami, Fla., June 14 to 16, 1978.

36. Yates, F. E., Ed., Driving rats to drink: dipsogenic effect of angiotensin II during continuous infusion into the third cerebral ventricle (CV3 infusion) for seven days, *Special Delivery, ALZET® Osmotic Minipump Tech. Bull.,* 1(3), 1, 1977.

37. Yum, S. I., Tillson, S. A., and Theeuwes, F., Miniaturized osmotic pump technology for control of experimentally induced diabetes, *Abstr. Short Communications and Poster Presentations, Vth International Congress of Endocrinology,* Hamburg, W. Germany, July 18 to 24, 1976, 366.

38. Patel, D. G., Rate of insulin infusion with a minipump required to maintain a normoglycemia in diabetic rats (41529), *Proc. Soc. Exp. Biol. Med.,* 172, 74, 1983.
39. Lopaschuk, G. D., Tahiliani, A. G., and McNeill, J. H., Continuous long-term insulin delivery in diabetic rats utilizing implanted osmotic minipumps, *J. Pharmacol. Methods,* 9, 71, 1983.
40. Rose, D. P. and Mountjoy, K. G., Influence of thyroidectomy and prolactin suppression on the growth of n-nitrosomethylurea-induced rat mammary carcinomas, *Cancer Res.,* 43, 2588, 1983.
41. Brown, J. G. and Millward, D. J., Dose response of protein turnover in rat skeletal muscle to triiodothyronine treatment, *Biochim. Biophys. Acta,* 757, 182, 1983.
42. Lynch, H. J., Rivest, R. W., and Wurtman, R. J., Artificial induction of melatonin rhythms by programmed microinfusion, *Neuroendocrinology,* 31, 106, 1980.
43. Lynch, H. J. and Wurtman, R. J., Control of rhythms in the secretion of pineal hormones in humans and experimental animals, in *Biological Rhythms and their Central Mechanism,* Suda, M., Hayaishi, O., and Nakagawa, H., Eds., Elsevier/North Holland, Amsterdam, 1979, 117.
44. Will, P. C., Cortright, R. N., and Hopfer, U., Polyethylene glycols as solvents in implantable osmotic pumps, *J. Pharm. Sci.,* 69, 747, 1980.
45. Morris, D. J. and Kenyon, C. J., Aldosterone and its metabolism in spontaneously hypertensive rats (SHR), *Clin. Exp. Hyper.-Theory Prac.,* A4, 1613, 1982.
46. Tam, C. S., Heersche, J. N. M., Murray, T. M., and Parsons, J. A., Parathyroid hormone stimulates the bone apposition rate independently of its absorptive action: differential effects of intermittent and continuous administration, *Endocrinology,* 110, 506, 1982.
47. Hefti, E., Trechsel, U., Fleisch, H., and Bonjour, J. P., Nature of calcemic effect of 1,25-dihydroxyvitamin D3 in experimental hypoparathyroidism, *Am. J. Physiol.,* 244, E313, 1983.
48. Ewing, L. L., Wing, T. Y., Cochran, R. C., Kromann, N., and Zirkin, B. R., Effect of luteinizing hormone on Leydig cell structure and testosterone secretion, *Endocrinology,* 112, 1763, 1983.
49. Schoenle, E., Zapf, J., and Froesch, E. R., Regulation of rat adipocyte glucose transport by growth hormone: no mediation by insulin-like growth factors, *Endocrinology,* 112, 384, 1983.
50. Fried, W., Barone-Varelas, J., Barone, T., and Anagnostou, A., Effect of angiotensin infusion on extrarenal erythropoietin production, *J. Lab. Clin. Med.,* 99, 520, 1982.
51. Kelinjans, J. C. S., Smits, J. F. M., Kasbergen, C. M., Vervoort-Peters, H. T. M., and Struyker-Boudier, H. A. J., Blood pressure response to chronic low-dose intrarenal noradrenaline infusion in conscious rats, *Clin. Sci.,* 65, 111, 1983.
52. Cervantes, M., Ruelas, R., and Beyer, C., Progesterone facilitation of EEG synchronization in response to milk drinking in female cats, *Psychoneuroendocrinology,* 4, 245, 1979.
53. Bochskanl, R. and Kirchner, C., Uteroglobin and the accumulation of progesterone in the uterine lumen of the rabbit, *Wilhelm Roue Arch. Entwicklungsmech. Org.,* 190, 127, 1981.
54. Clayton, R. N., Gonadotropin-releasing hormone modulation of its own pituitary receptors: evidence for biphasic regulation, *Endocrinology,* 111, 152, 1982.
55. Bear, M. F., Paradiso, M. A., Schwartz, M., Nelson, S. B., Carnes, K. M., and Daniels, J. D., Two methods of catecholamine depletion in kitten visual cortex yield different effects on plasticity, *Nature,* 302, 245, 1983.
56. Diz, D. I., Baer, P. G., and Nasjletti, A., Effect of norepinephrine and renal denervation of renal PGE2 and kallikrein in rats, *Am. J. Physiol.,* 241, F477, 1981.
57. Pratt, B. R., Butcher, R. L., and Inskeep, E. K., Effect of continuous intrauterine administration of prostaglandin E2 on life-span of corpora lutea of nonpregnant ewes, *J. Anim. Sci.,* 48, 1441, 1979.
58. Susa, J. B., McCormick, K. L., Widness, J. A., Singer, D. B., Oh, W., Admsons, K., and Schwartz, R., Chronic hyperinsulinemia in the fetal rhesus monkey, *Diabetes,* 28, 1058, 1979.
59. Elliott, M., Sehgal, P. K., Susa, J. B., Zeller, W. P., Widness, J. A., and Schwartz, R., Experimentally induced hyperinsulinemia in a fetus and newborn rhesus monkey *(Macaca mulatta), Lab. Anim. Sci.,* 31, 286, 1981.
60. Spencer, G. S. G., Hill, D. J., Garssen, G. J., Macdonald, A. A., and Colenbrander, B., Somatomedin activity and growth hormone levels in body fluids of the fetal pig: effect of chronic hyperinsulinemia, *J. Endocrinol.,* 96, 107, 1983.
61. Lorijn, R. H. W. and Longo, L. D., Clinical and physiologic implications of increased fetal oxygen consumptions, *Am. J. Obstet. Gynecol.,* 136, 451, 1980.
62. Lorijn, R. H. W., Nelson, J. C., and Longo, L. D., Induced fetal hyperthyroidism: cardiac output and oxygen consumption, *Am. J. Physiol.,* 239, H302, 1980.
63. Struyker-Boudier, H. A. J., The osmotic minipump: applications of a new tool in drug delivery to experimental animals, *Labo-Pharma Probl. Tech.,* 298, 373, 1980.
64. Struyker-Boudier, H. A. J., Rate-controlled drug delivery: pharmacological, therapeutic and industrial perspectives, *Trends Pharmacol. Sci.,* 3, 162, 1982.
65. Smits, J. F. M., van Essen, H., and Struyker-Boudier, H. A. J., Is the antihypertensive effect of propranolol caused by an action within the central nervous system?, *J. Pharmacol. Exp. Ther.,* 215, 221, 1980.

66. Struyker-Boudier, H. A. J. and van Essen, H., Chronic infusion of clonidine in the spontaneously hypertensive rat, *Naunyn-Schmiedebergs Arch. Pharmakol.,* 311 (Suppl.), R49, 1980.

67. Smits, J. F. M., Kasbergen, C. M., van Essen, H., Kleinjans, J. C., and Struyker-Boudier, H. A. J., Chronic local infusion into the renal artery of unrestrained rats, *Am. J. Physiol.,* 244, H304, 1983.

68. Kleinjans, J. C., Smits, J. F., van Essen, H., and Struyker-Boudier, H. A., Hemodynamic effects of intrarenal noradrenaline infusion in conscious rats, *Fed Proc. Fed. Am. Soc. Exp. Biol.,* 41, 1660, 1982.

69. Hosada, S., Hachiro, I., and Saito, T., *Praomys (Mastomys) natalensis:* animal model for study of histamine-induced duodenal ulcers, *Gasteroenterology,* 80, 16, 1981.

70. Szabo, S., Animal model: cysteamine induced acute and chronic duodenal ulcer in the rat, *Am. J. Pathol.,* 93, 273, 1978.

71. Tze, W. J., Wong, F. C., and Chen, L. M., Implantable artificial capillary unit for pancreatic islet allograft and xenograft, *Diabetologica,* 16, 247, 1979.

72. Greenberg, S. and Wilborn, W., Effect of clonidine and propranolol on venous smooth muscle from spontaneously hypertensive rats, *Arch. Int. Pharmacodyn.,* 258, 234, 1982.

73. Greenberg, S. and Wilborn, W., Effect of chronic administration of clonidine and propranolol on the myocardium of spontaneously hypertensive rats, *Arch. Int. Pharmacodyn. Ther.,* 255, 141, 1982.

74. Kleinjans, J., Kasbergen, C., Verwoort-Peters, L., Smits, J., and Struyker-Boudier, H. A. J., Chronic intravenous infusion of noradrenaline produces labile hypertension in conscious rats, *Life Sci.,* 29, 509, 1981.

75. Mills, D. E., Buckman, M. T., and Peake, G. T., A chronically hypoprolactinemic rat model: administration of lergotrile mesylate by osmotic minipump, *Proc. Soc. Exp. Biol. Med.,* 166, 438, 1981.

76. Gruppuso, P. A., Migliori, R., Susa, J. B., and Schwartz, R., Chronic maternal hyperinsulinemia and hypoglycemia, *Biol. Neonate,* 40, 113, 1981.

77. Tabakoff, B., Ritzmann, R. F., and Oltmans, G. A., The effect of selective lesions of brain noradrenergic systems on the development of barbiturate tolerance in rats, *Brain Res.,* 176, 327, 1979.

78. Wei, E., Enkephalin analogs: correlation of potencies for analgesia and physical dependence, in *Characteristics and Function of Opioids,* Van Ree, J. M. and Terenius, L., Eds., Elsevier/North Holland, Amsterdam, 1978, 445.

79. Wei, E. and Loh, H., Physical dependence on opiate-like peptides, *Science,* 193, 1262, 1976.

80. Volicer, L., Schmidt, W. K., Hartz, T. P., Klosowicz, B. A., and Meichner, R., Cyclic nucleotides and ethanol tolerance and dependence, *Drug Alcohol Depend.,* 4, 295, 1979.

81. Schmidt, W. K., and Way, E. L., Effect of a calcium chelator on morphine tolerance development, *Eur. J. Pharmacol.,* 63, 243, 1980.

82. Stewart, J. M., Chipkin, R. E., Channabasavaiah, K., Gay, M. L., and Krivoy, W. A., Inhibition of development of tolerance to morphine by a peptide related to ACTH, in *Neural Peptides and Neuronal Communication,* Costa, E. and Trabucchi, M., Eds., Raven Press, New York, 1980, 305.

83. Hetta, J. and Terenius, L., Prenatal naloxone affects survival and morphine sensitivity of rat offspring, *Neurosci. Lett.,* 16, 323, 1980.

84. Crawley, J. N. and Beinfeld, M. C., Rapid development of tolerance to the behavioural actions of cholecystokinin, *Nature (London),* 302, 703, 1983.

85. Schulz, R., Seidl, E., Wuster, M., and Herz, A., Opioid dependence and cross-dependence in the isolated guinea-pig ileum. *Eur. J. Pharmacol.,* 84, 33, 1982.

86. Wuster, M., Schulz, R., and Herz, A., The development of opiate tolerance may dissociate from dependence, *Life Sci.,* 31, 1695, 1982.

87. Schulz, R., Wuster, M., Krenss, H., and Herz, A., Lack of cross-tolerance on multiple opiate receptors in the mouse vas deferens, *Mol. Pharmacol.,* 18, 395, 1980.

88. Broccardo, M., Erspamer, V., Falconierierspamer, G., Improta, G., Linari, G., Melchiorri, R., and Montecucchi, P. C., Pharmacological data on dermorphins, a new class of potent opioid peptides from amphibian skin, *Br. J. Pharmacol.,* 73, 625, 1981.

89. Nielsen, E. B., Rapid decline of stereotyped behavior in rats during constant one week administration of amphetamine via implanted ALZET® osmotic minipumps, *Pharmacol. Biochem. Behav.,* 15, 161, 1981.

90. Nabeshima, T., Sivam, S. P., Tai, C. Y., and Ho, I. K., Development of dispositional tolerance to phenylcyclidine by osmotic minipump in the mouse, *J. Pharm. Method,* 7, 239, 1982.

91. Sun, C. L. J. and Hanig, J. P., Alteration of sensitivity of adrenergic vascular responses after prolonged exposure to agonists via osmotic minipump (41584), *Proc. Soc. Exp. Biol. Med.,* 172, 440, 1983.

92. Hauger, L. L., Aguilera, G., and Catt, K. J., Angiotensin II regulates its receptor sites in the adrenal glomerulosa zone, *Nature (London),* 271, 176, 1978.

93. Douglas, J. G., Potassium ion as a regulator of adrenal angiotensin II receptors, *Am. J. Physiol.,* 239, E317, 1980.

94. Aguilera, G., Menard, R. H., and Catt, K. J., Regulatory actions of angiotensin II on receptors and steroidogenic enzymes in adrenal glomerulosa cells, *Endocrinology*, 107, 55, 1980.

95. Douglas, J. G. and Brown, G. P., Effect of prolonged low dose infusion of angiotensin II and aldosterone on rat smooth muscle and adrenal angiotensin II receptors, *Endocrinology*, 111, 988, 1982.

96. Clayton, R. N., Gonadotropin-releasing hormone modulation of its own pituitary receptors: evidence for biphasic regulation, *Endocrinology*, 111, 152, 1982.

97. Zukin, R. S., Sugarman, J. R., Fitz-Syage, M. L., Gardner, E. L., Zukin, S. R., and Gintzler, A. R., Naltrexone-induced opiate receptor supersensitivity, *Brain Res.*, 245, 285, 1982.

98. Chang, R. S. L., Lotti, V. J., Martin, G. E., and Chen, T. B., Increase in brain ^{125}I-cholecystokinin (CCK) receptor binding following chronic haloperidol treatment, intracisternal 6-hydroxydopamine or ventral tegmental lesions, *Life Sci.*, 32, 871, 1983.

99. Levin, P., Haji, M., Joseph, J. A., and Roth, G. S., Effect of aging on prolactin regulation of rat striatal dopamine receptor concentrations, *Life Sci.*, 32, 1743, 1983.

100. Norstedt, G., Wrange, O., and Gustafsson, J. A., Multihormonal regulations of the estrogen receptor in rat liver, *Endocrinology*, 108, 1190, 1981.

101. Chan, V., Katikineni, M., Davies, T. F., and Catt, K. J., Hormonal regulation of testicular luteinizing hormone and prolactin receptors, *Endocrinology*, 108, 1607, 1981.

102. Norstedt, G., Mode, A., Eneroth, P., and Gustafsson, J. A., Induction of prolactin receptors in rat liver after the administration of growth hormone, *Endocrinology*, 108, 1855, 1981.

103. Aarons, R. D. and Molinoff, P. B., Changes in the density of beta adrenergic receptors in rat lymphocytes, heart and lung after chronic treatment with propranolol, *J. Pharmacol. Exp. Ther.*, 221, 439, 1982.

104. Norstedt, G., A comparison between the effects of growth hormone on prolactin receptors and estrogen receptors in rat liver, *Endocrinology*, 110, 2107, 1982.

105. Hagino, N., Nakamoto, O., Kunz, Y., Arimura, A., Coy, D. H., and Schally, A. V., Effect of D-Trp6-LH-RH on the pituitary-gonadal axis during the luteal phase in the baboon, *Acta Endocrinol.*, 91, 217, 1979.

106. Harwood, J. P., Clayton, R. N., Chen, T. T., Knox, G., and Catt, K. J., Ovarian gonadotropin-releasing hormone receptors. II. Regulation and effects on ovarian development, *Endocrinology*, 107, 414, 1980.

107. Huhtaniemi, I. and Martikainen, H., Rat testis LH/HCG receptors and testosterone production after treatment with GnRH, *Mol. Cell. Endocrinol.*, 11, 199, 1978.

108. Chang, H. Y., Klein, R. M., and Kunos, G., Selective desensitization of cardiac beta adrenoreceptors by prolonged *in vivo* infusion of catecholamines in rats, *J. Pharmacol. Exp. Ther.*, 221, 784, 1982.

109. Kenakin, T. P. and Ferris, R. M., Effects of *in vivo* β-adrenoceptor down-regulation on cardiac responses to prenalterol and pibuterol, *J. Cardovasc. Pharmacol.*, 5, 90, 1983.

110. Cohen, R. M., Aulakh, C. S., Campbell, I. C., and Murphy, D. L., Functional subsensitivity of α_2-adrenoceptors accompanies reductions in yohimbine binding after clorgyline treatment, *Eur. J. Pharmacol.*, 81, 145, 1982.

111. Cohen, R. M., Ebstein, R. P., Daly, J. W., and Murphy, D. L., Chronic effects of a monoamine oxidase-inhibiting antidepressant: decreases in functional α-adrenergic autoreceptors precede the decrease in norepinephrine-stimulated cyclic adenosine 3′:5′ monophosphate systems in rat brain, *J. Neurosci.*, 2, 1588, 1982.

112. Brown, H. S., Meltzer, G., Merrill, R. C., Fisher, M., Ferre, C., and Place, V. A., Visual effects of pilocarpine in glaucoma. Comparative study of administration by eyedrops or by ocular therapeutic systems, *Arch. Ophthalmol.*, 94, 1716, 1976.

113. Peng, Y. M., Alberts, D. S., Chen, H. S., Mason, N., and Moon, T. E., Antitumour activity and plasma kinetics of bleomycin by continuous and intermittent administrations, *Br. J. Canc.*, 41, 644, 1980.

114. Cotes, P. M., Bartlett, W. A., Das, R. E. G., Flecknell, P., and Termeer, R., Dose regimens of human growth hormone: effects of continuous infusion and of a gelatin vehicle on growth in rats and rate of absorption in rabbits, *J. Endocrinol.*, 87, 303, 1980.

115. Connors, J. M. and Hedge, G. A., Feedback effectiveness of periodic versus constant triiodothyronine replacement, *Endocrinology*, 106, 911, 1980.

116. Knobil, E., The neuroendocrine control of the menstrual cycle, *Recent Prog. Horm. Res.*, 36, 53, 1980.

117. Levy, G., Rowland, M., and Nau, H., Personal communications.

118. Coonely, G., Vugrin, D., La Monte, C., and Lacher, M. J., Bleomycin infusion: pulmonary toxicity, *Proc. Am. Assoc. Cancer Res.*, 22, 369, 1981.

119. Cooper, K. R. and Hong, W. K., Prospective study of the pulmonary toxicity of continuously infused bleomycin, *Cancer Treat. Rep.*, 65, 419, 1981.

120. Podbesek, R., Edouard, C., Meunier, P. J., Parsons, J. A., Reeve, J., Stevenson, R. W., and Zanelli, J. M., Effects of two treatment regimes with synthetic human parathyroid hormone fragment on bone formation and the tissue balance of trabecular bone in greyhounds, *Endocrinology,* 112, 1000, 1983.

121. Obie, J. F. and Cooper, C. W., Loss of calcemic effects of calcitonin and parathyroid hormone infused continuously into rats using the ALZET® osmotic minipump, *J. Pharmacol. Exp. Ther.,* 209, 422, 1979.

122. Smits, J. F. M., Coleman, T. G., Smith, T. L., Kasbergen, C. M., van Essen, H., and Struyker-Boudier, H. A. J., Antihypertensive effect of propranolol in conscious spontaneously hypertensive rats: central hemodynamics, plasma volume, and renal function during β-blockade with propranolol, *J. Cardiovasc. Pharmacol.,* 4, 903, 1982.

123. Abood, L. G., Lowy, K., and Booth, H., Acute and chronic effects of nicotine in rats and evidence for a noncholinergic site of action, in *Cigarette Smoking as a Dependence Process,* Krasnegor, N. A., Ed., NIDA Research Monograph 23, DHEW Pub. No. 79-800, 1979, 136.

124. Morgan, N. T., Vaughan, W. J., Rasband, W. S., Wehr, T. A., and Wirz-Justice, A., A computer-based system for collection and analysis of circadian rest-activity data, *Experientia,* 38, 1296, 1982.

125. Wirz-Justice, A. and Campbell, I. C., Antidepressant drugs can slow or dissociate circadian rhythms, *Experientia,* 38, 1301, 1982.

126. Christensen, S. and Agner, T., Effects of lithium on circadian cycles in food and water intake, urinary concentration and body weight in rats, *Physiol. Behav.,* 28, 635, 1982.

127. Wilson, C. G., Hardy, J. G., and Davis, S. S., Controlled release dosage forms, *Pharm. J.,* 231, 334, 1983.

Chapter 6

RATE-CONTROLLED INSULIN DELIVERY IN NORMAL PHYSIOLOGY AND IN THE TREATMENT OF INSULIN-DEPENDENT DIABETES

John C. Pickup and Ralph W. Stevenson

TABLE OF CONTENTS

I. INTRODUCTION

There can be few areas of pharmacology where the principles of rate-controlled drug delivery have been more extensively applied than in diabetes mellitus. This is partly because of the great clinical importance of diabetes: it is the commonest cause of blindness under the age of 65 years in the western world, and a major cause of mortality from renal failure.[1] About 2% of the population suffer from the disease and major efforts are therefore being expended on improvements in therapy and determining the etiology of the long-term diabetic tissue complications. In this respect, gathering evidence from animal studies and retrospective clinical data suggest that the progress of diabetic microvascular disease is related to the duration and severity of the metabolic disorder.[2] If control of blood glucose and other metabolic parameters could be improved and restored more toward normal there may be hope of slowing, arresting, or even reversing the complications associated with diabetes.

The second reason for the great interest in controlling the rate of drug delivery to the diabetic is the almost unique set of pharmacological problems presented by insulin. The short biochemical half-life of insulin in the circulation (3 to 4 min)[3,4] and the relatively short biological half-life (20 min or so) for glucose depression means that constant blood levels and maintained effect cannot be achieved by a single injection. The insulin must be infused, or injected as a delayed-release preparation. Secondly, insulin has a host of metabolic actions, e.g., inhibition of hepatic glycogenolysis, stimulation of glucose uptake in the periphery, stimulation of protein synthesis, etc. The dose-response curves for these effects are fairly distinct and cover a wide range of plasma insulin concentrations (Figure 1).[5-11] For example, switching from half-maximal inhibition of glycogenolysis to half-maximal stimulation of glucose uptake requires an almost tenfold increase in plasma insulin concentration.

The dose-response curves are also particularly steep, so that small changes in insulin produce large metabolic effects and are vitally important to the switching between catabolism and anabolism. Fine control of delivery is, therefore, necessary. Moreover, there are constantly fluctuating levels of substrate for insulin action (glucose, for example) which occur because of food intake and this makes maintenance of homeostasis complicated.

In normal physiology, a delicate balance is maintained by continuous pancreatic secretion of insulin, which can be altered in response to different stimuli and which can be regulated, at the level of the B cell, by glucose itself.

Figure 2 shows the plasma glucose and insulin levels throughout the day in a group of nondiabetics. Note the almost constant basal supply during the night and between meals, which maintains glucose levels by restraining and controlling hepatic glucose output. At mealtimes, glucose input from the gut increases and triggers a boost of insulin from the B cells of the islets of Langerhans. The augmented insulin level switches effect to the dose-response curves of glucose disposal in the periphery, protein synthesis, lipogenesis, etc. as well as inhibiting liver glucose output and increasing glycogen deposition (see Figure 1).

It must also be appreciated that insulin is delivered in the normal subject into the portal vein. This direct route to the liver may have advantages, in terms of metabolic control, for example, which cannot be achieved by peripheral administration (see below). In diabetic man, insulin is usually given into the subcutaneous tissue. Here the absorption and delivery rate into the general circulation is modified by a number of factors which are poorly understood, e.g., enzymatic degradation, changes in local blood flow, capillary permeability, sequestration, and tissue spread.

The aim of this review is first, to outline the impact of rate-controlled insulin administration in the treatment of diabetic man and elucidation of the causes of diabetic

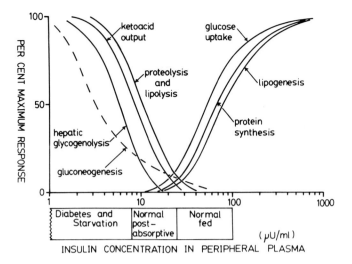

FIGURE 1. Estimated log dose-response curves for insulin in normal physiology and in untreated insulin-dependent diabetes. (Note: insulin concentrations in the portal vein exceed those in the peripheral circulation by approximately threefold.[131]

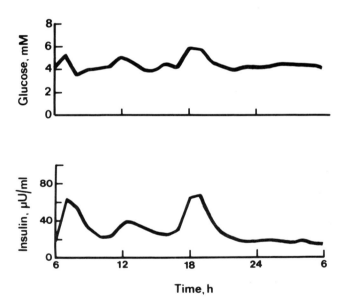

FIGURE 2. Diagram to illustrate mean plasma glucose (upper panel) and insulin (lower panel) concentrations throughout the day in normal healthy subjects.

tissue complications and second, to describe animal studies which complement and extend our knowledge of insulin physiology and pharmacology.

II. CLINICAL STUDIES

A. Control of Insulin Delivery by Conventional Injection Treatment

The available insulin preparations can be divided into three main groups: short, intermediate, and long-acting varieties.[12] Short-acting (i.e., soluble or regular insulin) is simply a solution of crystalline insulin in a diluting medium containing a preservative. The duration of action of short-acting insulin in the diabetic is not entirely clear and certainly varies enormously from day-to-day and person-to-person.[13] Part of the interpatient variability may be due to the variable presence of anti-insulin antibodies in most diabetics treated with animal insulins.[14] These antibodies are thought to modify the efficacy of insulin by binding and perhaps releasing insulin in the circulation and possibly also by altering absorption from the subcutaneous site of injection. However, even in nondiabetics (without antibodies) there is large patient-to-patient variation in absorption. Consequently, most published data on the duration of action and rate of absorption of short-acting (and other) insulins is obtained from experiments in nondiabetics.[15,16] and/or uses indirect means of measuring insulin delivery (e.g., disappearance of externally-counted radioactivity after the subcutaneous injection of ^{125}I-labeled insulin[146]). Values must be taken as a rough guide only.

Nevertheless, an average peak serum insulin at about 1 to 2 hr after subcutaneous injection of short-acting insulin indicates that this type of insulin is suitable for approximating the acute prandial boost of insulin secretion observed in the nondiabetic. The lag in subcutaneous insulin absorption compared to intravenous administration means that the insulin should be injected about 30 min before the start of the meal in the diabetic.

Intermediate-acting insulins represent an attempt to prolong the action of insulin as a depot injection preparation. Protamine insulin (Isophane) and protamine zinc insulin (PZI) have been available since the 1930s and produce prolongation of action by addition of the basic protein protamine and varying amount of zinc suspension to the formulation to slow absorption. In the 1950s, the lente or insulin zinc suspension insulins were introduced. Here, precipitated insulin containing zinc, but not added protein, is suspended in acetate buffer and remains relatively insoluble after injection. The duration of action is modified by the physical form of the suspension — semilente lasts longer than soluble insulin and ultralente at least one day and often much longer. Normal lente insulin is of intermediate duration and is a mixture of three parts of semilente to seven parts ultralente.

These intermediate and long-lasting insulins have been used to simulate the basal insulin secretion of the nondiabetic. A popular regimen, for example is injection of short and intermediate acting insulin (say soluble and isophane) before breakfast and again before the evening meal. However, while morning isophane provides a reasonable background supply during the day, its injection at about 18.00 hr frequently leads to declining plasma insulin and rising plasma glucose levels at about 0600 hr as the depot runs out.[17] Postponement of the evening intermediate-acting insulin to about 22.00 to 23.00 hr may lead to better support of the early morning insulin concentration in the circulation and control of the fasting plasma glucose.[18]

Several physicians now regard ultralente insulin as the optimal injection formulation for mimicking basal delivery.[19] Very good glycemic control has been achieved in a proportion of diabetics treated by ultralente once daily and short-acting insulin either before each meal (i.e., thrice daily) or in the morning and evening (Figure 3).

Apart from more optimized injection regimens, the other recent advance in conventional insulin delivery has been the revived interest in blood glucose self-monitoring.[20-22] Glucose concentration can be measured by the patient in finger-prick samples of capillary blood by spotting the drop of blood onto glucose oxidase reagent strips (e.g., Dextrostix, Boehringer). The color, which is proportional to the glucose concentration, can be estimated by comparison with color charts provided on the bottle or by a portable reflectance meter. The importance of blood glucose self-monitoring is not only that the patient can estimate his own blood glucose and relate the value to the

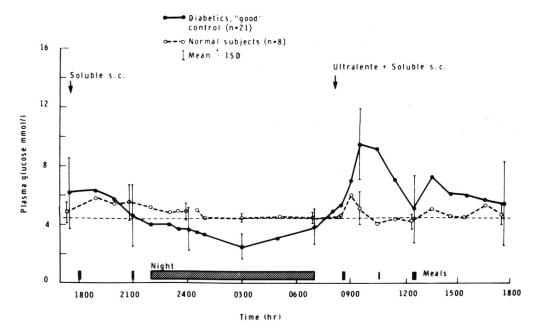

FIGURE 3. Mean circadian plasma glucose levels (±S.D.) in normal subjects (O---O) and insulin-dependent diabetics (●—●) treated by subcutaneous injection of ultralente in the morning and soluble insulin in the morning and evening (From Phillips, M. et al., *Q. J. Med.*, 48, 493, 1979. With permission.)

presence or absence of symptoms, but also that he can make appropriate adjustments in insulin dose and rate of delivery to the circulation, i.e., the patient can "close the loop."

B. Electromechanical Devices for Insulin Delivery
1. Closed-Loop Systems

Although prototype devices for continuous measurement of blood glucose and feedback control of insulin delivery were developed in the 1960s,[23] it was the work of Albisser and colleagues[24,25] and Pfeiffer et al.[26] in 1974 that developed and established the modern artificial endocrine pancreas (AEP). The device is commercially available (the "Biostator") and there are now many studies which have explored its potential in experimental and clinical diabetes and metabolism.

The details of the technology will not be described. The principle, however, is that venous blood is withdrawn from a peripheral vein in the subject and pumped to a bedside apparatus. Here the blood glucose concentration is continuously measured and the results fed to a computer which calculates how much insulin or glucose should be returned to the circulation of the subject to establish and maintain a given blood glucose concentration (usually euglycemia). The rules by which the computer relates glucose information to the appropriate insulin delivery rates are called algorithms. The two important variables are the absolute glucose level and the rate of change. The latter ensures rapid insulin delivery at meal times, reduces the insulin infusion rate when the glucose is falling (preventing hypoglycemia) and corrects for the delay between blood withdrawal and glucose measurement.

a. Applications of Closed-Loop Devices

The early publications[24-26] established that close to euglycemic control could be achieved and maintained in insulin-dependent diabetics for short periods of a few hours to a few days. These results have been confirmed many times (for reviews see References 27 and 28). Examination of the insulin infusion rates during the period of artificial pancreas treatment shows that the pharmacological principles discussed above are upheld by the automatic device — i.e., there is essentially a slow delivery between meals and at night with increased rates at meal times.

Several studies have examined the correlation of the short-term normoglycemia and improved insulin delivery with changes in blood levels of other intermediary metabolites and hormones which are known to be disordered in diabetes when treated by conventional insulin injections. Hanna et al.,[29] for example, examined a period of 10 hr of AEP control; branched chain amino acids as well as lysine and threonine were lower on AEP than for subcutaneous injections but also lower than for nondiabetics. Alanine concentrations also failed to normalize on the AEP. Nosadini et al.[30] found that blood lactate was higher in diabetics than nondiabetics over an 8-hr period of study, but that there was no difference between subcutaneous injection therapy and the AEP. During both treatments, levels of glycerol and free fatty acids were lower than normal and total ketone bodies remained significantly higher than in nondiabetics.

From both these studies, it is apparent that short-term normoglycemia on the AEP is not associated with a return to normal of several other metabolites. One explanation is the consistent demonstration of peripheral hyperinsulinemia during closed-loop control,[29,31] which would be expected to raise lactate and lower glycerol and free fatty acids. The raised plasma free insulin concentrations have been attributed to the route of insulin infusion — peripheral rather than portal.

Unexpectedly, though, when the AEP was used to clamp blood glucose at 10 to 12 mmol/ℓ rather than at 5 to 6 mmol/ℓ in a group of diabetics, and half the insulin infused as a result, there were no differences in blood levels of lactate, pyruvate, total ketone bodies, glycerol, and free fatty acids.[32] Only alanine concentrations were changed (elevated) during the hyperglycemic clamp.

As for hormones other than insulin, the inappropriately high blood glucagon concentrations seen in some diabetics have been shown to be lowered by the AEP.[33,34] In other work however, no difference could be detected between glucagon levels in normal subjects and diabetics treated by subcutaneous injections or the AEP.[30]

Another experimental use for the AEP is in the assessment of drug-action in diabetics. Somatostatin, for example has an antidiabetic, insulin-sparing action, largely because of its supression of glucagon and growth hormone. This effect can be measured by the lower insulin dose needed to maintain euglycemia in somatostatin-treated patients on the AEP.[35] The potency of various insulins or the pharmacokinetics of insulin absorption can be studied by using the AEP to clamp glycemic levels and therefore titrate glucose infusion against the appearance of insulin in the circulation and its subsequent biological effect (glucose lowering). Massi-Benedetti et al.,[36] for example, compared intravenous infusions of pork or human insulin (of recombinant DNA origin) in normal subjects and showed no significant difference in the amount of glucose needed to maintain euglycemia for each insulin.

The AEP has been used as an acute therapeutic tool in a number of circumstances where glycemic control in the diabetic is temporarily difficult with conventional insulin injections. Schwartz et al.,[37] for example, studied diabetics during major surgery. Blood glucose control was significantly better in diabetics on the AEP compared to diabetics or nondiabetics receiving an intraoperative intravenous glucose infusion. Other examples of short-term management by the AEP are during parturition[38] and during insulinoma resection.[39] In the latter case, the device is used essentially for variable glucose rather than insulin infusion, to avoid life-threatening hypoglycemia.

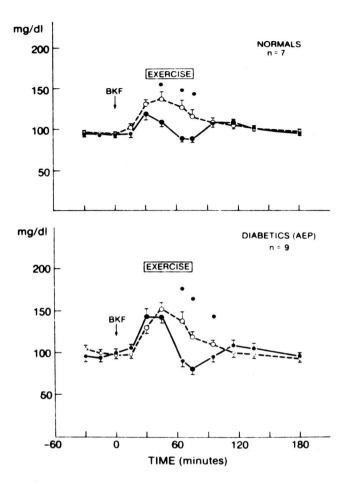

FIGURE 4.   Plasma glucose responses in normal (upper panel) and insulin-dependent diabetic (lower panel) subjects during breakfast (BKF) (O---O) and breakfast plus exercise (●—●). Diabetics were managed by AEP treatment. (From Nelson, J. D. et al., *Am. J. Physiol.*, 242, E309, 1982. With permission.)

It is well known that glycemic control is often very difficult to achieve during and after physical exercise in diabetics treated by conventional insulin injections.[40] Insulin deficiency exacerbates the metabolic disorder and insulin excess causes hypoglycemia (which frequently occurs because of increased subcutaneous insulin absorption during exercise, particularly if injected into the exercising part, such as the legs). The AEP almost completely normalizes metabolic responses to exercise, even in the immediate postprandial state.[41] As in the nondiabetic, insulin delivery is reduced, probably in response to falling glucose levels (certainly in the case of the AEP) and near-normoglycemia maintained (Figure 4).

Lambert et al.[42] have used the AEP as a therapeutic tool to determine the subcutaneous insulin requirements in diabetics. And on, perhaps, a more controversial therapeutic topic, Mirouze et al.[43] investigated the role of AEP-induced near-normoglycemia in newly diagnosed insulin-dependent diabetics and its effects on the so-called honeymoon remission. Short-lived "remissions" are often seen in the first few months after diagnosis in insulin-dependent diabetics and are characterized by decreasing insulin requirements, improved metabolic control, and temporarily increased endogenous insulin secretion (reflected by increased C-peptide concentrations). It has long been the notion that early in diabetes, there is a vicious circle of moderate insulin deficiency leading to hyperglycemia, which stimulates the B cell to secrete more insulin and leads to exhaustion and further hyperglycemia. If the B cell could be "rested" by a period of very good glycemic control at an early period, some recovery or preservation of B cell function may be possible. Mirouze and co-workers[43] showed that after 5 days of AEP treatment, a group of newly diagnosed diabetics had a significantly greater frequency (75%) of remissions compared to a group of diabetics treated by injections (11%). However, the long term benefits of these remissions on metabolic control and the effects of sustained glycemic normalization from diagnosis onwards, are unclear.

b. Disadvantages and Relative Merits of Closed-Loop Insulin Delivery Systems

The main disadvantages of the present closed-loop devices are the large size and complexity and the intravenous route of insulin delivery. The latter limits the duration of treatment, because of the risks of thrombosis and infection. The bulk restricts the device to virtually bedside use and also prevents long term experiments.

Miniaturization has been partly hampered by the lack of a suitable potentially implantable glucose sensor. This is an area of very active investigation and the reader is referred to recent reviews for discussion of technological progress.[27,28,44]

The further technological development, the clinical, and to some extent, the experimental use made of the AEP has been severely restricted by the topic reviewed in the next section: open-loop insulin delivery systems. In the early 1970s, Slama et al.[45] and Hepp and co-workers[46] showed that almost as good short-term glycemic control can be achieved by variable-rate intravenous infusion of insulin, without glucose sensing and feedback. Also, simple programs for the management of acute metabolic derangements of diabetes[47] (e.g., surgery, parturition, and ketoacidosis) were developed, often involving "open-loop" low dose intravenous insulin infusion (see diabetic ketoacidosis section). The great clinical success and simplicity of use have recommended these regimens to practicing physicians in preference to the expensive and complicated AEP.

2. Open-Loop Systems
a. Intravenous Delivery

Here the strategy is infusion of insulin at a variety of rates from a portable pump. Delivery is preprogrammed in the sense that the basal and prandial rates are decided by the operator and set for the individual patient, and not subject to feedback control by a glucose-sensing component.

It is well established that near-normal glycemic control can be achieved by open-loop devices over periods of a few days to many months.[45,46,48-51] Long-term infusions usually employ a central vein for administrations with subcutaneous tunneling of the cannula. Nevertheless, many investigators regard the threat of thrombosis and septicemia as still present and the system has not found wide clinical or experimental application. There are few studies in man of the correlation between glucose normalization and changes in metabolites, hormones, etc. during open-loop intravenous treatment of diabetics. (See below for comparisons of peripheral and portal venous infusions of insulin in animals.) However, there are several investigations of the intravenous insulin wave-forms necessary for control of prandial glucose excursions. It seems that complicated variations of infusion to mimic exactly the nondiabetic prandial profile are unnecessary. In dogs, rapid administrations of insulin within the first few minutes of a peripheral intravenous glucose infusion, followed by a lower rate of insulin infusion for a longer period achieves close to normal glucose concentrations.[52] In man, Horwitz et al.[53] used a hybrid AEP/open-loop intravenous system. High rate insulin infusion for the first 30 min of a meal, followed by closed-loop control achieved lower peak plasma glucose and free insulin levels than during AEP management alone.

b. Subcutaneous Delivery

Continuous subcutaneous insulin infusion (CSII) was introduced by Pickup et al.[54] to overcome the problems associated with the intravenous route of administration and to provide sufficiently long periods of strict metabolic near-normalization to examine the effect of good "control" on the incidence or progression of diabetic complications. The technology, procedures, and clinical management of patients on CSII have been extensively reviewed[55,56] and will not be discussed here. The technique has become the most widespread method of open-loop diabetic treatment using infusers and has already yielded considerable new information on the pathophysiology of diabetic complications and the associated metabolic abnormalities.

The system is simple to operate: a portable pump infuses insulin at basal and prandial rates into the subcutaneous tissue of the anterior abdominal wall. Mealtime boosts of insulin are, in fact, given about 30 min before meals to allow for absorption of effective concentrations of insulin. The site of infusion is commonly changed and rotated around the abdomen once every day or so and with this strategy infection and severe lipodystrophy are very rare.

Many patients have now been receiving CSII at home and work for up to 3 years or more.[57-60] Two recent prospective and randomized clinical trials[61-63] (The Steno Study Group, Copenhagen and the Kroc Study Group, U.K., U.S.A., and Canada) demonstrate the effectiveness of CSII compared to conventional injection treatment (CIT). In both studies, patients were randomly allocated to their usual unchanged injections or to CSII. Over 8 months (Kroc) and 1 year (Steno) glycemic control in the injected and infused groups was clearly separated as assessed by HbA_{1c} concentrations: values in the injection-treated patients remained high while those on CSII were near-normal throughout. (Figure 5).

Early studies[64,65] (see Figure 6) showed that short-term CSII-induced strict glucose control also restored other metabolites towards, but not exactly to, normal (e.g., lactate, pyruvate, 3-hydroxybutyrate, total cholesterol, and triglyceride). Raised glucagon levels on CIT were also lowered by 4 to 5 weeks of CSII[66] and the exaggerated growth hormone and catecholamine response during exercise on CIT was reduced by CSII.[67]

There is general agreement that profiles of plasma-free insulin levels during CSII mimic nondiabetic values, in that there are peaks with meals and constant levels during the night.[55,68] However, fasting or basal hyperinsulinemia is still a feature of CSII (as with the AEP). Its biological meaning (as discussed above) is uncertain.

The main experimental impact of CSII, however, has been on the understanding of the mechanisms of diabetic tissue complications — particularly microvascular disease. Shortly after the initial demonstration of the use of CSII to improve short-term blood glucose concentrations in diabetes, Viberti et al.[69] showed that 1 to 3 days of CSII also reduced or normalized the raised microalbuminuria of some diabetics treated by CIT. Microalbuminuria is the excretion of albumin in the urine at levels below that detectable by routine dipsticks (e.g., "Albustix"), and only measurable by sensitive methods such as radioimmunoassay. It is thought to be due to increased permeability of the glomerular capillaries, rather than to renal tubular damage. The reduced microalbuminuria on CSII occurred in such a short time as to indicate functional change (charge, pore size) rather than structural mechanisms (e.g., basement membrane thickening) for the permeability changes.

Although microalbuminuria may be a predictor of severe renal disease in the later stages of diabetes,[70] institution of good control by CSII in established diabetic renal failure (macroproteinuria, Albustix positive) is probably without effect. Viberti et al.[71]

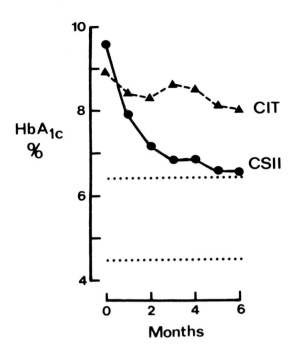

FIGURE 5.   Mean glycosylated hemoglobin (HbA$_{1c}$) concentrations in insulin-dependent diabetics managed by conventional insulin treatment (CIT) or continuous subcutaneous insulin infusion (CSII). Dotted lines: normal range
for HbA$_{1c}$. (Adapted from Pickup, J. C. et al., *Lancet*, 1,
121, 1982.)

showed that decline in glomerular filtration rate and albumin excretion was unaltered
by up to 2 years of CSII in six diabetics with advanced diabetic nephropathy. It is
postulated that at this stage of structural damage, the potentially reversible components are unable to alter the progress of the lesion, which has become essentially self-
maintaining. This is an argument, of course, for the start of strict control regimens at
the earliest possible stage of diabetes.

In the eye, a similar reversible index of capillary permeability exists in the leakage of
the fluorescent dye fluorescein into the vitreous humor. This is reduced by a short
period of CSII,[72] but its relationship to clinical diabetic retinopathy is now known.
Both the Steno and Kroc studies are examining patients with background retinopathy
randomly allocated to CSII or CIT. After 1 year of the protocol, the Steno group
reported[62] unexpectedly, a slight deterioration in the pump-treated patients compared
to the CIT diabetics. The long-term comparisons between the two regimens are not yet
known and are eagerly awaited.

As far as diabetic neuropathy is concerned, Pietri et al[73] showed a significant increase in motor nerve conduction (median and peroneal but not ulnar) in 10 patients
treated by CSII for 6 weeks. There was no change in sensory nerve conduction velocities. However, Boulton and his colleagues[74] could demonstrate a subjective improvement after CSII in patients with painful diabetic peripheral neuropathy.

A rare group of brittle or hyperlabile diabetics are not significantly improved on
CSII compared to ordinary injection treatment.[75] They are mostly young females, and
although some may be cheating by tampering with the device or their diet, definite
abnormalities of subcutaneous insulin handling are also suspected. Subcutaneous in-

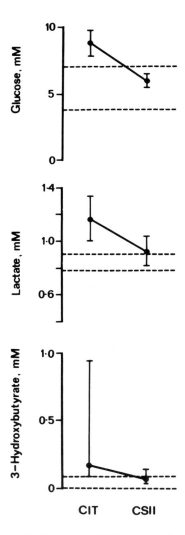

FIGURE 6. Daily mean (±SEM or range for 3-hydroxy-
butyrate) metabolite concentrations in diabetics treated by
CIT or CSII. Dotted line: normal ranges. (Data from Tamborlane, W. V. et al., *Lancet*, 1, 1258, 1979.)

sulin requirements are usually high and glycemic control markedly improved by continuous intramuscular insulin infusion.[75] This suggests a real or apparent barrier to insulin
absorption which is by-passed by the intramuscular route. Recently, Williams et al. [76]
demonstrated that in stable insulin-dependent diabetics and normal subjects, subcutaneous insulin injection produces a long-lasting local hyperemia. This is absent in some
brittle diabetics and may partly explain the difficulties in establishing glycemic control.

C. Intraperitoneal Delivery

In the last few years, there has been renewed interest in the intraperitoneal route,
largely because of the theoretical advantages of supplying insulin directly to the liver
and the probability that a proportion of intraperitoneal insulin is absorbed into the
portal vein. Peripheral blood glucose levels in man are intermediate between subcutaneous and intravenous delivery, but in some studies, plasma-free insulin concentrations

are lower than for s.c. or i.v. insulin.[77] There is very little information in man on the intermediary metabolite and hormonal changes associated with intraperitoneal insulin infusions.

From a practical point of view, the risk of peritonitis must be considered with this treatment option. However, it has been proposed that the peritoneum is an ideal site for insulin infusion from totally implanted pumps where infection may be less of a problem. Pilot studies with such devices have already begun, with encouraging initial results.[78]

D. Low-Dose Intravenous and Intramuscular Insulin Administration for the Treatment of Diabetic Ketoacidosis

The last decade has seen a move away from treatment of diabetic ketoacidosis by large doses of insulin given subcutaneously and or intravenously, towards low dose administration.[79] This came about partly because of better understanding of insulin physiology and pharmacology and the importance of rate of delivery on blood levels achieved. The dangers of overinsulinization were realized and low-dose regimens have become almost universally recognized as simple, relatively safe, and efficacious.

From the discussion of the dose-response curves and metabolic effects of insulin it can be appreciated that both hepatic glucose production and lipolysis/ketone body generation are very sensitive to inhibition by insulin (less than 30 μU/mℓ). This level of insulinization can be achieved by an intravenous insulin infusion of only about 1 U/ hr. In several centers, circulating levels of 80 to 120 μU/mℓ are aimed for, sufficient to inhibit liver glucose and ketone output, but not to precipitously lower blood glucose or potassium concentrations. Infusion rates of 4 to 8 U/hr are required for this, and Alberti et al.[80] gave intermittent intramuscular doses (a loading injection of 20 U followed by 5 U/hr) to simulate approximately the same circulating concentrations.

III. ANIMAL STUDIES

A. Comparison of Peripheral and Portal Insulin Infusions
1. Variable Rate Infusions

In freely mobile, normal dogs, intraportal administration of insulin at low infusion rates has been found to be less effective than peripheral administration in producing hypoglycemia, yet intraportal insulin appeared to have a greater effect on the liver.[81] A more comprehensive range of infusion rates has been tested in dogs made diabetic by selective destruction of the pancreatic beta cells using alloxan and streptozotocin.[82] During *peripheral* infusion of insulin at rates from 0.006 to 0.200 U·kg^{-1}·hr^{-1}, corresponding increases in immunoreactive insulin were measured in peripheral venous plasma (Figure 7).[83] The changes in blood levels of intermediary metabolites can virtually be predicted from Figure 1 on the basis of the plasma insulin concentrations achieved. Figure 8 shows the changes observed in blood lactate, alanine, glycerol, and 3-hydroxybutyrate.[83] In the absence of exogenous insulin, there tended to be increases in all the metabolites measured over the 150 min study period, and these rises presumably reflect increased proteolysis and lipolysis in muscle and fat, respectively. As the insulin infusion rate was increased, the falls in glycerol and 3-hydroxybutyrate were probably initially directly or indirectly due to an inhibition of lipolysis in adipocytes,[84,85] while at higher infusion rates, the greater fall in 3-hydroxybutyrate was probably the result of inhibition of hepatic output of ketone bodies. Although increasing the insulin infusion rate resulted in falls in plasma lactate and alanine, when the rate was increased further to 0.20 U·kg^{-1}·hr^{-1}, there were large increases in lactate and alanine, suggesting that increased production of both metabolites accompanied in-

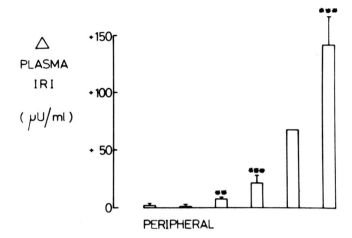

U kg⁻¹ h⁻¹   0.006 0.012 0.025 0.05   0.10   0.20

FIGURE 7. Changes in plasma immunoreactive insulin (IRI) (as mean changes from preinfusion levels ± SEM) in diabetic dogs during peripheral infusion of insulin at the rates shown (at top of figure). Significant differences from preinfusion levels are represented by asterisks (**$p < 0.01$, ***$p < 0.001$). (Adapted from Stevenson, R. W. et al., *Metabolism*, 30, 745, 1981.)

creased uptake and metabolism of glucose in muscle. In contrast, *intraportal* infusion of insulin produced reductions in all metabolites measured at infusion rates too low to increase insulin concentrations in peripheral blood.[83]

Peripheral infusion of insulin did not cause a significantly greater fall in peripheral blood glucose than intraportal insulin until the infusion rate was increased to 0.05 $U \cdot kg^{-1} \cdot hr^{-1}$. While peripheral infusion at this rate has been shown, using isotopically labeled glucose, to directly inhibit hepatic glucose production in diabetic man[91] and dog[92,93] this hepatic action probably does not account entirely for the reduction in blood glucose, as at first thought.[91,92] Indeed, a peripheral infusion rate as low as 0.006 $U \cdot kg^{-1} \cdot hr^{-1}$ can significantly lower blood glucose levels in diabetic dogs, not by inhibiting the already high hepatic glucose output (Figure 9) but by causing a small increase in glucose clearance[93] (which is a more direct indicator of hormonal modulation of glucose utilization than the rate of glucose disappearance). From Figure 1, one would not expect peripheral infusion of insulin to affect hepatic glucose production until a significant increase in plasma insulin concentration was detected, i.e., at 0.025 $U \cdot kg^{-1} \cdot hr^{-1}$ (Figure 7). In fact, only double this dose reduced glucose production in the diabetic dog to the levels observed in normal dogs (Figure 9). Intraportal infusion of insulin at this rate also normalized hepatic glucose output, but unlike peripheral administration, the eightfold lower infusion rate also caused significant inhibition of glucose output. This may explain why the fall in plasma glucose quickly reached a maximum as the intraportal infusion rate was increased from 0.006 to 0.05 $U \cdot kg^{-1} \cdot hr^{-1}$, and since hepatic extraction of insulin reduces the amount of insulin reaching peripheral tissues, may explain why the portal route of insulin administration caused a signficantly smaller fall in blood glucose than the peripheral route when insulin was infused at 0.05 $U \cdot kg^{-1} \cdot hr^{-1}$.[93]

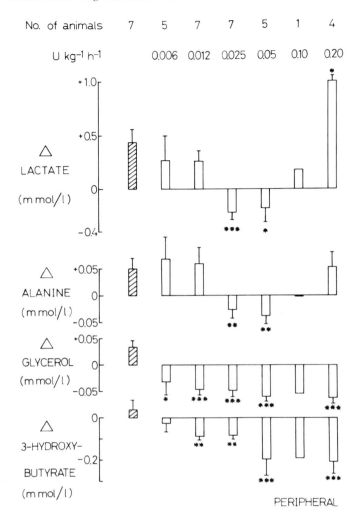

FIGURE 8.   Changes in plasma intermediary metabolites (as mean change from preinfusion levels ± SEM) by the end of infusions for 150 min in diabetic dogs during infusion of vehicle alone (hatched columns) or peripheral infusion of insulin at the rates shown (at top of Figure). Significant differences from the results of infusing vehicle alone are represented by asterisks (* $p < 0.05$, ** $p < 0.01$, *** $p < 0.001$). (From Stevenson, R. W. et al., *Metabolism*, 30, 745, 1981.)

Although glucose turnover could be normalized with peripheral insulin infusion at the latter rate, this was achieved at the expense of suppressed glucose recycling (i.e., recycling the products of glucose catabolism to glucose). Glucose recycling as determined by comparing the turnover of 3-^{3}H-glucose and 1-^{14}C-glucose[94] was found to be 19% in normal conscious dogs[93] and is similar to that in man.[30,94,95] A small increase in recycling to 24% was observed when the dogs were made diabetic, just as was found when glucose recycling was compared in normal and diabetic subjects,[95] but when glucose turnover in these dogs was normalized by peripheral insulin infusion, recycling was signficantly reduced to 11%.[93] This confirms the observations in insulin-dependent diabetic subjects of even more pronounced reductions in glucose recycling to 6 and 4% during relatively poor control of blood glucose by subcutaneous injection therapy and

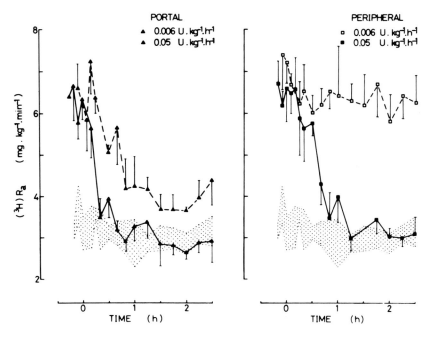

FIGURE 9. Effects of infusions of insulin for 150 min on mean (±SEM) hepatic glucose production (R_a) estimated using 3-³H-glucose in diabetic dogs. Left panel: *intraportal* infusion of insulin at 0.006 U·kg⁻¹·hr⁻¹ (△---△) and 0.05 U·kg⁻¹·hr⁻¹ (▲—▲). Right panel: *peripheral* infusion of insulin at 0.006 U·kg⁻¹·hr⁻¹ (□---□) and 0.05 U·kg⁻¹·ᵖ⁻¹ (■—■). Dotted portions represent mean R_a ± 2 SEM during infusion of vehicle alone to normal healthy dogs. (From Stevenson, R. W. et al., *Am. J. Physiol.*, 244, E190, 1983. With permission.)

during maintenance of normoglycemia by peripheral intravenous infusion of insulin using the artificial endocrine pancreas, respectively.[30]

A reduction in glucose recycling during peripheral administration of insulin may reflect diversion of radioactive glucose metabolites into other metabolic pathways, possibly resulting in extrahepatic glycogen formation or increased hepatic formation of lipid[96,97] at the same time as depressing gluconeogenesis.[98,99] Although lactate is preferred to glucose as a precursor for hepatic synthesis of fatty acids,[147,148] lactate availability is reduced during peripheral administration of insulin, as shown by the absence of a rise in lactate levels in hepatectomized rats given high doses of insulin,[149] and this action may partly explain the fall in blood lactate levels during peripheral infusion at 0.05 U·kg⁻¹·hr⁻¹ to diabetic dogs (Figure 8). Since the amounts of insulin reaching the periphery during intraportal insulin infusion are reduced by hepatic extraction of the hormone, production of lactate by peripheral tissues should be affected less than during peripheral insulin infusion and the Cori cycle will be more likely to operate normally. This was indeed found to be the case when insulin was infused into the portal vein at 0.05 U·kg⁻¹·hr⁻¹. Both glucose turnover (Figure 9) and glucose recycling (20%) were normalized simultaneously. The difference in Cori cycle activity in insulin-infused diabetics between the routes of insulin delivery suggests that there may be some metabolic derangement during insulin administration via the peripheral circulation, even when normoglycemia is maintained under fine control with a glucose-controlled insulin infusion system (artificial endocrine pancreas).

Therefore, it appears that in the diabetic animal, there are not only qualitative and quantitative differences in the metabolic responses to insulin administered peripherally and intraportally, but also in the responses to different infusion rates of insulin administered peripherally. Since the rates of peripheral insulin infusion shown to normalize fasting blood glucose levels in diabetic subjects using the artificial pancreas[86-89] and in the diabetic dog[90] lie in the range 0.01 to 0.03 $U \cdot kg^{-1} \cdot hr^{-1}$, it is evident that small changes in infusion rate within this range will have large metabolic consequences.

2. Metabolic and Hormonal Profiles During Fasting and Feeding in the Insulin-Infused Diabetic Animal

a. During Fasting

When normoglycemia was achieved by basal intraportal or peripheral intravenous infusion of insulin in dogs which had either been pancreatectomized[100] or had been made diabetic using alloxan alone[101,102] or alloxan plus streptozotocin,[90] there was simultaneous normalization of glucose turnover, plasma glucagon levels and blood lactate, pyruvate, and individual amino acids. Subcutaneous insulin infusion to diabetic dogs gave similar results.[103] However, blood levels of glycerol, nonesterified fatty acids, and 3-hydroxybutyrate were normalized only during intraportal administration of insulin[90,100](Table 1). The depressed levels of these three metabolites during peripheral administration of insulin to diabetic dogs was probably due to inhibition of lipolysis either directly or indirectly (in the case of 3-hydroxybutyrate) by the slightly higher plasma insulin concentration associated with this route of insulin delivery.[90,100,104] Blood alanine concentrations in dogs made diabetic chemically were also lower during normoglycemic infusions of insulin by the peripheral circulation than by the portal circulation[90,102] and may be the result of insulin inhibition of alanine production by muscle. In contrast, blood alanine levels in the pancreatectomized dog were about twice normal regardless of the route of insulin infusion. This latter finding may be the result of decreased hepatic uptake of alanine due to a lack of biologically active glucagon. Although the gut of the dog can produce glucagon similar to pancreatic glucagon,[105,106] the emergence of biologically active glucagon from extrapancreatic sources may have been inhibited if insulin therapy were started immediately after pancreatectomy. Thus, although near-normalization of most of the variables mentioned above can be achieved by both routes of insulin administration, adipose tissue metabolism in the diabetic animal appears to be somewhat abnormal during peripheral administration.

b. During Feeding and Glucose Loading

1. Pattern of Insulin Release or Infusion

In normal physiology, pancreatic release of insulin can occur in a biphasic manner depending on the type and magnitude of the stimulus and on the antecedent diet of the animal.[107] The biphasic secretion of insulin was first recognized in response to glucose, though it was soon observed in response to glucagon and other stimuli, and it is characterized by a brief but marked release of hormone followed by a more sustained but less elevated rate of release.[108,109] Cherrington and his colleagues[110,111] have investigated the relative metabolic consequences of each phase of insulin secretion in this case to counteract the effects of glucagon on glucose turnover and plasma glucose levels. This was accomplished by elevating plasma glucagon fourfold (by intraportal infusion) first in an uncontrolled conscious dog to establish the magnitude of both phases of insulin secretion and then during a "pancreatic clamp" in the presence of first, second, or combined first and second phase insulin release. The "pancreatic clamp" technique involves infusion of somatostatin to inhibit the endocrine pancreas and the infusion of basal amounts of insulin and glucagon to replace endogenous secretion of the pancreatic hormones. Both hormones were given intraportally so that normal portal-peripheral gradients of insulin and glucagon could be preserved. By the use of this tech-

Table 1

MEAN BASAL LEVELS (±SEM) OF THE VARIABLES MEASURED IN PERIPHERAL VENOUS BLOOD OF EIGHT FASTING NORMAL DOGS AND GROUPS OF SIX DIABETIC DOGS OFF INSULIN[a] OR MAINTAINED NORMOGLYCEMIC BY INTRAPORTAL OR PERIPHERAL INSULIN INFUSION

Insulin administration		Glucose (nmol/l)	Insulin (μU/ml)	Glucagon (pg/ml)	Lactate (mmol/l)	Alanine (mmol/l)	Glycerol (mmol)	NEFA (mmol/l)	3-Hydroxybutyrate (mmol/l)
Normal		5.3 ± 0.2	12.4 ± 1.8	49 ± 7	0.55 ± 0.04	0.229 ± 0.021	0.118 ± 0.013	0.88 ± 0.09	0.056 ± 0.010
Diabetic	Intraportal	5.5 ± 0.3	11.5 ± 1.2^{d}	65 ± 7	0.63 ± 0.04	0.236 ± 0.037	$0.109 \pm 0.013^{*}$	0.84 ± 0.09^{d}	$0.059 \pm 0.015^{*}$
	Peripheral	5.6 ± 0.6	16.4 ± 1.6	63 ± 5	0.54 ± 0.03	0.191 ± 0.008	0.074 ± 0.006^{c}	0.67 ± 0.04^{b}	0.018 ± 0.004^{c}
	Zero	15.5 ± 1.1	5.8 ± 1.6	184 ± 24	1.32 ± 0.16	0.302 ± 0.029	0.247 ± 0.035		0.536 ± 0.083

[a] 24 and 48 hours after the last injections of Actrapid and Ultralente insulin, respectively

[b] $p<0.05$; indicates significant differences between values in intraportally and peripherally infused diabetic dogs using paired t-test (n = 4)

[c] $p<0.01$; indicates significant differences between values in intraportally and peripherally infused diabetic dogs using paired t-test (n = 4)

[d] $p<0.05$; indicates significant differences between values in normal and diabetic dogs using paired t-test (n = 6)

* $p<0.01$; indicates significant differences between values in normal and diabetic dogs using paired t-test (n = 6)

nique plasma glucagon levels were raised by $\sim$220 pg/mℓ in the presence of simulated first phase (peak plasma insulin of 25 μU/mℓ at 5 min, basal by 30 min), second phase (peak plasma insulin of 19 μU/mℓ at 30 min and sustained thereafter), or first plus second phase (peak plasma insulin of 33 μU/mℓ at 5 min, 17 μU/mℓ at 30 min and sustained elevation thereafter) insulin release.

Optimal glycemic control required both first and second phase release while selective first phase deficiency resulted in a transient (90 min) worsening of the glucagon-induced hyperglycemia (i.e., twice the normal increment).[110] This defect was caused by a fourfold larger initial rise in hepatic glucose production (4 mg·kg^{-1}·min^{-1}) than that observed when both phases of insulin release were present. In addition, first phase insulin release by itself completely abolished the initial glucagon stimulation of gluconeogenesis (conversion of ^{14}C-alanine to ^{14}C-glucose) and even by 3 hr, gluconeogenesis was still inhibited by 70%.[111] Since the glucagon-induced increase in hepatic alanine extraction was unaffected, the first phase of insulin release must be important in inhibiting the effect of glucagon on intrahepatic gluconeogenesis. It is thus evident that the first phase of insulin release is vital to full regulation of the action of glucagon on glucose metabolism.

When considered in relation to the treatment of insulin-dependent diabetes by insulin infusion, it appears that a rapid initial priming or increase in infusion rate may be required for optimal glycemic and metabolic control during glucose loading. An early rise in insulin infusion rate by either the portal or peripheral circulation normalized the glycemic response to a glucose load introduced into the duodenum of diabetic dogs.[90] Plasma insulin levels rose faster than that found in normal dogs following the same glucose load and this may have replaced the relatively high first phase insulin release observed in normal animals.

The importance of an early increase in plasma insulin concentration, as was pointed out earlier, has also been demonstrated in the control of postprandial hyperglycemia in diabetic dog[100] and man.[53,112] Even use of the artificial endocrine pancreas, which reacts quickly to a rise in blood glucose by infusing more insulin, produced unacceptable hyperinsulinemia in insulin-dependent diabetic subjects during meals and this in turn prevented full metabolic normalization.[29,30,113] However, introduction of an early preprogrammed insulin infusion at the start of the meal with subsequent control by the artificial pancreas not only significantly reduced the insulin requirement and plasma insulin levels but also improved glycemic control. In this case, the anticipated preprogrammed insulin infusion may have reproduced normal physiology by simulating the early release of insulin by the intact pancreas due to stimulation by gastrointestinal hormones and the nervous system.

2. Metabolic Control

Complete metabolic normalization cannot be achieved in *fasting* diabetic dogs during peripheral administration of insulin (see earlier). On the other hand, *during a mixed meal,* it has recently been reported that there appears to be no practical advantage of portal compared to peripheral venous administration of insulin with respect to hepatic versus extrahepatic disposal of glucose in alloxan-diabetic dogs.[101,102] However, these authors did not ascertain the magnitude of the glycemic response to the same (liquid) mixed meal given to normal healthy dogs before attempting to control the glycemic excursion in the diabetic dogs by insulin infusion. The normal response to a (solid) mixed meal consists of no significant rise in blood glucose over an absorption period of 12 hr,[114] while in the above studies in diabetic dogs, blood glucose was allowed to rise by 2.2 mmol/ℓ (40 mg/dℓ) and 3.9 mmol/ℓ (70 mg/dℓ) respectively. Thus the lack of difference in whole body glucose appearance and disappearance rates after a meal when insulin was administered via a peripheral or the portal vein may not hold when the normal physiological response is reestablished.

When the normal glycemic responses to a mixed meal[100] and an intraduodenal glucose load[90] were recreated in diabetic dogs there were distinct differences in hormonal and metabolic responses between intraportal and peripheral infusion of insulin. In pancreatectomized dogs given a mixed meal, the major difference between the two routes of insulin administration was that plasma insulin levels were twofold higher during peripheral than intraportal infusion, the latter route producing insulin concentrations only slightly above those observed in normal dogs.[100] In the other series of studies, the hormonal and metabolic responses to an intraduodenal glucose load (0.5 g/kg) were first determined in conscious normal dogs before inducing diabetes (alloxan/streptozotocin) and then comparing the responses to the glucose load when normal plasma glucose profiles were recreated by preprogrammed infusion of insulin via the portal or peripheral circulations.[90] As in normal man and dog given glucose orally,[115-117] intraduodenal glucose to healthy dogs produced rises in blood lactate and alanine and falls in glycerol, nonesterified fatty acids (NEFA), and 3-hydroxybutyrate. During insulin infusions designed to normalize the glycemic response to the glucose load in diabetic dogs, the plasma glucagon response and all the metabolic responses were simultaneously normalized during intraportal infusion but depressed glycerol, NEFA, and 3-hydroxybutyrate responses resulted during peripheral infusion. As occurs during fasting, fat metabolism seems to be abnormal during glucose loading when insulin is infused via the peripheral circulation. This again probably relates to the marked hyperinsulinemia (103 μU/mℓ) common to this route of administration. Although the area under the plasma insulin curve was significantly greater in portally infused diabetic dogs than in normal dogs, this more physiological route of insulin delivery produced plasma insulin concentration not significantly higher than those achieved in the normal animals. Therefore, the metabolic abnormalities associated with the peripheral route of insulin delivery seem to be caused primarily by the elevated plasma insulin levels.

Since long-term insulin treatment of the insulin-dependent diabetic subject by the peripheral route, achieving near normal blood glucose levels, may arrest or even reverse some of the features associated with diabetic microangiopathy,[61] it seems possible that strict metabolic control by insulin delivered into the portal circulation may beneficially alter the course of the microvascular phenomena associated with diabetes even further. In particular it could have beneficial effects on macroangiopathy which may be related to peripheral hyperinsulinemia associated with the peripheral route of insulin administration.[118]

B. Hepatic Targeting of Insulin

In normal physiology, hepatic removal of insulin plays an important role in the regulation of both insulin and carbohydrate homeostasis. As discussed above, insulin exerts major effects on hepatic carbohydrate metabolism, even though the liver extracts 30 to 60% of the insulin delivered to it in a single passage.[110-121] It appears that hepatic insulin extraction may be modulated at the level of liver receptors,[122,123] and the possibility exists that hepatic receptor binding and biological activity of insulin and related peptides are proportional to their hepatic removal.[124,125] The percent hepatic extraction may even increase considerably during glucose ingestion.[126]

However, there is evidence for the existence of not one, but two degradative pathways of insulin. When insulin was infused into the portal vein of euglycemic dogs and somatostatin was infused to block endogenous insulin secretion, the relationship between steady-state plasma insulin concentration and plasma insulin disappearance rate (which equals the infusion rate under steady-state conditions) could be represented by

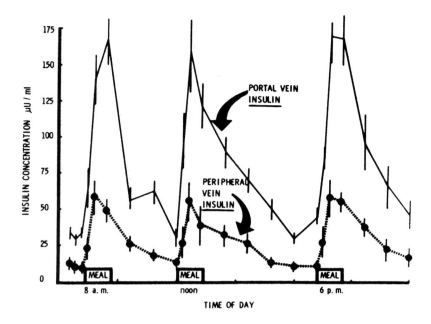

FIGURE 10.   Sequential estimation of portal vein insulin concentration relative to peripheral vein insulin concentration in normal healthy subjects throughout the day with ingestion of meals (750 cal) at 0800, 1200, and 0600 hr, respectively. Data shown are mean ±SEM. (From Eaton, R. P. et al., *Diabetes Care,* 3, 270, 1980. With permission.)

a straight line, at least over the peripheral plasma insulin range 0 to 100 μU/mℓ.[127] Insulin clearance decreased at higher insulin infusion rates which produced plasma concentrations in excess of 100 μU/mℓ. The results indicated the existence in the dog of a saturable and a virtually nonsaturable pathway of insulin degradation and these pathways are probably located in the liver and kidney, respectively.[128,129] It appeared that hepatic extraction of insulin may remain constant regardless of the amount reaching the liver up to insulin secretion rates ($\sim$0.2 U·kg^{-1}·hr^{-1}) producing peripheral insulin concentrations of about 100 μU/mℓ.

Normal insulin secretion rates into the portal vein of healthy man have been determined from analysis of plasma connecting peptide levels.[130,131] Examples of portal and peripheral plasma insulin concentrations before and after ingestion of three typical daily meals are shown in Figure 10. Mean basal portal vein levels in the preprandial state were 29 μU/mℓ with simultaneous peripheral levels of 9 μU/mℓ. The maximal portal levels of insulin were observed about 1 hr after the start of meal ingestion and the simultaneously measured peripheral levels (about 50 μU/mℓ) averaged only 32% of the portal concentration. Although the measurements were not made under steady-state conditions the possibility exists that fractional hepatic extraction may remain virtually constant in normal physiology during fasting and feeding.

Estimates of the basal insulin secretion rate in normal man[130,131] were between 0.010 and 0.015 U·kg^{-1}·hr^{-1}. These rates are somewhat lower than the intraportal infusion rates found to achieve normoglycemia in the diabetic dog studies discussed earlier and suggest that simulation of normal pancreatic secretion has not been fully achieved perhaps due to improper mixing before reaching the liver or inappropriate pulsatile delivery. Nevertheless, it is obvious that it would be difficult to simulate normal insulin secretion by infusion into the peripheral circulation. Since this route of delivery achieves slightly lower portal vein levels of insulin than those in the periphery (partly due to the renal degradative pathway) prandial portal vein insulin concentrations would be achieved at the expense of gross hyperinsulinemia. Since catheterization of the portal vein of diabetic man is not feasible, other means of insulin therapy are required to "target" insulin to the liver.

1. Oral Administration of Insulin

The potential of the oral route of insulin administration for direct delivery of insulin to the portal circulation as a means of controlling postprandial hyperglycemia has been extensively investigated. Early experiments suggested that absorption of insulin from the small intestine was favored by a high pH and could be enhanced by a variety of agents such as methyl salicylate and quinine.[132,133] However, only about 5% of the total dose was absorbed.

More recently, insulin has been entrapped in liposomes (phospholipid vesicles consisting of concentric lipid layers enclosing aqueous compartments[134]) in an attempt to protect insulin from proteolytic degradation in the gastrointestinal tract. Oral administration of insulin in liposomes was first shown to reduce the blood glucose level of diabetic rats.[135] Subsequently, the effectiveness of liposomes in aiding intestinal absorption of entrapped insulin was studied in normal and diabetic dogs.[136] Intraduodenal administration of 40 to 80 U insulin entrapped in liposomes of several lipid compositions to conscious normal dogs produced substantial rises in peripheral plasma immunoreactive insulin after 45 to 60 min. However, the magnitude of these rises was neither reproducible nor dose-dependent and no fall in plasma glucose could be observed. Administration of liposome-insulin to diabetic dogs produced similar results with the exception that a small fall in plasma glucose followed the rise in immunoreactive insulin. This glucose fall was also neither dose dependent nor was it related to the magnitude of the rise in plasma insulin immunoreactivity. It seems that administration of insulin in liposomes may allow absorption of partially degraded insulin but the amounts of biologically active insulin reaching the circulation are extremely low. Even if oral administration of insulin in liposomes eventually proves effective in allowing insulin access to the portal vein of diabetic subjects, the long delay in absorption of 45 to 60 min may prove unacceptable as a means of delivering insulin to control postprandial hyperglycemia.

2. Hepatic-Specific Insulin

Since liposomes are preferentially taken up by the liver,[137] parenteral administration of insulin-liposomes may be a useful means of controlling the rate of insulin delivery to the liver. The biological action of insulin entrapped in liposomes has been investigated following subcutaneous injection to diabetic dogs.[138] It appeared that the majority of the insulin absorbed into the circulation remained associated with intact liposomes and that the presence of intact liposomes persisted in the circulation for many hours after absorption had ceased. It was speculated that the prolonged hypoglycemic effect observed in diabetic dogs after subcutaneous injection reflected a direct hepatic action of insulin-liposomes. Therefore, peripheral administration of insulin entrapped in liposomes may allow delivery of insulin to the liver without allowing high concentrations of free insulin in the periphery.

3. Intraperitoneal Insulin Infusion

The intraperitoneal route of insulin delivery has been discussed as a possible means of reestablishing normal portal-peripheral insulin gradients in the insulin-dependent diabetic subject. Schade and Eaton have demonstrated that insulin is absorbed into the portal venous circulation from the peritoneum in dogs[140] and this route of insulin administration can be used successfully to control blood glucose in diabetic man.[139,141]

In unanesthetized swine, portal and peripheral venous insulin concentrations were measured following oral glucose or intramuscular and intraperitoneal administration (via a multiple side hole catheter) of insulin (1 U/kg).[142] Both glucose-stimulated endogenous insulin secretion and intraperitoneal insulin injection produced persistent positive portal-peripheral insulin differences while intramuscular injection led to higher systemic insulin concentrations. Peripheral insulin levels were about 60% and 40% lower than portal levels during intraperitoneal insulin administration and endogenous insulin secretion, respectively. Although not in steady state, the results imply that some insulin may have reached the systemic circulation from the peritoneum by by-passing the liver, uptake of insulin into lymph being one possible route of absorption.

On theoretical grounds, it seems probable that the site of the catheter tip in the peritoneum will determine the fraction of insulin absorbed into the portal circulation, and in practice, the volume of the insulin solution determines the rate of absorption.[140,150] Thus, although the peritoneal route of insulin delivery is a marked improvement over the peripheral route, it may not be possible to completely mimic the normal insulin secretory response.

4. Pancreatic Islet Transplantation

The first successful transplantation of islet tissue was in the peritoneal cavity of diabetic rats in 1972,[143] but administration of islets to the portal vein was found to be more effective in lowering blood glucose.[144] In a comparison of the peritoneal cavity, portal vein, and systemic vein as sites for islet transplants, it was concluded that access to a blood supply is important.[145] As the amount of tissue transplanted was decreased, significantly more rats remained normoglycemic during intraportal transplantation, suggesting that localization of the islets in the portal circulation is also important to graft survival.

Thus when the problems of tissue rejection and supply are overcome, pancreatic islet transplantation in insulin-dependent diabetic man may eventually prove to be the most efficient way of delivering the daily insulin requirement of about 45 U[131] into the portal circulation, even though neural control of release cannot be reestablished.

REFERENCES

1. WHO Expert Committee on Diabetes Mellitus, 2nd report, WHO Tech. Rep. Ser. No. 646, World Health Organization, Geneva, 1980.
2. Tchobroutsky, G., Relation of diabetic control to development of microvascular complications, *Diabetologia*, 15, 143, 1978.
3. Sonksen, P. H., Tompkins, C. V., Srivastava, M. C., and Nabarro, J. D. N., A comparative study on the metabolism of human insulin and porcine proinsulin in man, *Clin. Sci. Mol. Med.*, 45, 633, 1973.
4. Sherwin, R. S., Kramer, K. J., Tobin, J. D., Insel, P. A., Liljenquist, J. E., Berman, M., and Andres, R., A model of the kinetics of insulin in man, *J. Clin. Invest.*, 53, 1481, 1974.
5. Christensen, N. and Orskov, H., The relationship between endogenous serum insulin concentrations and glucose uptake in the forearm muscles of nondiabetics, *J. Clin. Invest.*, 47, 1262, 1968.
6. Cahill, G. F., Jr., Physiology of insulin in man, *Diabetes*, 20, 785, 1971.
7. Cahill, G. F., Jr., Insulin and glucagon, in *Peptide Hormones,* Parsons, J. A., Ed., MacMillan Press, London, 1976, chap. 6..
8. Schade, D. S. and Eaton, R. P., Dose response to insulin in man: differential effects on glucose and ketone body regulation, *J. Clin. Endocrinol. Metab.*, 44, 1038, 1977.
9. Rizza, R. A., Mandarino, L. J., and Gerich, J. E., Dose-response characteristics for effects of insulin on production and utilization of glucose in man, *Am. J. Physiol.*, 240, E630, 1981.

10. Cherrington, A. D. and Steiner, K. E., The effects of insulin on carbohydrate metabolism in vivo, *Clin. Endocrinol. Metab.*, 11, 307, 1982.
11. Thiebaud, D., Jacot, E., DeFronzo, R. A., Maeder, E., Jequier, E., and Felber, J.-P., The effect of graded doses of insulin on total glucose uptake, glucose oxidation, and glucose storage in man, *Diabetes*, 31, 957, 1982.
12. Sonksen, P. H., The evolution of insulin treatment, *Clin. Endocrinol. Metab.*, 6, 481, 1977.
13. Lauritzen, T., Faber, O. K., and Binder, C., Variation in ^{125}I insulin absorption and blood glucose concentrations, *Diabetologia*, 17, 291, 1979.
14. Kurtz, A. B. and Nabarro, J. D. N., Circulating insulin-binding antibodies, *Diabetologia*, 19, 329, 1980.
15. Berger, M., Cuppers, H. J., Hegner, H. et al., Absorption kinetics and biological effects of subcutaneously injected insulin preparations, *Diabetes Care*, 5, 77, 1982.
16. Galloway, J. A., Spradlin, C. T., Nelson, R. L., Wentworth, S. M., Davidson, J. A., and Swarner, J. L., Factors influencing the absorption, serum insulin concentration, and blood glucose responses after injections of regular insulin and various insulin mixtures, *Diabetes Care*, 4, 366, 1981.
17. Gale, E. A. M. and Tattersall, R. B., In search of the Somogyi effect, *Lancet*, 2, 279, 1980.
18. Francis, A. J., Home, P. D., Hanning, I., Alberti, K. G. M. M., and Tunbridge, W. M. G., Intermediate-acting insulin given at bedtime: effect on blood glucose concentrations before and after breakfast, *Br. Med. J.*, 286, 1173, 1983.
19. Phillips, M., Simpson, R. W., Holman, R. R., and Turner, R. C., A simple and rational twice daily insulin regime, *Q. J. Med.*, 48, 493, 1979.
20. Walford, S., Fale, E. A. M., Allison, S. P., and Tattersall, R. B., Self-monitoring of blood glucose, *Lancet*, 1, 732, 1978.
21. Sonksen, P. H., Judd, S. L., and Lowy, C., Home monitoring of blood glucose, *Lancet*, 1, 729, 1978.
22. Peacock, I. and Tattersall, R. B., Methods of self monitoring of diabetic control, *Clin. Endocrinol. Metab.*, 11, 485, 1982.
23. Kadish, A. H., Automation control of blood sugar, A servomechanism of glucose monitoring and control, *Trans. Am. Soc. Artif. Int. Organs*, 19, 363, 1963.
24. Albisser, A. M., Leibel, B. S., Ewart, T. G., Davidovac, Z., Botz, C. K., and Zingg, W., An artificial endocrine pancreas, *Diabetes*, 23, 389, 1974.
25. Albisser, A. M., Leibel, B. S., Ewart, T. G., Davidovac, A., Botz, C. K., Zingg, W., Schipper, H., and Gander, R., Clinical control of diabetes by the artificial pancreas, *Diabetes*, 23, 396, 1974.
26. Pfeiffer, E. F., Thum, C., and Clemens, A. H., The artificial beta cell — a continuous control of blood sugar by external regulation of insulin infusion (glucose controlled insulin infusion system), *Horm. Metab. Res.*, 487, 339, 1974.
27. Santiago, J. V., Clemens, A. H., Clarke, W. L., and Kipnis, D. M., Closed-loop and open-loop devices for blood glucose control in normal and diabetic subjects, *Diabetes*, 28, 71, 1979.
28. Soeldner, J. S., Treatment of diabetic mellitus by devices, *Am J. Med.*, 70, 183, 1981.
29. Hanna, A. K., Zinman, B., Nakhooda, A. F., Minuk, H. L., Stokes, E. F., Albisser, A. M., and Marliss, E. B., Insulin, glucagon, and amino acids during glycemic control by the artificial pancreas in diabetic man, *Metabolism*, 29, 321, 1980.
30. Nosadini, R., Noy, G. A., Nattrass, M., Alberti, K. G. M. M., Johnston, D. G., Home, P. D., and Orskov, H., The metabolic and hormonal response to acute normoglycaemia in type I (insulin-dependent) diabetes: studies with a glucose controlled insulin infusion system (artificial endocrine pancreas), *Diabetologia*, 23, 220, 1982.
31. Horwitz, D. L., Zeidler, A., Goner, B., and Jaspan, J. B., Hyperinsulinism complicating control of diabetes mellitus by an artificial beta-cell, *Diabetes Care*, 3, 274, 1980.
32. Nosadini, R., Noy, G. A., Alberti, K. G. M. M., Hodson, A., and Orskov, H., The metabolic response to hyperglycaemic clamping in insulin-dependent diabetes, *Diabetologia*, 20, 113, 1981.
33. Schichiri, M., Kawamori, R., and Abe, H., Normalisation of the paradoxic secretion of glucagon in diabetics who were controlled by the artificial beta cell, *Diabetes*, 28, 272, 1979.
34. Horwitz, D. L., Gonen, B., Jaspan, J. B., Langer, B. G., Rodman, D., and Zeidler, A., An "artificial beta cell" for control of diabetes mellitus: effect on plasma glucagon levels, *Clin. Endocrinol. (Oxford)*, 11, 639, 1979.
35. Meissner, C., Thum, C., Beischer, W., Winkler, G., Schroder, K. E., and Pfeiffer, E. F., Antidiabetic action of somatostatin — assessed by the artificial pancreas, *Diabetes*, 24, 988, 1975.
36. Massi-Benedetti, M., Burrin, J. M., Capaldo, B., and Alberti, K. G. M. M., A comparative study of the activity of biosynthetic human insulin and pork insulin using the glucose clamp technique in normal subjects, *Diabetes Care*, 4, 163, 1981.
37. Schwartz, S. S., Horwitz, D. L., Zehfus, B., Langer, B., Moosa, A. R., Ribeiro, G., Kaplan, E., and Rubenstein, A. H., Use of a glucose controlled insulin infusion system (artificial beta cell) to control diabetes during surgery, *Diabetologia*, 16, 157, 1979.

38. Nattrass, M., Alberti, K. G. M. M., Dennis, K. J., Gillibrand, P. N., Letchworth, A. T., and Buckle, A. L., A glucose-controlled insulin infusion system for diabetic women during labour, *Br. Med. J.,* 2, 599, 1978.

39. Duncan, W. E., Duncan, T. G., DeLaurentis, D. A., Kryston, L., Kaminski, K., and Paskin, D. L., Artificial pancreas as an aid during insulinoma resection, *Am. J. Surg.,* 142, 528, 1981.

40. Vranic, M. and Berger, M., Exercise and diabetes mellitus, *Diabetes,* 28, 147, 1979.

41. Nelson, J. D., Poussier, P., Marliss, E. B., Albisser, A. M., and Zinman, B., Metabolic response of normal man and insulin-infused diabetics to postprandial exercise, *Am. J. Physiol.,* 242, E309, 1982.

42. Lambert, A. E., Buysschaert, M., and Lamotte, L., Use of an artificial pancreas as a tool to determine subcutaneous insulin doses in juvenile diabetes, *Diabetes Care,* 2, 256, 1979.

43. Mirouze, J., Selam, J. L., Pham, T. C., and Orsetti, A., The external artificial pancreas: an instrument to induce remissions in severe recent juvenile diabetes. Comparison with a preprogrammed insulin infusion system, *Horm. Metab. Res.,* 8 (Suppl.), 141, 1979.

44. Soeldner, J. S., Symposium on potentially implanted glucose sensors, *Diabetes Care,* 5, 147, 1982.

45. Slama, G., Hautcouverture, M., Assan, R., and Tchobroutsky, G., One to five days of continuous insulin infusion on seven diabetic patients, *Diabetes,* 23, 732, 1974.

46. Hepp, K. D., Renner, R., VonFunke, H. J., Mehnert, H., Haerten, R., and Kresse, H., Intravenous insulin therapy under conditions imitating physiological profiles, *Diabetologia,* 11, 349, 1975.

47. Leslie, R. D. and Mackay, J. D., Intravenous insulin infusion in diabetic emergencies, *Br. Med. J.,* 2, 1343, 1978.

48. Deckert, T. and Lorup, B., Regulation of brittle diabetes by a preplanned infusion programme, *Diabetologia,* 12, 573, 1976.

49. Service, F. J., Normalisation of plasma glucose of unstable diabetes: studies under ambulatory, fed conditions with pumped intravenous insulin, *J. Lab. Clin. Med.,* 91, 480, 1978.

50. Hanna, A. K., Minuk, H. L., Albisser, A. M., Marliss, E. B., Leibel, B. S., and Zinman, B., A portable system for continuous insulin delivery: Characteristics and results in diabetic patients, *Diabetes Care,* 3, 1, 1980.

51. Irsigler, K. and Kritz, H., Long-term continuous intravenous insulin therapy with a portable insulin dosage-regulating apparatus, *Diabetes,* 28, 196, 1979.

52. Botz, C. K., Marliss, E. B., and Albisser, A. M., Blood glucose regulation using closed- and open-loop insulin delivery systems, *Diabetologia,* 17, 45, 1979.

53. Horwitz, D. L., Granger, J. F., Nattrass, M., Martin, M. J., and Ash, S. L., Combined preprogrammed and feedback-controlled insulin administration with an artificial beta cell, *Diabetes,* 28, 376, 1979.

54. Pickup, J. C., Keen, H., Parsons, J. A., and Alberti, K. G. M. M., Continuous subcutaneous insulin infusion: an approach to achieving normoglycemia, *Br. Med. J.,* 1, 204, 1978.

55. Pickup, J. C., Keen, H., Viberti, G. C., White, M. C., Kohner, E. M., Parsons, J. A., and Alberti, K. G. M. M., Continuous subcutaneous insulin infusion in the treatment of diabetes mellitus, *Diabetes Care,* 3, 290, 1980.

56. Pickup, J. C. and Keen, H., Continuous subcutaneous insulin infusion: a developing tool in diabetes research, *Diabetologia,* 18, 1, 1980.

57. Tamborlane, W. V., Sherwin, R. S., Genel, M., and Felig, P., Reduction to normal of plasma glucose in juvenile diabetes by subcutaneous administration of insulin with a portable infusion pump, *N. Engl. J. Med.,* 300, 573, 1979.

58. Tamborlane, W. V., Sherwin, R. S., Genel, M., and Felig, P., Outpatient treatment of juvenile-onset diabetes with a preprogrammed portable subcutaneous insulin infusion system, *Am. J. Med.,* 68, 190, 1980.

59. Champion, M. C., Shepherd, G. A. A., Rodger, N. W., and Dupre, J., Continuous subcutaneous insulin supression in the management of diabetes mellitus, *Diabetes,* 29, 106, 1980.

60. Pickup, J. C., White, M. C., Keen. H., Kohner, E. M., Parsons, J. A., and Alberti, K. G. M. M., Long-term continuous subcutaneous insulin infusion in diabetics at home, *Lancet,* 2, 870, 1979.

61. Steno Study Group, Effect of 6 months of strict metabolic control on eye and kidney function in insulin-dependent diabetics with background retinopathy, *Lancet,* 1, 121, 1982.

62. Lauritzen, T., Frost-Larsen, K., Larsen, H. W., Deckert, T., and the Steno Study Group, Effect of 1 year of near-normal blood glucose levels on retinopathy in insulin-dependent diabetics, *Lancet,* 1, 200, 1983.

63. Kroc Collaborative Study Group, Near normal glycemic control does not slow progression of mild diabetic retinopathy, *Diabetes,* 32, (Suppl. 1), 10A, 1983.

64. Tamborlane, W. V., Sherwin, R. S., Genel, M., and Felig, P., Restoration of normal lipid and amino acid metabolism in diabetic patients with a portable insulin-infusion pump, *Lancet,* 1, 1258, 1979.

65. Pickup, J. C., Keen, H., Parsons, J. A., Alberti, K. G. M. M., and Rowe, A. S., Continuous subcutaneous insulin infusion: improved blood glucose and intermediary metabolite control in diabetics, *Lancet,* 1, 1255, 1979.

66. Raskin, P., Pietri, A., and Unger, R. H., Changes in glucagon levels after four to five weeks of glucoregulation by portable insulin infusion pumps, *Diabetes*, 28, 1033, 1979.

67. Tamborlane, W. V., Sherwin, R. S., Koivisto, V., Hendler, R., Genel, M., and Felig, P., Normalization of the growth hormone and catecholamine response to exercise in juvenile-onset diabetic subjects treated with a portable insulin infusion pump, *Diabetes*, 28, 785, 1979.

68. Rizza, R. A., Gerich, J. E., Haymond, M. W., Westland, R. E., Hall, L. D., Clemens, A. H., and Service, F. J., Control of blood sugar in insulin-dependent diabetes: comparison of an artificial endocrine pancreas, continuous subcutaneous insulin infusion and intensified conventional insulin therapy, *N. Engl. J. Med.*, 303, 1313, 1980.

69. Viberti, G. C., Pickup, J. C., Jarrett, R. J., and Keen, H., Effect of control of blood glucose on urinary excretion of albumin and β_2 microglobulin in insulin-dependent diabetes, *N. Engl. J. Med.*, 300, 638, 1979.

70. Viberti, G. C., Hill, R. D., Jarrett, R. J., Argyropoulos, A., Mahmud, U., and Keen, H., Microalbuminuria as a predictor of clinical nephropathy in insulin-dependent diabetes mellitus, *Lancet*, 1, 1430, 1982.

71. Viberti, G. C., Bilous, R. W., Mackintosh, D., Bending, J. J., and Keen, H., Long-term correction of hyperglycaemia and progression of renal failure in insulin dependent diabetes, *Br. Med. J.*, 286, 598, 1983.

72. White, N. H., Waltman, S. R., Krupin, T., Lebandoski, L. D., Flavin, K., and Santiago, J. V., Comparison of long-term intensive conventional therapy and pumped subcutaneous insulin on diabetic control, ocular fluorophotometry, and nerve conduction velocities, in *Artificial Systems for Insulin Delivery*, Serono Symposia Publications, Vol. 6, Brunetti, P., Alberti, K. G. M. M., Albisser, A. M., Hepp, K. D., Massi Benedetti, M., Eds., Raven Press, New York, 1983, 217.

73. Pietri, A., Ehle, A. L., and Raskin, R., Changes in nerve conduction velocity after six weeks of glucoregulation with portable insulin infusion pumps, *Diabetes*, 29, 668, 1980.

74. Boulton, A. J. M., Drury, J., Clarke, B., and Ward, J. D., Continuous subcutaneous insulin infusion in the management of painful diabetic neuropathy, *Diabetes Care*, 5, 386, 1982.

75. Pickup, J. C., Home, P. D., Bilous, R. W., Keen, H., and Alberti, K. G. M. M., Management of severely brittle diabetes by continuous subcutaneous and intramuscular insulin infusions: evidence for a defect in subcutaneous insulin absorption, *Br. Med. J.*, 282, 347, 1981.

76. Williams, G., Clark, A. J. L., Cooke, E., Bowcock, S., Pickup, J. C., and Keen, H., Local changes in subcutaneous blood flow around insulin injection sites measured by photoelectric plethysmography, *Diabetologia*, 21, 516, 1981.

77. Schade, D. S., Eaton, R. P., Friedman, N. M., and Spencer, W. J., Intraperitoneal delivery of insulin by a portable microinfusion pump, *Metabolism*, 29, 699, 1980.

78. Schade, D. S., Eaton, R. P., Spencer, W. J., Edwards, W. S., and Doberneck, R., Implantation of a remotely controlled insulin pump in diabetic man, *Diabetes*, 30 (Suppl. 1), 15A, 1981.

79. Alberti, K. G. M. M. and Hockaday, T. D. R., Diabetic coma: a reappraisal after five years, *Clin. Endocrinol. Metab.*, 6, 421, 1977.

80. Alberti, K. G. M. M., Hockaday, T. D. R., and Turner, R. C., Small doses of intramuscular insulin in the treatment of diabetic coma, *Lancet*, 2, 515, 1973.

81. Stevenson, R. W., Parsons, J. A., and Alberti, K. G. M. M., Insulin infusion into the portal and peripheral circulation of unanaesthetized dogs, *Clin. Endocrinol. (Oxford)*, 8, 335, 1978.

82. Stevenson, R. W. and Parsons, J. A., Chemical induction of diabetes in the dog and restoration of fasting normoglycaemia by insulin minipump implanted subcutaneously, *Diabetologia*, 20, 675, 1981.

83. Stevenson, R. W., Parsons, J. A., and Alberti, K. G. M. M., Comparison of the metabolic responses to portal and peripheral infusions in diabetic dogs, *Metabolism*, 30, 745, 1981.

84. Zierler, Z. L. and Rabinowitz, D., Effect of very small concentrations of insulin in forearm metabolism. Persistence of its action on potassium and free fatty acids without its effect on glucose, *J. Clin. Invest.*, 43, 950, 1964.

85. O'Connell, R. C., Morgan, A. P., Aoki, T. T., Ball, M. R., and Moore, F. D., Nitrogen conservation in starvation: graded responses to intravenous glucose, *J. Clin. Endocrinol. Metab.*, 39, 555, 1974.

86. Slama, G., Hautecouverture, M., Assan, R., and Tchobroutsky, G., One to five days of continuous insulin infusion on seven diabetic patients, *Diabetes*, 23, 732, 1974.

87. Albisser, A. M., Leibel, B. S., Zinman, B., Murray, F. T., Zingg, W., Botz, C. K., Denoga, A., and Marliss, E. B., Studies with an artificial endocrine pancreas, *Arch. Intern. Med.*, 137, 639, 1977.

88. Mirouze, J., Selam, J. L., Pham, T. C., and Cavadore, D., Evaluation of exogenous insulin homeostasis by the artificial pancreas in insulin-dependent diabetes, *Diabetologia*, 13, 273, 1977.

89. Nattrass, M., Alberti, K. G. M. M., Buckle, A. L. J., Cluett, B., Jaspan, J. B., Noy, G. A., Stubbs, W. A., and Walton, R., Metabolic studies during normoglycaemic clamping of insulin-dependent diabetics using a glucose controlled insulin infusion system. *Horm. Metab. Res.*, Suppl. 8, 86, 1979.

90. Stevenson, R. W., Orskov, H., Parsons, J. A., and Alberti, K. G. M. M., Metabolic responses to intraduodenal glucose loading in insulin-infused diabetic dogs, *Am. J. Physiol.,* 245, E200, 1983.

91. Brown, P. M., Tompkins, C. V., Juul, S., and Sonksen, P. H., Mechanism of action of insulin in diabetic patients; a dose-related effect on glucose production and utilisation, *Br. Med. J.,* 1, 1239, 1978.

92. Issekutz, B., Jr., Issekutz, T. B., Elahi, D., and Borkow, I., Effect of insulin infusion on glucose kinetics in alloxan-streptozotocin diabetic dogs, *Diabetologia,* 10, 323, 1974.

93. Stevenson, R. W., Parsons, J. A., and Alberti, K. G. M. M., Effect of intraportal and peripheral insulin on glucose turnover and recycling in diabetic dogs, *Am. J. Physiol.,* 244, E190, 1983.

94. Streja, D. A., Steiner, G., Marliss, E. B., and Vranic, M., Turnover and recycling of glucose in man during prolonged fasting, *Metabolism,* 26, 1089, 1977.

95. Reichard, G. A., Jr., Moury, N. F., Jr., Hochella, N. J., Patterson, A. L., and Weinhouse, S., Quantitative estimation of the Cori cycle in the human, *J. Biol. Chem.,* 238, 495, 1963.

96. Jansen, G. R., Hutchinson, C. F., and Zanetti, M. E., Studies on lipogenesis in vivo. Effect of dietary fat or starvation on conversion of [^{14}C]glucose into fat and turnover of newly synthesized fat, *Biochem J.,* 99, 323, 1966.

97. Edar, H. A., Novikoff, P. M., Novikoff, A. B., Yan, A., Beyer, M., and Gidez, L. I., Biochemical and morphologic studies on diabetic rats: effects of sucrose-enriched diet in rats with pancreatic islet transplants, *Proc. Natl. Acad. Sci. U.S.A.,* 11, 5905, 1979.

98. Jennings, A. S., Cherrington, A. D., Liljenquist, J. E., Keller, U., Lacy, W. W., and Chiasson, J.-L., The role of insulin and glucagon in the regulation of gluconeogenesis in the postabsorptive dog, *Diabetes,* 26, 847, 1977.

99. Hall, S. E. H., Saunders, J. and Sonksen, P. H., Glucose and free fatty acid turnover in normal subjects and in diabetic patients before and after insulin treatment, *Diabetologia,* 16, 297, 1979.

100. Goriya, Y., Bahoric, A., Marliss, E. B., Zinman, B., and Albisser, A. M., The metabolic and hormonal responses to a mixed meal in unrestrained pancreatectomised dogs chronically treated by portal or peripheral insulin infusion, *Diabetologia,* 21, 58, 1981.

101. Rizza, R. A., Westland, R. E., Hall, L. D., Patton, G. S., Haymond, M. W., Clemens, A. H., Gerich, J. E., and Service, F. J., Effect of peripheral versus portal venous administration of insulin on postprandial hyperglycemia and glucose turnover in alloxan-diabetic dogs, *Mayo Clin. Proc.,* 56, 434, 1981.

102. Fischer, U., Rizza, R. A., Hall, L. D., Westland, R. E., Haymond, M. W., Clemens, A. H., Gerich, J. E., and Service, F. J., Comparison of peripheral and portal venous insulin administration on postprandial metabolic responses in alloxan-diabetic dogs, *Diabetes,* 31, 579, 1982.

103. Campbell, E. A., Burrin, J. M., Parsons, J. A., and Stevenson, R. W., Metabolic normalisation in diabetic dogs using a new miniature insulin infuser, *Diabetologia,* 22, 383, 1982.

104. Botz, C. K., Leibel, B. S., Zingg, W., Gander, R. E., and Albisser, A. M., Comparison of peripheral and portal routes of insulin infusion by a computer controlled insulin infusion system (artificial endocrine pancreas), *Diabetes,* 25, 691, 1976.

105. Sasaki, H., Rubalclava, B., Baetens, D., Blazquez, E., Srikart, C. B., Orci, L., and Unger, R. H., Identification of glucagon in the gastrointestinal tract, *J. Clin. Invest.,* 56, 135, 1975.

106. Muller, W. A., Girardier, L., Seydoux, J., Berger, M., Renold, A. E., and Vranic, M., Extrapancreatic glucagon and glucagon-like immunoreactivity in depancreatized dogs, *J. Clin. Invest.,* 63, 124, 1978.

107. Fujita, Y., Chacra, A. R., Herron, A. L., and Smeltzer, H. S., Influence of carbohydrate intake on the biphasic insulin response to intravenous glucose, *Diabetes,* 24, 1072, 1975.

108. Grodsky, G. M., A threshold distribution hypothesis for packet storage of insulin and its mathematical modeling, *J. Clin. Invest.,* 51, 2047, 1972.

109. Grodsky, G. M., Secretion of insulin in *Handbook of Experimental Pharamcology,* Vol. 32, No. 2, Hasselblatt, A. and Bruchhausen, F. V., Eds., Springer-Verlag, Berlin, 1975, 1.

110. Steiner, K. E., Mouton, S. M., Bowles, C. R., Williams, P. E., and Cherrington, A. D., The relative importance of first- and second-phase insulin secretion in countering the action of glucagon on glucose turnover in the conscious dog. *Diabetes,* 31, 964, 1982.

111. Steiner, K. E., Williams, P. E., and Cherrington, A. D., First phase insulin release as a regulator of gluconeogenesis, *Diabetes,* 30 (Suppl. 1), 46A, 1981.

112. Calabrese, G., Bueti, A., Zega, G., Biomboline, A., Bellomo, G., Antonella, M. A., Massi-Benedetti, M., and Brunetti, P., Improvement of artificial endocrine pancreas (Biostator; GCIIS) performance combining feedback controlled insulin administration with a pre-programmed insulin infusion, *Horm. Metab. Res.,* 14, 505, 1982.

113. Albisser, A. M., Leibel, B. S., Zinman, B., Murray, F. T., Zingg, W., Botz, C. K., Denoga, A., and Marliss, E. B., Studies with an artificial endocrine pancreas, *Arch. Int. Med.,* 137, 639, 1977.

114. Goriya, Y., Bahoric, A., Marliss, E. B., Zinman, B., and Albisser, A. M., Diurnal metabolic and hormonal responses to mixed meals in healthy dogs, *Am. J. Physiol.,* 240, E54, 1981.

115. Huckabee, W. E., Relationships of pyruvate and lactate during anaerobic metabolism. I. Effects of infusion of pyruvate or glucose and of hyperventilation, *J. Clin. Invest.,* 37, 244, 1958.

116. Doar, J. W. H., Cramp, D. G., Maw, D. S. J., Seed, M., and Wynn, V., Blood pyruvate and lactate levels during oral and intravenous glucose tolerance tests in diabetes mellitus, *Clin. Sci.,* 39, 259, 1970.

117. Felig, P., Wahren, J., and Hendler, R., Influence of oral glucose ingestion on splanchnic glucose and gluconeogenic substrate metabolism in man, *Diabetes,* 24, 468, 1975.

118. Stout, R. W., Diabetes and atherosclerosis — role of insulin, *Diabetologia,* 16, 141, 1979.

119. Madison, L. L. and Kaplan, N., The hepatic binding of labeled insulin in human subjects during a single transhepatic circulation, *J. Lab. Clin. Med.,* 52, 927, 1958.

120. Samols, E. and Ryder, J. A., Studies on tissue uptake of insulin in man using a differential immunoassay for endogenous and exogenous insulin, *J. Clin. Invest.,* 40, 2092, 1961.

121. Kaden, M., Harding, P., and Field, J. B., Effect of intraduodenal glucose administration on hepatic extraction of insulin in the anesthetized dog, *J. Clin. Invest.,* 52, 2016, 1973.

122. Terris, S., Hofmann, C., and Steiner, D. F., Mode of uptake and degradation of labeled insulin by isolated hepatocytes and H4 hepatoma cells, *Can. J. Biochem.,* 57, 459, 1979.

123. King, A. C. and Cuatrecasas, P., Peptide hormone-induced receptor mobility, aggregation and internalization, *N. Engl. J. Med.,* 305, 77, 1981.

124. Kitabchi, A. E., Proinsulin and C-peptide. A review, *Metab. Clin. Exp.,* 26, 547, 1977.

125. Jaspan, J. and Polonsky, K., Glucose ingestion in dogs alters the hepatic extraction of insulin. In vivo evidence for a relationship between biologic action and extraction of insulin, *J. Clin. Invest.,* 69, 516, 1982.

126. Field, J. B., Rojdmark, S., Harding, P., Ishida, T., and Chou, M. C. Y., Role of liver in insulin physiology, *Diabetes Care,* 3, 255, 1980.

127. Stevenson, R. W., Cherrington, A. D., and Steiner, K. E., The relationship between plasma concentration and disappearance rate of immunoreactive insulin in the dog, *Horm. Metab. Res.,* in press.

128. Ooms, H. A., Brunengraber, H., and Franckson, J. R. M., Hepatic influence on labeled insulin metabolism, *Acta Diabetol. Lat.,* 5, 162, 1968.

129. Franckson, J. R. M. and Ooms, H. A., The catabolism of insulin in the dog: evidence for the existence of two catabolic pathways, *Postgrad. Med. J.,* 49, 931, 1973.

130. Waldhausl, W., Bratusch-Marrain, P., Gasic, S., Korn, A., and Nowotny, P., Insulin production rate following glucose ingestion estimated by splanchnic C-peptide output in normal man, *Diabetologia,* 17, 221, 1979.

131. Eaton, R. P., Allen, R. C., Schade, D. S., and Standefer, J. C., "Normal" insulin secretion: the goal of artificial delivery systems, *Diabetes Care,* 3, 270, 1980.

132. Driver, R. L. and Murlin, J. R., Factors in the absorption of insulin from the alimentary tract, *Am. J. Physiol.,* 132, 182, 1941.

133. Hanzlik, P. J. and Cutting, W. C., Agents promoting gastrointestinal absorption of insulin, *Endocrinology,* 28, 368, 1941.

134. Bangham, A. D., Standish, M. M., and Watkins, G. C., Diffusion of univalent ions across the lamellae of swollen phospholipids, *J. Mol. Biol.,* 13, 238, 1965.

135. Patel, H. M. and Ryman, B. E., Oral administration of insulin by encapsulation within liposomes, *FEBS Lett.,* 62, 60, 1976.

136. Patel, H. M., Stevenson, R. W., Parsons, J. A., and Ryman, B. E., Use of liposomes to aid intestinal absorption of entrapped insulin in normal and diabetic dogs, *Biochim. Biophys. Acta,* 716, 188, 1982.

137. Gregoriadis, G. and Ryman, B. E., Fate of protein-containing liposomes injected into rats. An approach to the treatment of storage diseases, *Eur. J. Biochem.,* 24, 485, 1972.

138. Stevenson, R. W., Patel, H. M., Parsons, J. A., and Ryman, B. E., Prolonged hypoglycemic effect in diabetic dogs due to subcutaneous administration of insulin in liposomes, *Diabetes,* 31, 506, 1982.

139. Schade, D. S., Eaton, R. P., Friedman, N. M., and Spencer, W. J., Normalization of plasma insulin profiles with intraperitoneal insulin infusion in diabetic man, *Diabetologia,* 19, 35, 1980.

140. Schade, D. S., Eaton, R. P., Davis, T., Akiya, F., Phinney, E., Kubica, R., Vaughn, E. A., and Day, P. W., The kinetics of peritoneal insulin absorption, *Metabolism,* 30, 149, 1981.

141. Schade, D. S., Eaton, R. P., Friedman, N. M., Spencer, W. J., and Standefer, J. C., Five-day programmed intraperitoneal insulin delivery in insulin-dependent diabetic man, *J. Clin. Endocrinol. Metab.,* 52, 1165, 1981.

142. Nelson, J. A., Stephen, R., Landau, S. T., Wilson, D. E., and Tyler, F. H., Intraperitoneal insulin administration produces a positive portal-systemic blood insulin gradient in unanesthetized, unrestrained swine, *Metabolism,* 31, 969, 1982.

143. Ballinger, W. F. and Lacy, P. E., Transplantation of intact pancreatic islets in rats, *Surgery,* 72, 175, 1972.

144. Kemp, C. B., Knight, M. J., Scharp, D. W., Ballinger, W. F., and Lacy, P. E., Effect of transplantation site on the results of pancreatic islet isografts in diabetic rats, *Diabetologia,* 9, 486, 1973.

145. Matas, A. J., Payne, W. D., Grotting, J. C., Sutherland, D. E. R., Steffes, M. W., Hertel, B. F., and Najarian, J. S., Portal versus systemic transplantation of dispersed neonatal pancreas, *Transplantation,* 24, 333, 1977.

146. Joiner, C. L., Rate of clearance of insulin labelled with ^{131}I from the subcutaneous tissues in normal and diabetic subjects, *Lancet,* 1, 964, 1959.

147. Clark, D. G., Rognstad, R., and Katz, J., Lipogenesis in rat hepatocytes, *J. Biol. Chem.,* 249, 2028, 1974.

148. Salmon, D. M. W., Bowen, N. L., and Hems, D. A., Synthesis of fatty acids in the perfused mouse liver, *Biochem. J.,* 142, 611, 1974.

149. Blackshear, P. J., Holloway, P. A. H., and Alberti, K. G. M. M., The effects of starvation and insulin on the release of gluconeogenic substrates from the extrasplanchnic tissues in vivo, *FEBS Lett.,* 48, 310, 1974.

150. Lewis, B. M. and Hayes, T. M., Intraperitoneal insulin: a comparison of various doses and dilutions with subcutaneous insulin, *Diabetologia,* 21, 511, 1981.

Chapter 7

RATE-CONTROLLED CARDIOVASCULAR DRUG ADMINISTRATION AND ACTION

H. A. J. Struyker-Boudier, J. C. S. Kleinjans, L. M. L. le Noble,
H. M. N. Nievelstein, and J. F. M. Smits

TABLE OF CONTENTS

I. INTRODUCTION

Cardiovascular diseases are the major source of morbidity and mortality in western society. The important advance in life expectancy during this century as a consequence of improved control of infectious diseases, amongst others, has unmasked a vast health problem related to cardiovascular diseases in the later decades of life. In fact, in the aged (>70 years) cardiac failure is the most prominent cause of death, whereas of the adult population approximately 15% suffers from high blood pressure.

In recent years, some progress has been made in the control of cardiovascular diseases. The influence of life style, especially dietary habits, on the occurrence of cardiovascular risk factors such as plasma cholesterol levels has been recognized. Diagnostic procedures for early detection of vascular abnormalities, including those of the coronary circulation, have greatly improved. The beneficial effects of coronary by-pass surgery and drug induced secondary prevention of coronary diseases are the subject of thorough scientific investigation right now. Probably, the most important improvement of the last 2 decades has been the development of effective drug therapy for hypertension. Almost all patients with elevated blood pressure can now be treated effectively with a variety of antihypertensive drugs.

There is a reverse side to the medal of modern pharmacotherapeutic tools for the treatment of cardiovascular diseases. Very often, such drugs have to be administered on a lifelong basis. Effective treatment of heart failure and hypertension can usually only be achieved with chronic daily administration of drugs. Also, long-term exposure to drugs seems necessary in the treatment of angina pectoris, certain cardiac arrhythmias, and peripheral vascular diseases. A major effort has been made to develop drugs with relatively few side effects. Still, the traditional routes of administration expose the body to widely fluctuating drug levels. Drug-related toxicities may occur whenever drug levels rise above a certain value, although in other instances the opposite may be true, e.g., the rebound phenomena upon withdrawal of centrally acting antihypertensives or beta-adrenoceptor blockers. This chapter will give a survey of how modern technology, using rate-controlled methods of drug administration, can overcome some of these problems through optimized schedules of drug application.

A second aspect of this chapter will be the pharmacodynamic consequences of rate-controlled cardiovascular drug administration. It is generally assumed that there is a close relationship between the concentration of a drug in plasma or the receptor compartment and its biological effect. Recent studies have indicated that this may not always be true. An illustrative example in cardiovascular research is the study by Smits et al.[1] who showed that upon a bolus injection of propranolol in conscious hypertensive rats, the maximum fall in blood pressure occurs when there is hardly any drug left in the body. Only after prolonged continuous infusion of propranolol could a relationship between plasma levels and effects be noticed.[2] Urquhart et al.[3] recently reviewed a number of studies in different fields of pharmacology that showed a dependence of the biological effect upon the schedule of administration of a drug. Other reviews outside the cardiovascular field are given in different chapters in this book.

We shall focus here on the impact of different schedules of administration on the dynamics of the responses to cardiovascular drugs. We shall first briefly review how the cardiovascular system and its control mechanisms operate. This is essential for a full understanding of the dynamics of cardiovascular drug action. We shall then discuss in more detail the rate-controlled action of the major classes of cardiovascular drugs.

II. THE CARDIOVASCULAR SYSTEM AND ITS CONTROL MECHANISMS

The cardiovascular system is aimed at providing an adequate blood flow to different

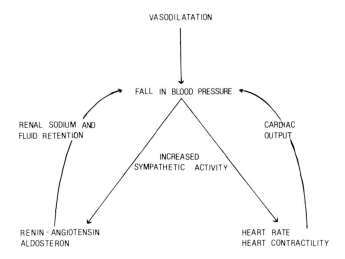

FIGURE 1. Cardiovascular regulatory mechanisms that oppose an initial fall in blood pressure after the administration of an arteriolar vasodilator.

tissues in the body in order to supply these tissues with nutrients and to remove waste products. The cardiovascular system consists of a pump (the heart), an arterial — high pressure — conduction system ending in a number of parallel vascular beds, and a venous — low pressure — conduction system. The parallel vascular beds have widely different blood flow needs, e.g., certain tissues, such as the myocardium and brain, require a constant blood flow, whereas others, such as skeletal muscle or skin, show a wide range of blood flows depending upon the actual need. The blood flow through an exercising muscle may be 20- to 50-fold higher than that through a resting muscle. A number of mechanisms contribute to an optimal control of the cardiovascular system. Certain variables, e.g., arterial blood pressure, are held amazingly constant throughout life, whereas others vary at different time scales. A detailed discussion of cardiovascular control mechanisms can be found in the monograph by Guyton.[4]

The aim of pharmacotherapy of cardiovascular diseases is usually to alter the steady-state value of one or more variables. In the treatment of hypertension, this variable is arterial blood pressure; the treatment of heart failure aims at a permanent improvement of the relationship between venous return of blood to the heart and cardiac output; the primary goal of treatment of angina pectoris is to alter the relationship between cardiac blood supply and myocardial oxygen consumption. On a more cellular level, the aim of treating atherosclerosis is to reverse structural changes of blood vessels, whereas on a molecular level anticoagulants are given chronically to alter the steady state of the prothrombin complex activity or other coagulation factors. In each case a drug, or combination of drugs, is given to go from one (abnormal) steady state to a new (hopefully normal) steady state. The ultimate success of this attempt is determined by (a) the primary molecular or cellular mechanisms of action of the drug and (b) the reactions of the cardiovascular systems and its control mechanisms to the disturbance caused by the primary effect of the drug.

In the past, drug treatment for cardiovascular diseases was designed primarily on the basis of only the first of these two factors. An illustrative example is the administration of an arteriolar vasodilator to lower blood pressure (Figure 1). Most forms of hypertension are characterized by an increased peripheral vascular resistance. Vasodilators thus seem a logical approach to treat hypertension. The primary effect of these

Table 1

MAJOR NEURAL MECHANISMS INVOLVED IN CARDIOVASCULAR CONTROL

Control mechanism	Stimuli for activation	Effector mechanisms
Sinoaortic baroreceptor reflex	Arterial blood pressure Cardiac output	Autonomic nervous system
Cardiopulmonary baroreceptor reflex	Atrial and pulmonary vein pressure Blood volume	Autonomic nervous system Antidiuretic hormone
Chemoreceptor reflex	Chemoreceptor blood flow Chemical factors in blood (e.g., pO_2) Plasma catecholamines	Autonomic nervous system
CNS ischemia reflex	CNS blood flow	Autonomic nervous system
Somatic afferent reflex	Somatic (pain?) stimuli	Autonomic nervous system
Renal afferent reflex	Chemical factors in renal blood (e.g., bradykinin) Renal arterial pressure	Autonomic nervous system

drugs is arteriolar vasodilatation with a subsequent fall in arterial blood pressure. However, the fall in blood pressure triggers an immediate baroreceptor-reflex mediated rise in sympathetic nerve activity.[5,6] This leads to a rise in heart rate and cardiac output. In the long term, the rise in plasma renin activity due to the increased sympathetic activity, as well as the fall in renal perfusion pressure, causes renal retention of fluid. Ultimately, the original fall in blood pressure will have disappeared almost completely due to the short- and long-term actions of cardiovascular control mechanisms. This explains why a seemingly logical pharmacological approach to the treatment of hypertension is not very successful in the long run.

Therefore, for a full understanding of the dynamics of cardiovascular drug action, it is necessary to consider potential interferences by cardiovascular control mechanisms. The control mechanisms interfering with the ultimate effect of a cardiovascular drug can be distinguished in neural, endocrine, renal, and vascular (including structural) mechanisms. We shall only briefly review these mechanism here. A detailed description of cardiovascular control mechanisms and their responses to cardiovascular drugs can be found elsewhere.[4,7,8]

A. Neural Mechanisms

A summary of neural mechanisms involved in cardiovascular control is given in Table 1.

The most prominent neural reflex mechanism is the sinoaortic baroreceptor reflex. This reflex is a powerful, rapidly acting buffer against acute changes in blood pressure. It is a negative feedback control mechanism, e.g., a fall in blood pressure leads to an afferent reflex activation and an increase in sympathetic and a decrease in parasympathetic activity, thus bringing blood pressure back to values close to those before the original disturbance. Recent studies show that the baroreceptor reflex may not only sense changes in arterial pressure, but also in cardiac output.[9,10]

The sinoaortic baroreceptor reflex is primarily involved in short-term control of blood pressure. Its activity wanes rapidly during a sustained change in blood pressure. This has important implications for the effects of cardiovascular drugs, as will be discussed in more detail later.

Another important nervous reflex mechanism is the cardiopulmonary baroreceptor reflex. The stretch-sensitive receptors for this reflex are located in the low pressure

Table 2
MAJOR ENDOCRINE MECHANISMS INVOLVED IN CARDIOVASCULAR CONTROL

Control mechanism	Stimuli for activation	Effector mechanisms
Adrenal catecholamines	Activity in parts of CNS (?)	Adrenal catecholamine secretion
Renin-angiotensin system	Sympathetic nerve activity Afferent arteriolar transmural pressure Macula densa chemoreceptors Prostaglandins	Local renal and systemic angiotensin-II concentration
Aldosterone	ACTH plasma concentration Angiotensin-II plasma concentration Extracellular K^+ concentration	Adrenal aldosterone secretion
Antidiuretic hormone	Extracellular osmotic pressure Baroreceptors (sinoaortic and cardiopulmonary) Activity in parts of CNS	ADH release from hypophysis
Prostaglandins	Regional blood flow (?) Angiotensin-II plasma concentration(?)	Local prostaglandin release
Kallikreins-kinins	Plasma activators	Local kinin release
Atriopeptins	Unknown	Cardiac atriopeptin release

Note: ACTH = adrenocorticophic hormone; ADH = antidiuretic hormone.

parts of the cardiovascular system, viz., the pulmonary blood vessels and the atria of the heart. The afferent signal for this reflex seems primarily a change in the degree of filling of the low pressure side of the circulation. On the efferent side, this reflex operates predominantly through a change in the central release of antidiuretic hormone (vasopressin) and sympathetic nerve activity, especially to the kidneys.

Further — very special — neural reflex mechanisms are the chemoreceptor reflex and the CNS ischemic reflex. These reflexes do not play an important role in the normal control of arterial blood pressure. Chemoreceptor reflexes are activated by changes in the chemical constitution of blood, including blood oxygen and carbon dioxide concentration. Although the chemoreceptor reflex serves a primary purpose in the control of respiration, it may affect the cardiovascular system through changes in autonomic nerve activity. The CNS ischemic reflex is only activated when CNS blood flow falls below a critical level. It is then a powerful mechanism to induce sympathetic hyperactivity.

A final group of nervous control mechanisms are the somatic afferent reflexes. Stimulation of afferent nerves from several sites influences the cardiovascular system through changes in efferent sympathetic nerve activity. An especially important mechanism in this respect is the renal afferent nervous reflex control of the cardiovascular system.[11-13] Activation of renal afferents through either chemical (e.g., adenosine,[12] bradykinin[13]) or mechanical (e.g., reduced renal blood flow) stimuli strongly influences the cardiovascular system. Recent studies have provided evidence for an important role of renal afferents in the development of several forms of experimental hypertension.[11,14,15] The role of this reflex in the dynamics of action of cardiovascular drugs has not yet been investigated.

B. Endocrine Mechanisms

Table 2 summarizes the most important endocrine mechanisms involved in cardiovascular control.

The stimuli for the release of adrenal catecholamines are not yet fully understood.

Once released, circulating catecholamines are able to activate adrenoceptors, especially the alpha-2 and beta-2 adrenoceptors.[16] These receptors are located both pre- and post-synaptically. Activation of presynaptic alpha-2 receptors inhibits noradrenaline release from sympathetic nerves whereas beta-2 receptor stimulation causes facilitation. Post-synaptic alpha-2 receptor stimulation leads to several effects, including constriction of arterioles and veins. Beta-2 receptor stimulation has an opposite effect.

The renin-angiotensin system is of importance for the control of intra- as well as extrarenal hemodynamics. Renin is synthesized and released from the juxtaglomerular cells in the kidney, although renin-like enzyme activity has been reported in other tissues, including blood vessel wall and brain.[17] The release of renin from the kidney is controlled by sympathetic nerve activity, transmural pressure in the afferent arterioles at the level of the juxtaglomerular cells and macula densa chemoreceptors sensitive to the rate of delivery and content of tubular fluid. Intrarenal prostaglandins also affect renin release.[18] Renin acts upon a glycoprotein, from which after several converting steps angiotensin II is formed. This substance is the primary efferent limb of the renin-angiotensin system. It acts as a powerful systemic as well as intrarenal vasoconstrictor; it influences the renal excretion of sodium and water both directly and indirectly through stimulation of aldosterone synthesis and release; it enhances vascular permeability and increases sympathetic nerve activity by both a CNS and a peripheral presynaptic effect.[17]

Aldosterone is an adrenal hormone participating in the control of body fluid volumes. Its release from the adrenal gland is determined by plasma adrenocorticotrophic hormone, circulating angiotensin II and extracellular potassium. Aldosterone plays a role in cardiovascular control by its effects on sodium and potassium excretion in the distal part of the kidney tubules.

Antidiuretic hormone is involved in the control of both body fluid volumes and vascular resistance. Its release from neurohypophysis is controlled by hypothalamic osmoreceptors and baroreceptor — both sinoaortic and cardiopulmonary — reflex mechanisms. Antidiuretic hormone influences body fluid volumes by its effects on tubular water reabsorption. Moreover, it has an effect on arteriolar resistance.

Several chemical factors involved in cardiovascular control act as "tissue hormones". The most prominent of these are the prostaglandins and the kallikrein-kinin system. Prostaglandins are released from endothelial cells to adjust local blood flow to changing metabolic requirements of tissues.[19] Such effects of prostaglandins have now been described in different tissues. In the kidney, this is expressed as a contribution to the regulation of renal blood flow and its zonal distribution.

Prostaglandins also affect intrarenal renin release and tubular salt and water reabsorption. A similar action has been proposed for the kallikrein-kinin system.[20] Kinins are formed from plasma substrates called kininogens by the action of kallikrein. They act as potent vasodilators. Smits and Brody[13] recently proposed a possible role of bradykinin in cardiovascular control by virtue of its ability to stimulate renal afferent nerves. In the kidney, Muirhead et al.[21] have described another potential tissue hormone. They proposed that the renal medulla contains lipid-like substances with vasodilatory activity.

A final group of chemical, possible endocrine, factors involved in cardiovascular control are the recently described natriuretic factors. De Wardener[22] already suggested a number of years ago the existence of a circulating natriuretic hormone, released upon a rapid expansion of extracellular fluid volume. Thus far, it has not been possible to trace the endogenous source of this hormone or characterize its chemical structure. Recent studies have suggested that the substance may act as an endogenous inhibitor of Na^+/K^+ activated ATPase, thus interfering with transmembrane sodium transport.[23]

This activity would lead to an enhanced tubular sodium excretion and to a constriction of blood vessels. Another natriuretic factor has recently been described in the atria of a number of species. Although the endocrine activity of this substance has not yet been proven, its chemical structure has been resolved.[24] In fact, a group of peptides is involved, now referred to as atriopeptins.[25] Some of these substances are potent natriuretic and diuretic agents, whereas one analog also acts as a vasodilator. The physiological role nor the effects by drugs on these natriuretic factors have yet been studied in any detail.

C. Renal Mechanisms

The kidney has a unique role in cardiovascular control. It is the source of afferent nervous reflex mechanisms as well as some endocrine agents involved in cardiovascular control (vide supra). Apart from these mechanisms, the kidney is essential in controlling body fluid volumes and their composition. Guyton and co-workers[4,26] have pointed out the important relationship between renal control of fluid volumes and cardiovascular control. This relationship is determined by the effect of renal perfusion pressure (under normal conditions equal to arterial pressure) on renal fluid output. An increase in arterial pressure of just a few millimeters of Hg can cause a massive renal excretion of fluid, a phenomenon usually referred to as pressure diuresis. Over a prolonged period of time, the fluid loss reduces the extracellular fluid volume, cardiac output, and ultimately, arterial pressure. Thus, the renal fluid control mechanism operates as a negative feedback system. In a quantitative analysis, Guyton and co-workers[4,26] indicated that, although acting slowly, this mechanism is a highly effective controller of blood pressure. In fact, the gain of this negative feedback control system is infinite, e.g., upon a disturbance blood pressure will be brought back all the way to its original value through the renal fluid control mechanism. In short-term situations, neural and endocrine mechanisms almost completely achieve the same effect. However, long-term disturbances of blood pressure are controlled predominantly by the renal fluid control mechanism. This concept has important implications for the pharmacological treatment of hypertensive disease. It implies that a new steady-state blood pressure level can only be achieved if the antihypertensive drug or drug combination causes a permanent shift of the pressure-diuresis relationship towards a lower pressure level. We have extensively discussed these implications elsewhere.[7]

D. Vascular Mechanisms

A final form of cardiovascular control is exerted by local vascular mechanisms. We should distinguish between mechanisms aimed at the short-term control of blood flow and long-term mechanisms reflected in the structural design of vascular beds.

Short-term vascular control usually serves the maintenance of blood flow ("auto-regulation"). It involves myogenic mechanisms related to stretch of the vascular wall and chemical factors, such as oxygen, adenosine, or prostaglandins. Different tissues in the body have a variable degree of autoregulatory control of their blood flow. Also, the chemical factors involved may differ per tissue.

Long-term vascular control can be exerted by the structural design of vascular beds. In several forms of hypertension, a prolonged increase in blood pressure is associated with a gradual increase in the wall-to-lumen ratio of precapillary resistance vessels.[27] It has been speculated that the hypertrophy of these vessels may occur independently of blood pressure elevation per se. Trophic chemical factors may be involved to induce an abnormal pattern of cell division in vascular smooth muscle.[28] Whatever the cellular mechanisms involved, the hypertrophy causes an enhanced resistance to flow. A second long-term control mechanism is the degree of vascularity. During development as well as during aging, there is a continuous dynamic process of capillary growth and

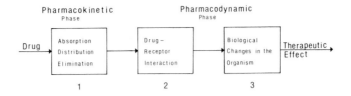

FIGURE 2. Major steps involved in drug action.

disappearance. The physical or chemical factors controlling angiogenesis are not yet known. However, this aspect of structural design of vascular beds is also of great importance in the control of flow and resistance to flow.

There is very little known about the influence of cardiovascular drugs on the structural design of the microcirculation. Such studies are urgently needed, since a primary goal of treatment of diseases like essential hypertension, angina pectoris or atherosclerosis, should be the reversal of structural vascular changes.

III. KINETICS OF CARDIOVASCULAR DRUG RESPONSES

The science of pharmacology aims at providing a quantitative prediction of drug effects on the basis of a given drug input. Usually in this process, a distinction is made between the pharmacokinetic and pharmacodynamic phase of drug action (Figure 2). Pharmacokinetics provides a description of the quantitative relationships between drug input functions and plasma (or other tissue) concentration as a function of time. Elsewhere in this volume, Van Rossum et al. and Smits and Thijssen give detailed descriptions of the influence of different types of drug input functions on plasma and tissue concentrations. Pharmacodynamics should provide a quantitative description of the relationship between plasma or tissue concentration and drug effects, again as a function of time. However, the dimension of time is not usually considered in pharmacodynamics. The central paradigm of pharmacodynamics is the dose or concentration-response curve. This paradigm originates from the classical methodologies used in pharmacodynamics, *in casu* the use of isolated organs to quantify drug effects.[29-31] It is obvious that time plays no important role in in vitro pharmacodynamic analyses. However, the foregoing discussion on the cardiovascular sytem and its control mechanisms stresses that in vivo drug-induced cardiovascular effects in man or experimental animals have a strong time dependency. Dose or concentration-effect curves are not sufficient to quantify the dynamics of drug action in these cases. An example from the work of O'Reilly[32] may illustrate this point. O'Reilly has attempted to quantify the relationship between the concentrations of R(+) and S(−) enantiomers of warfarin and their anticoagulant effects, expressed as prothrombin time. Such a relationship was difficult to establish because of the complications caused by the time course of coagulation factor synthesis and degradation. Only by using the areas under the log prothrombin time vs. time and warfarin concentration vs. time after a single dose of each enantiomer, O'Reilly obtained a linear model to determine the relative potencies. (Figure 3).

Thus far, no general theory has been developed to account for the nonlinear, timevarying dynamics of drug action, in contrast to the established general pharmacokinetic theories. In pharmacokinetics, the law of conservation of mass is the basis of the mathematical models to explain the kinetic behavior of drugs in the body. Such models may be based on classical compartment analysis or, more recently, upon a detailed physiological description of the major systems in the body involved in drug distribution and elimination[33,34] (cf. also Smits and Thijssen, Chapter 4). In Chapter 3, Van Ros-

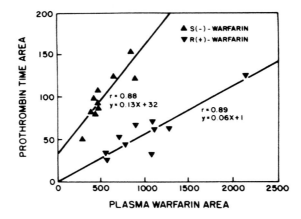

FIGURE 3. Linear model of the areas under the warfarin concentration versus time and the log prothrombin-time versus time after a single dose of the S(−) and R(+) isomers of warfarin in man. (From O'Reilly, R. A., *Clin. Pharmacol. Ther.*, 16, 348, 1974. With permission.)

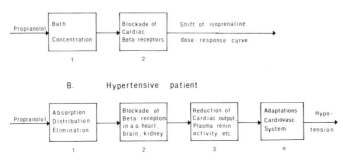

FIGURE 4. Major steps involved in propranolol's effects on (A) the isoprenaline dose-response curve in an isolated heart and (B) blood pressure in a hypertensive patient.

sum et al. present an even more advanced mathematical treatment of pharmacokinetics, using principles from dynamic systems theory. The situation is fundamentally different when trying to develop a mathematical framework for the dynamic, time-dependent aspects of drug action. In the last decades, it has been possible to develop mathematical models for drug-receptor interactions.[29-31] However, as was argued before, such models in general do not take into account the variation of drug responses in time. In these models, it is generally assumed that drug-receptor interactions create a "stimulus" that causes the effect(s) of the drug. The relationship between the stimulus and the effect is governed by the dynamic behavior of molecular, cellular, and tissue structures in the body. An illustration of such a sequence of events may be the blood-pressure-lowering effect of a beta-blocker (Figure 4). The blockade of cardiac beta-adrenoceptors on the basis of the competitive receptor antagonism by the beta-blocker, causes a reduced sensitivity of the heart to the positive inotropic and chronotropic effects of the sympathetic neurotransmitter noradrenaline. This leads — via several steps involving the excitation-contraction mechanisms of cardiac muscle — to a reduction of cardiac output, the time course of which parallels the dynamics of the cardiac beta-adrenoeceptor blockade.[1,2] However, due to the baroreceptor reflex activation of the sympathetic nervous system, total peripheral resistance increases, thus opposing an early fall in blood pressure.[10] Within several hours, the baroreceptor reflex adapts to the prevailing level of cardiac output. This leads to a delayed, gradual fall in blood pressure. The dynamics of the blood pressure lowering effect of propranolol is not only caused by the time course of cardiac beta-adrenoceptor blockade, but — even more importantly — by the dynamic behavior of the cardiovascular system and its control mechanisms.

This example illustrates that on a more integrated level than isolated organs, pharmacodynamic theory should incorporate time-dependent events taking place beyond the receptor level. The lack of detailed understanding of many of these events has thus far hampered the development of such theories. Dynamic systems analysis can provide a conceptual tool for quantifying drug responses as a function of time. Elsewhere we have given a detailed description of a systems analysis approach to the dynamics of cardiovascular drug action.[7] Also, a recent review by Greenway[36] contains a quantitative description of time-dependent cardiovascular drug action based on principles from dynamic systems theory.

The incorporation of the dimension time in pharmacodynamic analyses has important implications for the study of the influence of schedules of drug administration on drug responses. The traditional pharmacodynamic theory — or "pharmacostatics", a term coined by Yates[37] in view of the absence of the the dimension time — supposes a time-independent relationship between receptor occupancy, stimulus formation and biological effect. This view implicates that the influence of different drug input functions are only reflected in the kinetic pattern of drug concentration in plasma or other tissues. However, there is ample evidence now that the rate of drug administration as such can affect pharmacological responses. This phenomenon has been recognized in the field of hormone action for a long time already.[38] Some endocrine responses depend on the rate of change of hormone concentrations rather than on their absolute level. Chapter 10 contains a number of such examples from the endocrine field, as well as a theoretical framework to understand how different rates of delivery of endocrine agents may affect their responses.

We shall provide examples of different cardiovascular responses that depend on the rate of their administration in the following paragraphs. We shall discuss the major groups of cardiovascular drugs from the point of view of both pharmacokinetic and pharmacodynamic consequences of rate-controlled drug administration.

IV. ANTIHYPERTENSIVE DRUGS

A. Time Course of the Development of Hemodynamic Effects

In the preceding paragraphs, the dynamics of the antihypertensive effect of beta-blockers was used to illustrate the lack of correlation between drug input functions and subsequent pharmacokinetics in the organism on the one hand and drug responses on the other. Smits et al.[12] have performed a series of studies to carefully measure the time course of the major cardiovascular changes following a bolus (Figure 5) or constant rate infusion (Figure 6) of propranolol in conscious spontaneously hypertensive rats (SHR). Similar studies have been performed in hypertensive patients.[39,40]

A major conclusion from these studies is that upon acute administration of propranolol, there is a close relation between the kinetics of distribution and elimination of propranolol and its effects on cardiac beta-adrenoceptors. Thus, parallel to the time course of propranolol in plasma and cardiac tissue, the beta-adrenoceptors in the heart are blocked. This leads to a fall in heart rate and cardiac output. However, there is a

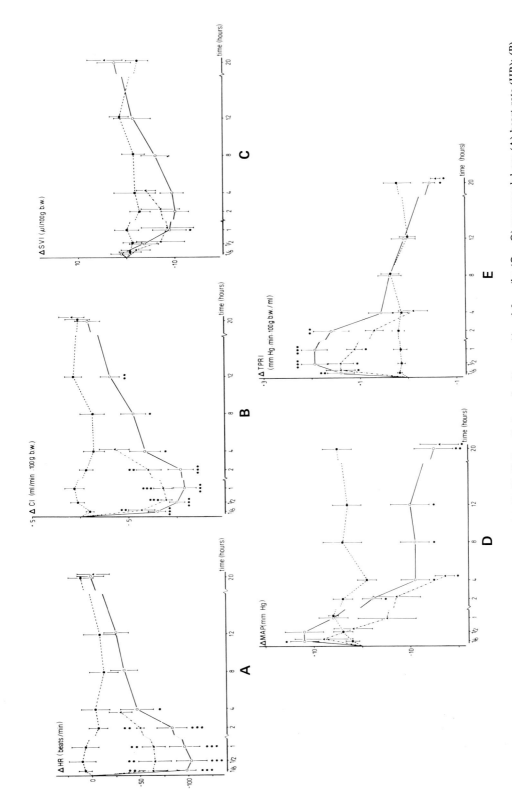

FIGURE 5. Acute effects of s.c. injections of 0.9% NaCl (●——●), 1 mg/kg (▲—·—▲) and 5 mg/kg (O——O) propranolol on: (A) heart rate (HR); (B) cardiac index (CI); (C) stroke volume index (SVI); (D) mean arterial pressure (MAP), and (E) total peripheral resistance index (TPRI) in conscious SHR.

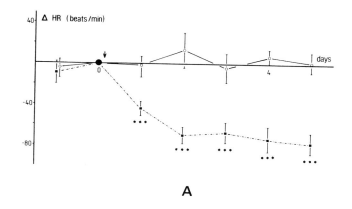

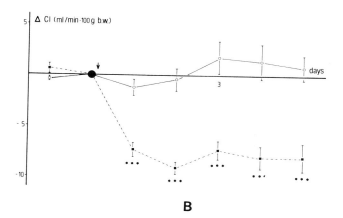

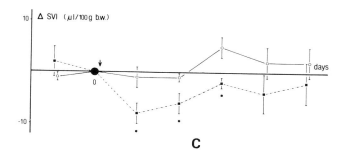

FIGURE 6.   Long-term effects of s.c. continuous osmotic mini-pump infusion of 0.9% NaCl (O--O) and 5 mg/kg/day propranolol (■—·—■) in conscious SHR. Abbreviations: see legend to Figure 5.

delay of several hours in the blood-pressure-lowering effect, primarily as a consequence of the activation of nervous reflex mechanisms. In the rat, the opposing activity of the sinoaortic baroreflex mechanisms disappears within approximately 4 to 6 hr following a bolus injection of propranolol. During continuous, zero-order delivery of propranolol, there is a much more gradual fall in blood pressure over the course of 1

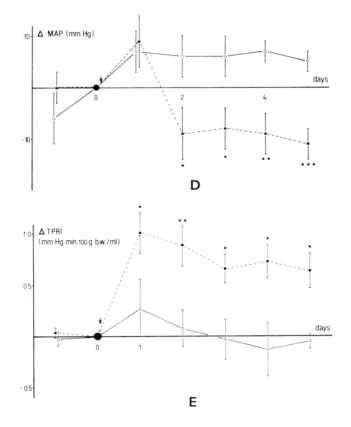

FIGURE 6 continued

to 2 days, even though the plasma half-life of propranolol in the rat is 50 to 70 min and a steady-state plasma level is reached within 1 day. The data by Smits et al.[2] suggest that baroreflex adaptation occurs much more slowly during continuous propranolol administration than during a bolus delivery of one dose. The possible mechanisms underlying this rate-sensitive form of reflex control have not yet been investigated.

The propranolol studies in the SHR illustrate another important point. The antihypertensive activity of beta-blockers was discovered by coincidence in careful clinical studies.[41] The traditional animal screening techniques in pharmaceutical companies did not reveal an antihypertensive effect of beta-blockers. In fact, it was a long-held belief that beta-blockers do not have antihypertensive activity whatsoever in many experimental models of hypertension. However, the traditional screening methods only observe acute hypotensive activity. The studies by Smits et al.[2] show that the most important blood-pressure-lowering effect occurs much later, at a moment when most propranolol has been cleared from plasma and other tissues.

Similar time-dependent actions may be anticipated for other antihypertensives as well. Figures 7 to 9 show the influence of the rate of administration of a vasodilator on important hemodynamic variables in the SHR as a function of time. The drug used was endralazine, a hydralazine-like classical vasodilator.[5,42] The bolus administration (Figure 7) of this drug causes a large fall in mean arterial pressure and total peripheral resistance, similar to the effects of hydralazine. Heart rate and cardiac output increase, due to the baroflex activation of sympathetic nerve activity.[5] If endralazine is infused at constant rates over a 6-day period, using osmotic minipumps, its antihypertensive

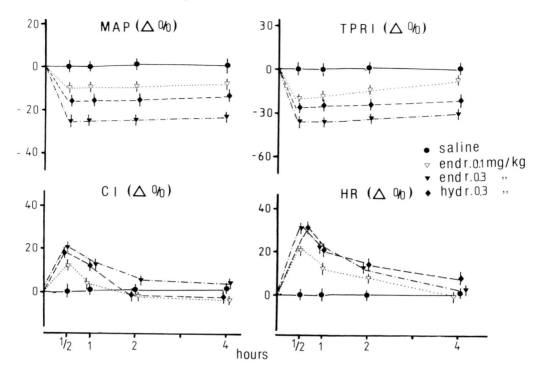

FIGURE 7.   Acute effects of intra-arterial bolus injections of 0.9% NaCl, 0.1 and 0.3 mg/kg endralazine and 0.3 mg/kg hydralazine in conscious SHR. Abbreviations: see legend to Figure 5.

effect gradually decreases somewhat (Figure 8). The early fall in blood pressure and peripheral resistance trigger a baroreflex-mediated increase in sympathetic activity. This leads to an initial rise in heart rate and cardiac output and also to a gradual renal retention of sodium and fluid (cf. Figure 1). These mechanisms compensate for the original effects of endralazine. However, a different effect is obtained if endralazine is administered at gradually increasing rates. Figure 9 shows what happens if the drug is given at stepwise increasing rates with 2-day intervals to increase the rate of adminis-tration. During the first 2 days, a subactive rate was administered. Thereafter, blood pressure gradually decreased, this time without a concurrent baroreflex-mediated rise in cardiac output and heart rate. Apparently, the gradual rise in endralazine delivery rates and parallel gradual fall in blood pressure is a less effective stimulus for barore-flex activation than administration of the full antihypertensive dose at once. We do not yet know the physiological mechanisms underlying this complex drug action, but the clinical implications are obvious. Clinical studies have indicated that some of the severe side effects of vasodilators, such as prazosin, during the early phases of their administration are related to reflex mechanisms triggered by the acute reduction in blood pressure. It is now generally accepted that the dose of prazosin should be in-creased gradually during the first week(s) of therapy.[43] Similar considerations may be true for other vasodilators.

McNay[44] analyzed the time course of the blood pressure lowering effect of different vasodilators in man as a function of the dose administered. Neither the moment of maximal effect nor the time course of return to baseline correlated with corresponding kinetic profiles of the drugs in plasma. In fact, McNay[44] suggested that intensity and time course of the blood pressure lowering effect was inversely related to the sensitivity of the baroreceptor reflex. Brubak and Bathan[45] came to a similar conclusion in a

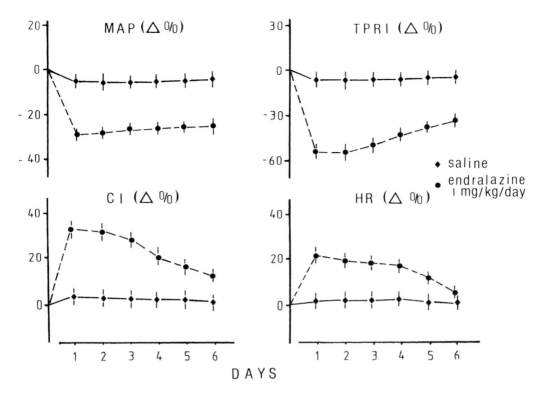

FIGURE 8. Long-term effects of i.v. continuous osmotic minipump infusion of 0.9% NaCl and 1 mg/kg/day endralazine in conscious SHR. Abbreviations: see legend to Figure 5.

clinical study to investigate the hemodynamic actions of the vasodilator diazoxide in hypertensive patients. By use of a simulation model, these authors showed that the compliance of the aorta is the main factor determining baroreflex sensitivity, and thus the time course and size of the antihypertensive action of diazoxide.[45]

B. Dosing Schedules of Antihypertensive Drugs

The above-discussed lack of relationship between the pharmacokinetic behavior of antihypertensives and their time course of action, has important implications for the design of dosage regimens. Pharmacokinetic variables may be of little value in the design of such regiments.[44] Clinical studies have confirmed this conclusion. Thus, whereas the plasma half-life of propranolol is only 3 to 5 hr, twice and even once daily administration of this drug may already provide adequate blood pressure control.[46,47] Similar observations were made for hydralazine and other vasodilators.[48] These observations throw some doubt on the value of some recently introduced "long-acting" slow-release delivery forms of antihypertensive drugs. Although the pharmacokinetic behavior of the drug contained in these release forms can be changed, the consequences thereof may be very little for the therapeutic efficacy. Probably the main advantage is related to a reduction in the amount and size of the side effects.

C. Rebound Phenomena after Withdrawal of Antihypertensive Drugs

The sudden withdrawal of antihypertensive drugs that were previously given on a continuous basis often leads to rebound phenomena. In a series of studies, Thoolen et al.[49-51] showed that acutely stopping continuous minipump infusions of clonidine and

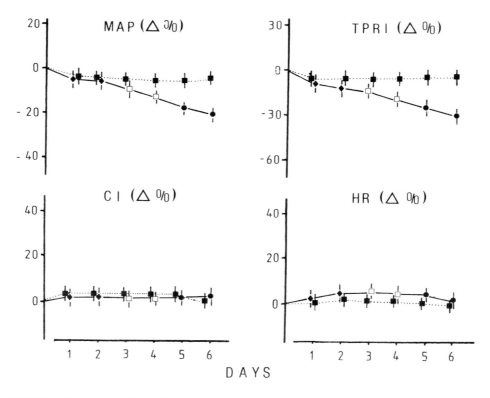

FIGURE 9.   Long-term effects of i.v. osmotic minipump infusion of 0.9% NaCl and increasing rates of endralazine in conscious SHR. Endralazine was infused at a rate of 0.1 mg/kg/day during the first two days (◆—◆) 0.3 mg/kg during days 3 and 4 (□—□) and 1 mg/kg/day during days 5 and 6 (●-●). Abbreviations: see legend to figure 5. Note the absence of reflex increases in cardiac index and heart rate during this infusion protocol.

related centrally acting antihypertensives leads to a hyperactivity of the sympathetic nervous system, a tachycardia and irregular patterns of large increases of blood pressure. The blood pressure pattern is similar to that observed during chronic continuous intravenous noradrenaline infusion.[52] Thoolen et al.[51] furthermore showed that intraperitoneal administration of the alpha$_2$-adrenoceptor blocker yohimbine on the 12th day of clonidine infusion can precipitate the withdrawal syndrome. This effect was not observed if yohimbine was injected before the 5th day of infusion, again showing a time factor in the development of this cardiovascular drug response pattern.

An important phenomenon — possibly involved in some of the rebound effects — occurring during the continuous presence of many drugs or hormones is the regulation of receptor populations. There is abundant evidence now for increasing ("up-regulation") or decreasing receptor populations ("down-regulation") during long-term continuous exposure to different receptor antagonists and agonists, respectively. Long-term continuous exposure to the beta-blocker propranolol is associated with an increased number of beta-adrenoreceptors in, amongst others, lymphocytes, heart, and lungs.[53] The possible influence of receptor up- or down-regulation during long-term exposure to different rate-controlled schedules of antihypertensive drugs has not yet been thoroughly investigated.

D. Rate-Controlled Administration and the Site of Antihypertensive Drug Action

Antihypertensive drugs can act at a number of sites in the body, including the brain, the heart, vascular smooth muscle, the sympathetic nervous system, or the kidneys. Sometimes the major site of antihypertensive action is obvious from the molecular mechanisms of action. Thus, a renal site of action of some diuretics can be concluded on the basis of their effects on sodium transport mechanisms. An interference with vascular smooth muscle contraction seems likely as a primary site of antihypertensive action of vasodilators. However, for the majority of antihypertensives, it is not possible to draw such conclusions. Traditionally, the site and subsequent mechanism of antihypertensive action is deduced indirectly from in vitro observations or from the in vivo hemodynamic profile of activity of the antihypertensive. A more direct approach is the application of the drug at or near its sites of supposed antihypertensive activity. An example is the direct application of presumed centrally acting antihypertensives into the arterial blood supply of the brain, the cerebral ventricles or the direct microperfusion of brain tissue.[54] Elsewhere in this volume, Smits and Thijssen reviewed the limitations of bolus or short-term administration of drugs via such routes as a method to draw conclusions on their potential sites of actions. They also discussed the advantages and limitations of long-term rate-controlled administration of drugs into the arterial bloodstream of the organ of assumed primary activity.

The literature now contains several examples of application of long-term rate-controlled localized administration to conclude on the sites of antihypertensive drug action. The first example is the study of the presumed central nervous system site of action of propranolol. Smits et al.[55] performed a series of studies to discriminate between central and peripheral sites of action of propranolol in conscious, unrestrained SHR. A 5-day intracerebroventricular infusion only caused an antihypertensive effect at rates of delivery comparable to rates active upon subcutaneous infusion. In the case of intracerebroventricular infusions, brain concentrations in steady state were obtained that were 100- to 600-fold higher than those achieved during subcutaneous infusions at equal rates, whereas the plasma concentrations were approximately the same. When intracerebroventricular infusion rates were reduced so as to produce brain concentrations comparable to those during subcutaneous infusion, the antihypertensive effect disappeared. Smits et al.[55] concluded from these studies that the view of a central site of action of propranolol can no longer be supported. Using a similar approach, we were able to show that the long-term antihypertensive action of clonidine in SHR is, in contrast to that of propranolol, caused by a central nervous system effect.[56,57] When comparing rate of infusion-response curves, the intracerebroventricular curve is shifted to the left compared to the subcutaneous curve by a factor of 10 to 30 (Figure 10).

Kleinjans et al.[58] used rate-controlled infusions of noradrenaline into the arterial blood supply of the kidneys of normotensive rats to investigate the hypothesis that a localized renal vasoconstriction can cause a long-term increase in blood pressure. They infused different rates of noradrenaline into a cannula placed in the suprarenal artery with its tip at the bifurcation with the renal artery to avoid obstruction of renal blood flow.[59] The data indicate that intrarenal noradrenaline infusion causes chronic hypertension at much lower rates of administration than intravenous infusion (Figure 11). Moreover, the chronic form of hypertension caused by intrarenal noradrenaline infusion is characterized by an elevated total peripheral resistance, the size of which depends upon the rate of infusion.[58] This approach allows further unraveling of nephrogenic mechanisms involved in the pathogenesis and treatment of hypertension. There is already preliminary evidence that selective vasodilatation of the kidneys is a novel antihypertensive mechanism of action of certain drugs.[60]

E. Rate-Controlled Antihypertensive Drug Preparations for Clinical Use

In the last years, a number of new delivery forms have been designed to optimize the administration of antihypertensive drugs. One class is the "long-acting" or "slow-

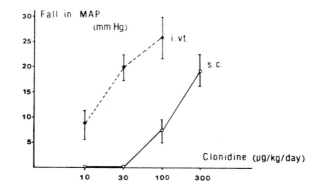

FIGURE 10.   Fall in mean arterial pressure (MAP) induced during 5-day continuous osmotic minipump infusion of different rates of clonidine by the subcutaneous (s.c.) or intracerebroventricular (i.vt.) route in conscious SHR.

release" forms of many agents, including beta-blockers, vasodilators, and centrally acting antihypertensives. These delivery forms do not provide a rate-controlled delivery in a strict sense (cf. Chapter 1 and Chapter 2). There is good evidence for a different kinetic profile of the drugs contained in these delivery forms when compared to classical delivery systems. However, as was argued before, the lack of correlation between the pharmacokinetic behavior and the antihypertensive effect implies that the "long-acting" forms do not necessarily provide an advantage with respect to the therapeutic actions. The main advantage of the "slow-release" forms may be enhanced patient compliance and a reduced incidence of side effects. However, systematic studies showing such effects are not yet available.

A more controlled form of release is obtained by the OROS (oral osmotic therapeutic system). These systems have the appearance of a normal tablet. However, the system employs osmotic pressure obtained by body fluid uptake through a rate-controlling semipermeable membrane as a source of energy for the controlled release of the drug. Recently, OROS-release forms of the antihypertensive beta-blockers metoprolol and oxprenolol were introduced. These beta-blockers have a relatively short plasma half-life. Studies with the OROS forms have shown a near constant plasma level throughout the period of treatment.[61]

Another recent rate-controlled antihypertensive delivery system is the clonidine transdermal therapeutic system (Clonidine TTS). In a TTS, an adhesive drug-containing film delivers a drug to the surface of the skin, e.g., behind the ear or on the upper arm, at a preprogrammed rate. The rate of delivery is determined by the membrane between the drug reservoir and the adhesive (cf. Chapter 2). This device allows the maintenance of a steady-state blood level for a prolonged period of time. The pharmacokinetics and pharmacodynamics of clonidine TTS was recently compared with standard clonidine tablets as well as a slow-release form of clonidine.[62] This study indicated that a once weekly application of clonidine TTS delivering approximately 0.2 mg/day was comparable to multiple oral doses of clonidine tablets 0.15 mg b.i.d., or clonidine slow-release 0.2 mg once daily. The daily fluctuations in drug plasma concentrations were minimized during clonidine TTS application, whereas the intensity of the side effects was reduced when compared to oral administration of clonidine. Arndts and Arndts[62] conclude from their study that "the side effects produced by clonidine are correlated more with the rate of increase than with the absolute plasma concentra-

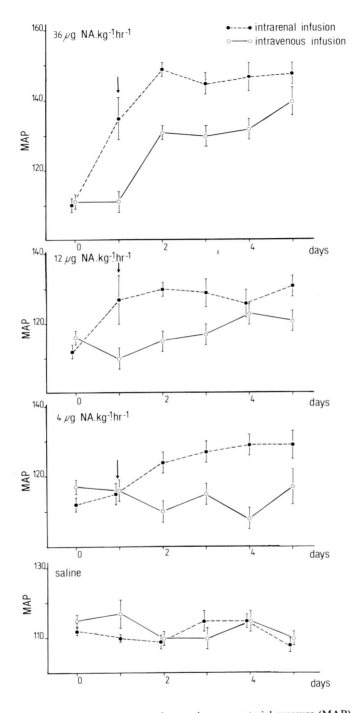

FIGURE 11. Long-term changes in mean arterial pressure (MAP) induced by a 5-day continuous osmotic minipump infusion of 0.9% NaCl and 4, 12 and 36 μg/kg/day noradrenaline by the intravenous and intrarenal route in conscious normotensive rats. The arrows indicate the moments from which on the difference in effects following the two infusion routes was significantly different upon analysis of variance for the whole curves.

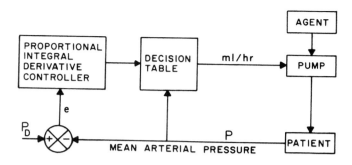

FIGURE 12.   Schematic block diagram of the control loop used in the computer controlled infusion of vasodilators in patients. (With permission from *Ann. Biomed. Eng.,* Vol. 8, Sheppard, L. C., Computer control of the infusion of vasoactive drugs, Copyright 1980, Pergamon Press, Ltd.).

tion of the drug". Future placebo-controlled, double-blind cross-over clinical trials in larger groups of patients should confirm this interesting observation.

F. Computer-Controlled Vasodilator Infusion

One of the oldest forms of rate-controlled drug administration is the intravenous infusion of vasodilators, e.g., sodium nitroprusside or diazoxide, in patients with a hypertensive emergency. Especially sodium nitroprusside is often used in these cases, since its effect has a rapid onset and is reversed within a few minutes of stopping the infusion. The rate of infusion is usually determined by the hypotensive response. During prolonged infusion, signs of cyanide intoxication may occur. This toxicity is related to the rate of infusion rather than to the total amount infused.[63]

Recently, several attempts have been made to develop computer-controlled vasodilator infusion systems for optimal control of blood pressure.[64-66] One of these systems is the IMED digitally controlled infusion pump interfaced with a proportional-integrative-derivative (PID) controller algorithm[64] (see Figure 12). In this sytem, the infusion rates are revised at 1-min intervals by computing the incremental increase or decrease in blood pressure proportional to the corrective action derived by the PID controller algorithm. In a study of more than 1100 patients, it was shown that computer control exhibits approximately half the variation observed during manual control.[67] Other automated drug administration systems to regulate the mean blood pressure have been described for experimental animals as well as humans (cf. the review by Jelliffe[68]). These closed-loop drug administration systems with microprocessor-based control may represent early examples for future trends of automated drug delivery systems.

V. DRUGS USED IN THE TREATMENT OF CARDIAC FAILURE

A. Pathophysiology and Drug Treatment of Cardiac Failure

Cardiac failure is a situation in which a defect in the heart reduces the ability of the heart to pump blood. A number of causes can lead to this reduced ability, e.g., a diminished blood supply through the coronary arteries, damage to the heart valves, cardiac muscle disease, or a long-term elevation of arterial blood pressure. The most common clinical cause of heart failure is a diminished coronary blood flow.

The acute effect of a moderate cardiac failure is a reduction of cardiac output and an increased blood content in the venous system. This leads to a baroreflex activation, causing a rise in sympathetic nerve activity. The increased activity of the sympathetic nervous system has a positive inotropic (and chronotropic) effect, whereas it also leads to an increased venous return of blood to the heart because of the rise in venous tone. Over a prolonged period of time, the kidneys retain fluid as a consequence of the elevated sympathetic activity, a decreased glomerular filtration rate and an increase in the activity of the renin-angiotensin-aldosterone system. Ultimately, the originally reduced cardiac output in cardiac failure is compensated for by the renal retention of fluid.

In situations of a more severely damaged heart, the sympathetic hyperactivity and renal fluid retention can no longer compensate for the original reduction of cardiac output. In the case of a decompensated failure, a patient will progressively retain more and more fluid. The condition of the myocardium itself will deteriorate in this case due to decreased blood supply to the heart and the edema buildup in heart muscle (cf. Guyton[69]).

The pharmacological treatment of cardiac failure is based upon the following principles: (1) increasing the contractility of the myocardium by administration of digitalis-like agents or other positive inotropic drugs; (2) reducing the extracellular fluid content of the body by administration of diuretics; (3) decreasing the preload and especially the afterload (the arteriolar vascular resistance) of the heart by administration of vasodilators. From the foregoing discussion it is clear that the responses to each of these groups of drugs depend on the dynamics of the cardiovascular control mechanisms. Thus far, relatively little attention has been given to the dynamics of drug action in cardiac failure. *A fortiori*, little is known about the influence of different schedules of administration of these drugs on their therapeutic responses. Clinically, the influence of different schedules of administration of cardiac glycosides has been studied mainly from a pharmacokinetic point of view. Only recently, some interesting observations were made on the hemodynamic effects of different schedules of administration of the positive inotropic drug dobutamine.

B. Schedules of Digitalis Administration

The small therapeutic index of cardiac glycosides necessitates careful control of the schedule of administration of these agents. Several decades ago, Gold[70] developed the concept of two types of doses of digitalis. The first, the digitalizing (or loading) dose, represents the dose schedule needed for rapid recovery from cardiac failure; the second, the maintenance dose, maintains a properly functioning myocardium. More recently, with the development of assays for digitalis-type glycosides, refined schedules of administration were proposed. Jelliffe[68,71,72] even developed computer programs for designing loading and maintenance dosage regimens for the cardiac glycosides, adjusted to patient variables such as body weight and renal function. The use of these programs has assisted in reducing the incidence of digitalis toxicity.[72] More recent versions of this computer program also include a quantitative description of the competition between digitalis and potassium, allowing an estimation of the quantitative contribution of each factor to the risk of cardiac arrhythmias.[68] Another new development is the employment of two-compartment pharmacokinetic models in which the therapeutic effect resides in a peripheral compartment. With these programs, loading and maintenance regimens can be designed to achieve optimal concentrations in the peripheral compartment.[68]

All these models presume a linear and time-independent relationship between the concentration of the glycoside in plasma or the peripheral compartment and its hemodynamic effects. There are no systematic studies to support or deny this concept, although a recent preliminary study contains some evidence that signs of adequate cardiac function are maintained far beyond the time of presence of glycosides in plasma.[73] Also, the old pre-digoxin protocol of treating cardiac failure with intermittent intra-

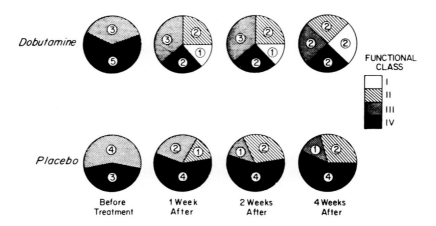

FIGURE 13.   Percentage of patients falling into New York Heart Association functional classes I to IV before and at different times after 72 hr infusion of either dobutamine or dextrose (placebo). The absolute number of patients in each class is indicated by a circled numeral. (From Liang, C. S. et al., *Circulation,* 69, 113, 1984. By permission of the American Heart Association, Inc.)

venous strophantin, contains some evidence for effects beyond the time of presence of the glycoside. However, these protocols have not been the study of systematic investigation. Clearly, further pharmacodynamic studies are needed to elaborate these observations.

C. Rate-Controlled Administration and Action of Dobutamine

Dobutamine is a synthetic sympathomimetic amine capable of increasing cardiac contractility at rates of administration that have little or no effect on heart rate.[74] It has a predominant effect on cardiac beta$_1$-adrenoceptors. Chemically, dobutamine is a racemic mixture of a (+) and (−) isomer. Ruffolo et al.[75] recently showed that the racemate and the (−) isomer are potent partial agonists at alpha-adrenoceptors, whereas the (+) isomer lacks alpha-agonist activity, but is a potent competitive alpha-blocker. Both stereoisomers are agonists at beta-adrenoceptors, the (+) isomer being the most potent agonist in this respect.

Continuous short-term infusion of dobutamine in man causes a sustained improvement of cardiac function, measured as left ventricular ejection fraction and cardiac index, in the failing heart 30 min after termination of the infusion. These improved parameters of left ventricular function in patients with chronic congestive cardiomyopathy were sustained for several months after infusion of dobutamine.[76] This original observation was recently confirmed in two independent studies.[77,78] In one study, 15 patients with congestive cardiomyopathy were either infused with 5% dextrose in water (n = 7) or with dobutamine (15 to 35 μg/kg/min, n = 8) for 3 days.[77] Cardiac function was measured 1, 2, and 4 weeks after stopping the infusion. Both functional class (New York Heart Association classification of the degree of cardiac failure) and cardiac function variables were significantly better after 4 weeks in the dobutamine group (Figure 13).[77] The second study was performed in 23 patients with congestive cardiomyopathy.[78] All patients received a 3-day infusion of an average dose of 11.1 ± 3.4 μg/kg/min (mean ± S.D.), whereas no control group was included in this study. All patients experienced subjective (functional class) and objective (cardiac hemodynamics) improvements during the dobutamine infusion. After stopping the infusion, the condition of an increasing number of patients gradually deteriorated. However, even after

2 months, 11 patients still had a better condition than before the dobutamine infusion.[78]

The mechanisms underlying this important clinical observation are still unknown. Dobutamine does not only lead to an improved hemodynamic condition, but also corrects the metabolic abnormalities including hyponatremia and azotemia.[78] The improved performance is associated with decreased swelling of subendocardial mitochondria. The improvements are consistent with long-term increased subendocardial blood flow. Additional studies are needed to investigate the mechanism underlying this fascinating phenomenon. Such studies should include rate-controlled administration of individual stereoisomers of dobutamine as well as other positive inotropic agents.

D. Drug Synergism in the Treatment of Cardiac Failure

The chronic treatment of cardiac failure often implies the combined use of drugs with different mechanisms of action, e.g., positive inotropic, diuretic, and vasodilator agents. The schedules of combination of these agents are still largely empirical. Several authors have recently attempted to quantitatively study the synergism obtained by using rate-controlled administration of drugs with different mechanisms of action.[79,80] Awan et al.[79] compared the effects of intravenous nitroglycerin (average 267 μg/min) and dobutamine (average 7.7 μg/min) infusion as well as the combined administration of these agents to patients with left ventricular failure after acute myocardial infarction. Nitroglycerin achieved lowering of the abnormally elevated left ventricular filling pressure, whereas dobutamine augmented left ventricular pump function. The combined infusion of the two agents was very effective in decreasing preload and enhancing pump performance.[79] In a similar study Loeb et al.[80] showed the beneficial effects of intravenous infusions of dopamine (4.5 $\pm$ 0.3 μg/kg/min) combined with nitroglycerin (3.2 $\pm$ 0.3 μg/kg/min) in patients with severe left ventricular failure. This synergism is specially interesting in view of the possibility to reduce the rate of dopamine administration. There is evidence now that with increasing rates of administration of dopamine its alpha-adrenoceptor stimulating properties will dominate, leading to peripheral vasoconstriction and limiting the usefulness of the drug as an inotropic.[80,81]

VI. ANTIARRHYTHMIC DRUGS

Many drugs used in the treatment of cardiac arrhythmias have narrow therapeutic index and variable pharmacokinetics. In recent years, great emphasis has been put on the design of dosage schedules to maintain optimal kinetics throughout the treatment period. In general, this has stimulated the design of regimens or delivery systems for maintaining a near constant plasma level. A first approach has been the development of a number of long-acting delivery forms, mostly based upon sustained-release principles. There are now such delivery forms for many antiarrhythmics, including quinidine, disopyramide, verapamil, bepridil, and mexiletine. However, these delivery forms do not provide a true rate-controlled form of delivery and some represent only small biopharmaceutical differences relative to the conventional form.

Much recent research has been published on intravenous rate-controlled administration of the antiarrhythmic lidocaine. This agent is the first line drug for the hospital management of ventricular arrhythmias following an acute myocardial infarction, and it is the only drug which has been shown to reduce the incidence of primary ventricular fibrillation when given prophylactically.[82] Since lidocaine has a limited bioavailability upon oral administration and a relatively short elimination half-life, it is usually given by the intravenous route. Arrhythmia control without toxicity usually occurs at plasma concentrations between 1.5 and 5.5 mg/ℓ.[82] Such levels can be obtained by infusing lidocaine at a constant rate. However, in view of the half-life of 1 to 2 hr it would take several hours before this level is obtained. On the other hand, in the past, the major lidocaine toxicity was due to the rapid intravenous infusion of loading doses.[83] A number of authors have recently described alternative regimens based upon either serial bolus injections or rapid short-term infusions of low doses of lidocaine.[83-86] Riddell et al.[84] have recently reviewed the different schedules of rate-controlled lidocaine administration.

Collins and Arzbaecher[87] have described an automated control system for cardiac arrhythmias in experimental animals. This system is based upon the detection of ventricular premature beats which triggers a computer-controlled release of lidocaine. Lidocaine is infused on a rate-controlled basis using a two-compartment model to describe its pharmacokinetic behavior. In the meantime, algorithms have been developed for other antiarrhythmics as well.[68] Recently, these computer programs were used for rate-controlled delivery of lidocaine to patients who had suffered from a myocardial infarct.[68] These programs are still used in an open-loop manner, i.e., the arrhythmias as such are not used to alter the rate of lidocaine release. However, if future technological developments allow accurate measurement of arrhythmias, the development of closed-loop computer controlled delivery of antiarrhythmics can be anticipated.

Anderson et al.[88] have described the use of a totally implanted drug delivery system for long-term administration of the antiarrhythymics procainamide and bretylium in dogs. They used the Infusaid®, model 100, vapor-pressure powered pump which has also been used for the administration of insulin, heparin, and cytostatics (see elsewhere in this volume). Delivery of lidocaine was limited by the high viscosity of this drug and the corrosion of steel elements within the pump.[88] The use of this implantable drug delivery system in patients needing antiarrhythmics remains to be established.

Studies on the electrophysiological effects of antiarrhythmic agents have thus far concentrated on the steady-state effects of these agents. It is generally assumed that there is a close correlation between plasma levels and electrophysiological effects. However, Nattel and Bailey[89] recently provided evidence that upon start or discontinuation of antiarrhythmic drug administration the electrophysiological effects are sensitive to the rate of change of drug concentration. They showed that both the onset and washout of the effects of quinidine, disopyramide, and lidocaine in the isolated dog heart are independent of absolute drug concentration.[89] Although the mechanisms determining the rate of antiarrhythmic drug action are not yet known, this observation may have important clinical implications. The treatment of episodic cardiac arrhythmias is based upon steady-state maintenance therapy. This creates problems of patient compliance and increased risks of adverse side effects. Already there is some evidence that intermittent antiarrhythmic drug therapy in which the medication is only taken at the onset of an episode of arrhythmia, may be of clinical use.[90] More studies, using different rate-controlled schedules of antiarrhythmic drug administration should be performed to investigate this possibility further.

VII. ANTIANGINAL DRUGS

A. Pathophysiology and Treatment of Angina Pectoris

Angina pectoris occurs if there is a discrepancy between the oxygen demand and the oxygen supply of the myocardium. The most frequent cause of angina pectoris is atherosclerosis of coronary vessels. Other causes include spasms of the coronary vasculature or obstructions due to thrombocyte aggregation.

The treatment of angina pectoris is based upon a number of nonpharmacological and pharmacological approaches. The nonpharmacological approaches include coronary by-pass surgery, angioplasty, and electrical carotid sinus nerve stimulation. The most important groups of drugs used in the treatment of angina pectoris are nitroglycerin and related nitrates, beta-adrenoceptor blocking drugs, and calcium entry-blockers. The beneficial effects of these agents are based upon their hemodynamic effects. Nitrates dilate both arteriolar and venous blood vessels, including the coronary vasculature. Their primary effect in angina pectoris is the reduction of oxygen need of the myocardium, since both preload and afterload are reduced. The increased blood (and oyxgen) supply to the heart following dilatation of the coronary vessels may also contribute to their therapeutic effect. Beta-blockers reduce cardiac output and systemic blood pressure, thereby reducing the oxygen need of the myocardium. Moreover, they block the cardiac effects of sympathetic stimulation during conditions of stress. The beneficial effects of calcium entry blockers in angina pectoris have not yet been fully investigated. Some of these agents (e.g., verapamil) act predominantly on the myocardium to reduce oxygen demand, whereas others (e.g., nifedipine) strongly reduce peripheral vascular resistance. Some of the newer calcium entry blockers may have an additional dilatory effect on the coronary blood vessels.

The drug treatment of angina pectoris is largely based upon empirical observations on the clinical conditions of patients. With the exception of some new delivery forms of the nitrates the drugs are given sublingually or orally with dosing schedules based upon either the clinical need (subjective complaints of angina pectoris) or pharmacokinetic considerations. Recently, a number of long-acting, slow-release forms of several antianginal drugs have been developed for alternative dosing schedules. Although these delivery forms may provide a more optimal pharmacokinetic pattern of the antianginal drugs, it is not yet clear whether the therapeutic response is controlled better. Thus far, only some of the newer nitroglycerin delivery forms have been studied from a point of view of temporal control of their hemodynamic effects.

B. Pharmacokinetic-Hemodynamic Studies of Nitroglycerin

A number of authors have recently studied the relationship between different rates of intravenous nitroglycerin administration and the hemodynamic effect.[91-94] Sorkin et al.[95] have reviewed a number of these studies. Due to its extremely short elimination half-life in plasma of 1 to 3 min, nitroglycerin rapidly reaches steady-state concentrations upon intravenous infusion. It has been difficult to correlate the infusion rate with steady-state plasma concentrations due to large interindividual variation in the pharmacokinetic behavior of nitroglycerin and difficulties in the assay procedure.[95] There is also little correlation between plasma concentration and hemodynamic response. Imhof et al.[92] showed that the decrease in blood pressure induced by nitroglycerin was still present 15 min after the end of the infusion, when no drug was detectable in plasma. The hemodynamic effects appeared related to rates of infusion rather than absolute plasma concentration.[95] At low rates of nitroglycerin administration, venodilatation dominates whereas higher infusion rates dilate both arterial and venous blood vessels.[96] The decreases in mean arterial blood pressure are correlated with the infusion rate of nitroglycerin. At the higher rates of infusion, a reflex tachycardia is sometimes observed in normal subjects, but not in patients with heart failure. The lack of reflex tachycardia has been suggested to result from the gradual lowering, rather than a precipitous decrease, in blood pressure.[97] Most studies on the effects of intravenous nitroglycerin infusions on coronary blood flow and oxygen consumption have been performed in the dog. It was generally noted that nitroglycerin causes a redistribution of myocardial flow in favor of blood delivery to the subendocardium.[98] In man, Sethna et al.[99] found that total coronary blood flow remains unchanged at rates which significantly decreased preload and afterload. No firm conclusion can be drawn yet on the myocardial oxygen supply during nitroglycerin infusion.

Intravenous nitroglycerin infusions are not only used for the treatment of pain attacks during unstable angina pectoris. Recently, several studies have suggested a limitation of cardiac ischemia following intravenous nitroglycerin infusion in acute myocardial infarction.[95,100,101] Preliminary studies indicate a possibly favorable effect on early and late mortality.[101]

A recent approach to the early treatment of myocardial infarction has been the local infusion of vasodilators (e.g., nitroglycerin) or thrombolytic (e.g., streptokinase) agents into the coronary artery. The relatively low blood flow through the coronary arteries favors a localized action of these drugs in the coronary circulation. However, other factors — tissue binding, systemic clearance — also determine the gain to be obtained by intra-arterial infusion (cf. Chapter 4). Thus far, only limited attempts have been made to compare the intracoronary and intravenous or sublingual routes of administration.[102] An interesting agent to include in such studies would be prostacyclin, in view of its high clearance, its potent vasodilating properties, and its favorable effects on platelet aggregation.

C. Rate-Controlled Antianginal Drug Preparations for Clinical Use

We previously mentioned the development of a number of slow-release forms of beta-blockers, nitrates, and calcium entry-blockers. True rate-controlled delivery systems for antianginal drugs have been designed for nitroglycerin. A number of intravenous infusion preparations have been developed, including Nitroglycerin IV (Abbott), Tridil® (American Critical Care), Nitro-Bid® (Marion Laboratories) and Nitrostat-IV® (Parke Davis). These intravenous delivery systems allow careful titration of the nitroglycerin dose on the basis of the observed hemodynamic effects of the drug.[95]

Recently, several transdermal delivery systems were developed for the controlled release of nitroglycerin (Nitro-Disc®, Searle and Nitro-Dur®, Key Pharmaceuticals). A true rate-controlled transdermal delivery of nitroglycerin is only obtained with the nitroglycerin transdermal therapeutic system (Nitroderm TTS®, Ciba-Geigy/Alza). Recent studies by Chien et al.[103] indicate that nitroglycerin penetrates through the skin at a rate profile which can be described by zero-order kinetics. Moreover, constant plasma nitroglycerin concentrations are reached throughout the period of application of Nitroderm TTS® (cf. Figure 14). The plasma concentration is directly proportional to the contact surface. The cutaneous tolerability of this system is good.[104,105]

Another new release form of nitroglycerin is the buccal controlled release system.[106-108] Such buccal nitroglycerin systems contain nitroglycerin impregnated into an inert polymer-matrix (Synchron, Forest Laboratories).[108] The tablet is placed in the buccal cavity between the upper lip and teeth. The surface of the tablet quickly develops a gel-like coating which makes the tablet adhere to the mucosal surface of the mouth. The polymer matrix then provides continuous release of nitroglycerin into the buccal cavity so long as some of the tablet remains intact. Nitroglycerin release may continue up to 6 hr.[106,107]

VIII. ANTICOAGULANT DRUGS

Anticoagulant drugs are used in the treatment of several diseases involving abnormal blood coagulation such as thrombophlebitis and pulmonary embolism. Moreover, these agents are widely used following different types of surgery in postmyocardial infarction patients and in the treatment of cerebrovascular disease. The classical anticoagulant is heparin, which can be used by intravenous or subcutaneous routes of administration. It acts promptly and is preferred in acute thromboembolic diseases. Orally active anticoagulants include the vitamin K antagonistic coumarin derivatives warfarin, acenocoumarol, and phenprocoumon. These drugs suppress the synthesis of the vitamin K-dependent clotting factors II (prothrombin), VII, IX, and X.

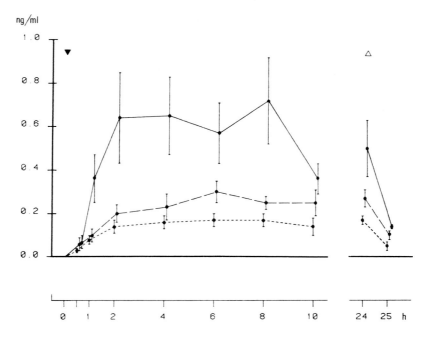

FIGURE 14. Concentration of nitroglycerin in plasma after application of the transdermal therapeutic system for the administration of nitroglycerin. The following systems were each applied to 6 patients: 1 NTG-TTS (●...●), 2 NTG-TTS (●–●) and 4 NTG-TTS(●–●). Δ: removal of the system. (From Müller, P. et al., *Eur. J. Clin. Pharmacol.*, 22, 473, 1982. With permission.)

For systemic anticoagulation with heparin given by s.c. injection regimen, the protocol usually consists of an initial loading dose (e.g., 5000 units by i.v. injection followed by 10,000 to 20,000 units s.c. of a concentrated solution) followed by intermittent injections every 8 or 12 hr. The drug is also given intravenously either by continuous infusions or intermittent (every 4 to 6 hr) injections. The dosage in each case is adjusted according to the patient's coagulation test results. Such tests are performed frequently, thus allowing a very precise control of the rate of administration of heparin. Recently, implantable refillable pumps have been studied for heparin infusion in patients with severe thromboembolic disease refractory to treatment with oral anticoagulants.[109-111] Some patients received continuous heparin infusions for longer than 3 years. Because heparin can be administered in concentrated format low pump flow rates, periods of 70 to 80 days are reached between refills.[109,110]

The use of oral anticoagulants is complicated by wide variations in the individuals' responses to these drugs, with periods of underdosing with increased risks of thrombosis or overdosing with increased risk of hemorrhage. It has been estimated that a patient taking oral anticoagulants is within the therapeutic range of only 55 to 65% of the time.[112] Other authors reported that in large groups of patients treated with oral anticoagulants at any given time only 65 to 70% were within the therapeutic range.[113,114] An early attempt to improve the dosing schedules was made by Routledge et al.[115] These authors found a correlation between the time required to reach a specified level of anticoagulation during the loading phase of an oral anticoagulant with the ultimately required maintenance dose. Another approach to improve the reliability of warfarin therapy is based upon mathematical models describing the time course of the anticoagulant effects of the drugs.[114,116-118] These mathematical models describe the kinetics of plasma concentration of the anticoagulant as well as the time course of its effect on the prothrombin complex activity. It is assumed that the inhibition of the active prothrombin complex synthesis can be described by an enzyme-substrate model and, hence, a Michaelis-Menten type of equation. This suggestion is consistent with the mechanism of action of the vitamin K antagonists. Thus on the basis of repeated measurements of the prothrombin time (i.e., the Quicktest) predictions are made on the dosage schedule to be given. By repeated adjustment of the dose to the measured prothrombin time, an optimized schedule is obtained. These computer-assisted calculations have indeed led to significant increases in the percentage of patients on oral anitcoagulant therapy within the therapeutic range.[114] Although the effectiveness of this approach has been indicated for once daily administration of warfarin (plasma half-life approximately 40 hr), it is not certain that this approach leads to optimal rates of administration of any orally given anticoagulant. The coumarin derivatives inhibit the synthesis of other vitamin K-dependent coagulation factors than prothrombin as well. Thijssen and Hemker[119] recently pointed out that the half-life of plasma disappearance after synthesis inhibition of prothrombin is 70 to 100 hr, whereas that of factor VII is only 4 to 6 hr. This implies a much larger degree of potential fluctuation of plasma concentration of factor VII than of prothrombin during treatment with coumarin derivatives. Factor VII initiates the extrinsic coagulation pathway which plays an important role in thrombus formation, Hence, an optimal control of factor VII concentration in plasma should be an important goal of anticoagulant therapy. With once daily oral administration of coumarin derivatives with a short half-life (e.g., acenocouramol with a half-life of 8 to 10 hr), this control of factor VII may not be optimal.[119] Clearly, other patterns of administration of these agents should be investigated in the light of the complex kinetics of synthesis and degradation of the various coagulation factors. Ultimately, one may envisage the development of closed-loop computer-controlled systems of administration of anticoagulants sensitive to changes in the activity in the different clotting factors in plasma.

IX. CONCLUSIONS

The cardiovascular system operates as a closed hydraulic loop. An optimal function of this system depends upon accurate detection of appropriate signals and properly acting effector mechanisms. Cardiovascular drugs can be regarded as tools to optimize the function of the circulatory system in conditions when it fails. Thus far, these drugs have been used almost exclusively in an open-loop manner: the drugs are administered on the basis of clinical experience of the physician or limited measurements of relevant variables in the patient. When compared to the vast progress made over the last decades in cardiovascular diagnostic technology, this approach to therapy seems rather primitive.

In recent years, some progress has been made in the development of technology to optimize the administration of cardiovascular drugs. However, these attempts were almost exclusively aimed at an improvement of the pharmacokinetic profile of the active ingredient of the drug and to reduce the incidence of its adverse effects. Systematic studies to optimize drug input on the basis of an analysis of the dynamics of cardiovascular drug action are still lacking. Some of the recent clinical studies with dobutamine and several of the animal studies discussed in this chapter represent early examples of such an approach to pharmacodynamics. It is highly interesting to note that these studies indicate that a constant, zero-order administration of a drug — an ideal for many drug designers with a predominant pharmacokinetic perspective — is not always the most optimal solution from pharmacodynamic point of view. The new delivery systems providing rate-controlled drug release are important tools for further investigation of optimal design of drug input functions.

Optimal cardiovascular control on the basis of drug therapy may in the future be based upon the use of closed-loop systems. An early form of closed-loop cardiovascular control for therapeutic purposes is the intra-aortic balloon counterpulsation.[120-122] This system assists a seriously failing heart in patients suffering from cardiogenic shock who are refractory to drug therapy. A balloon is placed in the aorta and assistance to ventricular ejection is obtained by reducing aortic pressure. An appropriate amount of balloon inflation and deflation and proper timing of synchronization with respect to cardiac cycle are essential for effective assistance.

Another example of closed-loop cardiovascular control is the computer-aided vasodilator therapy, In this case, the rate of administration of a vasodilator is determined by the blood pressure level. Further knowledge of the dynamic behavior of the circulatory system and the effects exerted by cardiovascular drugs may lead to other more refined forms of therapy.

REFERENCES

1. Smits, J. F. M., VanEssen, H., and Struyker-Boudier, H. A. J., Propranolol in conscious spontaneously hypertensive rats. I. Cardiovascular effects after subcutaneous and intracerebroventricular administration, *Naunyn Schmiedebergs Arch. Pharmacol.*, 309, 13, 1979.
2. Smits, J. F. M., Coleman, T. G., Smith, T. L., Kasbergen, C. M., VanEssen, H., and Struyker-Boudier, H. A. J., Antihypertensive effect of propranolol in conscious SHR; central hemodynamics, plasma volume, and renal function during beta-blockade, *J. Cardiovasc. Pharmacol.*, 4, 903, 1982.
3. Urquhart, J., Fara, J. W., and Willis, K. L., Rate-controlled delivery systems in drug and hormone research, *Ann. Rev. Pharmacol. Toxicol.*, 24, 199, 1984.
4. Guyton, A. C., *Arterial Pressure and Hypertension*, W. B. Saunders, Philadelphia, 1980.
5. Struyker-Boudier, H. A. J., VanEssen, H., and Smits, J. F. M., Hemodynamic effects of the arteriolar vasodilators hydralazine, dihydralazine and endralazine in the conscious spontaneously hypertensive rat, *Eur. J. Pharmacol.*, 95, 151, 1983.
6. Struyker-Boudier, H. A. J. and Smits, J. F. M., Systemic and regional hemodynamic effects of vasodilators in hypertension, *Neth. J. Med.*, 27, 146, 1984.
7. Struyker-Boudier, H. A. J., Dynamic systems analysis as a basis for drug design: application to antihypertensive drug action, in *Drug Design*, Vol. 10, Adriens, E. J., Ed., Academic Press, New York, 1980, 146.
8. Struyker-Boudier, H. A. J., The interaction of antihypertensive drugs with mechanisms of blood pressure regulation, in *Handbook of Hypertension*, Vol. 3, van Zwieten, P. A., Ed., Elsevier, Amsterdam, 1984, 46.
9. Charlton, J. D. and Baertschi, A. J., Responses of aortic baroreceptors to changes of aortic blood flow and pressure in rat, *Am. J. Physiol.*, 242, H529, 1982.
10. Struyker-Boudier, H. A. J., Smits, J. F. M., and VanEssen, H., The role of the baroreceptor reflex in the cardiovascular effects of propranolol in the conscious spontaneously hypertensive rat, *Clin. Sci.*, 56, 163, 1979.
11. Moss, N. G., Renal function and renal afferent and efferent nerve activity, *Am. J. Physiol.*, 243, F425, 1982.
12. Katholi, R. E., Renal nerves in the pathogenesis of hypertension in experimental animals and humans, *Am. J. Physiol.*, 245, F1, 1983.
13. Smits, J. F. M. and Brody, M. J., Activation of afferent renal nerves by intrarenal bradykinin in conscious rats, *Am. J. Physiol.*, in press, 1984.
14. Katholi, R. E., Naftilan, A. J., and Oparil, S., Importance of renal sympathetic tone in the development of DOCA-salt hypertension in the rat, *Hypertension*, 2, 266, 1980.
15. Katholi, R. E., Whitlow, P. L., Winternitz, S. R., and Oparil, S., Importance of the renal nerves in established two-kidney one-clip Goldblatt hypertension, *Hypertension*, 4 (Suppl. 2), 166, 1982.
16. Ariëns, E. J. and Simonis, A. M., Physiological and pharmacological aspects of adrenergic receptor classification, *Biochem. Pharmacol.*, 32, 1539, 1983.
17. Swales, J. D., Renin-angiotensin system in hypertension, *Pharmacol. Ther.*, 7, 173, 1979.
18. Yun, J. C. H., On the control of renin release, *Nephron*, 23, 72, 1979.

19. McGiff, J., Prostaglandins, prostacyclin, and thromboxanes, *Ann. Rev. Pharmacol. Toxicol.*, 21, 479, 1981.
20. Schachter, M., Kallikreins (kininogenases) — a group of serine proteases with bioregulatory actions, *Pharmacol. Rev.*, 31, 1, 1980.
21. Muirhead, E. E., Byers, L. W., Desiderio, D. M., Brooks, B., and Brosius, W. M., Antihypertensive lipids from the kidney: alkyl ether analogs of phosphatidylcholine, *Fed. Proc. Fed. Am Soc. Exp. Biol.*, 40, 2285, 1981.
22. DeWardener, H. E., Natriuretic hormone, *Clin. Sci. Mol. Med.*, 53, 1, 1977.
23. DeWardener, H. E. and McGregor, G. A., Dahl's hypothesis that a saluretic substance may be responsible for a sustained rise in arterial pressure: its possible role in essential hypertension, *Kidney Int.*, 18, 1, 1980.
24. Thibault, G., Garcia, R., Cantin, M., and Genest, J., Atrial natriuretic factor characterization and partial purification, *Hypertension,* 5 (Suppl. 1), I-75, 1983.
25. Currie, M. G., Geller, D. M., Cole, B. R., Siegel, N. R., Fox, K. F., Adams, S. P., Enbanks, S. R., Gallupi, G. R., and Needleman, P., Purification and sequence analysis of bioactive atrial peptides (atriopeptins), *Science,* 223, 67, 1984.
26. Guyton, A. C., Coleman, T. G., and Granger, H. J., Circulation: overall regulation, *Annu. Rev. Physiol.*, 34, 13, 1972.
27. Folkow, B., Cardiovascular structural adaptation: its role in the initiation and maintenance of primary hypertension, *Clin. Sci. Mol. Med.*, 55, 3, 1978.
28. Schwartz, S. M., Cellular proliferation in atherosclerosis and hypertension, *Proc. Soc. Exp. Biol. Med.*, 173, 1, 1983.
29. Ariëns, E. J. and Simonis, A. M., A molecular basis for drug action, *J. Pharm. Pharmacol.*, 27, 137, 1964.
30. Holford, N. H. G. and Sheiner, L. B., Kinetics of pharmacologic response, *Pharmacol. Ther.*, 16, 143, 1982.
31. VanRossum, J. M., *Kinetics of Drug Action,* Springer-Verlag, Berlin, 1977.
32. O'Reilly, R. A., Studies on the optical enantiomorphs of warfarin in man, *Clin. Pharmacol. Ther.*, 16, 348, 1974.
33. Bischoff, K. B., Dedrick, R. L., Zaharko, D. S., and Longstreith, J. A., Methotrexate pharmacokinetics, *J. Pharm. Sci.*, 60, 1128, 1971.
34. Bischoff, K. B., Current applications of physiological pharmacokinetics, *Fed. Proc. Fed. Am. Soc. Exp. Biol.*, 39, 2456, 1980.
35. Smits, J. F. M. and Struyker-Boudier, H. A. J., The mechanism of antihypertensive action of beta-adrenergic receptor blocking drugs, *Clin. Exp. Hypert.*, A4, 71, 1982.
36. Greenway, C. V., Mechanisms and quantitative assessment of drug effects on cardiac output with a new model of the circulation, *Pharmacol. Rev.*, 33, 213, 1982.
37. Yates, F. E., Integrative pharmacology — beyond structure activity relationships into pharmacolinguistics, *Am. J. Physiol.*, 6, R251, 1979.
38. Yates, F. E., Analysis of endocrine signals: the engineering and physics of biochemical communication systems, *Biol. Reprod.*, 24, 73, 1981.
39. VanHooff, M. E. J., Does, R. J. M. M., Rahn, K. H., and VanBaak, M. A., Time course of blood pressure changes after intravenous administration of propranolol or furosemide in hypertensive patients, *J. Cardiovasc. Pharmacol.*, 5, 773, 1983.
40. Fagan, T. C., Walle, T., Corns-Hurwitz, R., Conradi, E. C., Privitera, P., Harmon, G., Degenhart, W., and Gaffney, T. E., Time course of development of the antihypertensive effect of propranolol, *Hypertension,* 5, 852, 1983.
41. Prichard, B. N. C., Hypotensive action of pronethalol, *Br. Med. J.*, 1, 1227, 1964.
42. Salzman, R., Burki, H., Chu, D., Clark, B., Marbach, P., Markstein, R., Reinert, H., Siegl, H., and Waite, R., Pharmakologische Wirkungen des Antihypertensivums 6-Benzoyl-3-hydrazino-5,6,7,8-tetrahydropyrido [4,3-C]-pyridazin (BQ 22-708, Endralazine), *Arzneim. Forsch.*, 29, 1843, 1979.
43. Brogden, R. N., Heel, R. C., Speight, T. M., and Avery, G. S., Prazosin: a review of its pharmacological properties and therapeutic efficacy in hypertension, *Drugs,* 14, 163, 1977.
44. MacNay, J. L., Dose response studies with vasodilator antihypertensive drugs, *Clin. Exp. Hypert.*, 4, 61, 1982.
45. Brubakk, A. O. and Bathen, J., Use of a simulation model to study the acute hemodynamic effects of diazoxide in man, *Eur. J. Clin. Pharmacol.*, 15, 73, 1979.
46. VandenBrink, G., Boer, P., VanAsten, P., Dorhout Mees, E. J., and Geyskes, G. G., Once and three doses of propranolol a day in hypertension, *Clin. Pharmacol. Ther.*, 27, 9, 1980.
47. Coelho, J. B., Dvornik, D., Mullane, J. F., Kaufman, J., Simon, J., Krantz, K. D., Lee, T. Y., Perdue, H. A., and Weidler, D., Dynamics of propranolol dosing schedules, *Clin. Pharmacol. Ther.*, 34, 440, 1983.

48. Silas, J. H., Ramsay, L. E., and Freestone, S., Hydralazine once daily in hypertension, *Br. Med. J.,* 284, 1602, 1982.

49. Thoolen, M. J. M. C., Timmermans, P. B. M. W. M., and VanZwieten, P. A., Withdrawal syndrome after continuous infusion of clonidine in the normotensive rat, *J. Pharm. Pharmacol.,* 33, 232, 1981.

50. Thoolen, M. J. M. C., Timmermans, P. B. M. W. M., and VanZwieten, P. A., Discontinuation syndrome after continuous infusion of clonidine in the spontaneously hypertensive rat, *Life Sci.,* 28, 2103, 1981.

51. Thoolen, M. J. M., Timmermans, P. B. M. W. M., and VanZwieten, P. A., Cardiovascular effects of withdrawal of some centrally acting antihypertensive drugs in the rat, *Br. J. Clin. Pharmacol.,* 15, 491S, 1983.

52. Kleinjans, J., Kasbergen, C., Vervoort-Peters, L., Smits, J., and Struyker-Boudier, H. A. J., Chronic intravenous infusion of noradrenaline produces labile hypertension in conscious rats, *Life Sci.,* 29, 509, 1981.

53. Aarons, R. D. and Molinoff, P. B., Changes in the density of beta-adrenergic receptors in rat lymphocytes, heart and lung after chronic treatment with propranolol, *J. Pharmacol. Exp. Ther.,* 221, 439, 1982.

54. VanZwieten, P. A., Antihypertensive drugs with a central action, *Prog. Pharmacol.,* 1, 1, 1975.

55. Smits, J. F. M., VanEssen, H., and Struyker-Boudier, H. A. J., Is the antihypertensive effect of propranolol caused by an action within the central nervous system?, *J. Pharmacol. Exp. Ther.,* 215, 221, 1980.

56. Struyker-Boudier, H. A. J. and VanEssen, H., Chronic infusion of clonidine in the SHR, *Naunyn Schmiedebergs Arch. Pharmacol.,* 311 (Suppl.), R49, 1980.

57. Struyker-Boudier, H. A. J., The osmotic minipump: applications of a new tool in drug delivery to experimental animals, *Labo Pharma,* 298, 373, 1980.

58. Kleinjans, J. C. S., Smits, J. F. M., Kasbergen, C. M., VanEssen, H., and Struyker-Boudier, H. A. J., Blood pressure response to chronic low-dose intrarenal noradrenaline infusion in conscious rats, *Clin. Sci.,* 65, 111, 1983.

59. Smits, J. F. M., Kasbergen, C. M., VanEssen, H., Kleinjans, J. C. S., and Struyker-Boudier, H. A. J., Chronic infusion into the renal artery of unrestrained rats, *Am. J. Physiol.,* 244, H304, 1983.

60. Smits, J. F. M., Hofbauer, K. G., Fuhrer, W., and Struyker-Boudier, H. A. J., Preferential renal vasodilatation by CGP 22 979A as compared to hydralazine and CGP 18 137A, *Fed. Proc. Fed. Am. Soc. Exp. Biol.,* 43, 553, 1984.

61. Kendall, M. J., Jack, D. B., Woods, K. L., Langher, S. J., Quarterman, C. P. and John, V. A., Comparison of the pharmacokinetic profiles of single and multiple doses of a commercial slow-release metroprolol formulation with a new OROS delivery system, *Br. J. Clin. Pharmacol.,* 13, 393, 1982.

62. Arndts, D. and Arndts, K., Pharmacokinetics and pharmacodynamics of transdermally administered clonidine, *Eur. J. Clin. Pharmacol.,* 26, 78, 1984.

63. Anonymous, Controlled intravascular sodium nitroprusside treatment, *Br. Med. J.,* II, 784, 1978.

64. Sheppard, L. C., Computer control of the infusion of vasoactive drugs, *Ann. Biomed. Eng.,* 8, 431, 1980.

65. Auer, L. M. and Rodler, H., Microprocessor-control of drug infusion for automatic blood pressure control, *Med. Biol. Eng. Comput.,* 19, 171, 1981.

66. Koivo, A. J., Larnard, D., and Gray, R., Digital control of mean arterial pressure in dogs by injecting a vasodilator drug, *Ann. Biomed. Eng.,* 9, 185, 1981.

67. Sheppard, L. C., Shotts, J. F., Roberson, N. F., Wallace, F. D., and Kouchoukos, N. T., Computer controlled infusion of vasoactive drugs in post cardiac surgical patients, IEEE/1979 Frontiers in Engineering in Health Care, 280-282, 1979.

68. Jelliffe, R. W., Computer-controlled administration of cardiovascular drugs, *Prog. Cardiovasc. Dis.,* 26, 1, 1983.

69. Guyton, A. C., *Medical Physiology,* Saunders, Philadelphia, 1981.

70. Gold, H., Digitalis: its action and usage, *Med. Ann.,* DC10, 127, 1941.

71. Jelliffe, R. W., A mathematical analysis of digitalis kinetics in patients with normal and reduced renal function, *Math. Biosci.,* 1, 305, 1967.

72. Jelliffe, R. W., Buell, J., and Kalaba, R., Reduction of digitalis toxicity by computer-assisted glycoside dosage regimens, *Ann. Intern. Med.,* 77, 891, 1972.

73. Griffiths, B. E., Penny, W. J., Leuris, M. J., and Henderson, A. H., Maintenance of the inotropic effect of digoxin on long-term treatment, *Br. Med. J.,* 284, 1819, 1982.

74. Tuttle, R. R. and Mills, J., Dobutamine: development of a new catecholamine to selectively increase cardiac contractility, *Circ. Res.,* 36, 185, 1975.

75. Ruffolo, R. R., Spraklin, R. A., Pollock, D., Waddell, J. E., and Murphy, P. J., Alpha and beta-adrenergic effects of the stereo-isomers of dobutamine, *J. Pharmacol. Exp. Ther.,* 219, 447, 1981.

76. Leier, C. V., Webel, J., and Bush, C. A., The cardiovascular effects of continuous infusion of dobutamine in patients with severe heart failure, *Circulation,* 56, 468, 1977.

77. Liang, C. S., Sherman, L. G., Doherty, J. U., Wellington, K., Lee, V. W., and Hood, W. B., Sustained improvement of cardiac function in patients with congestive heart failure after short-term infusion of dobutamine, *Circulation*, 69, 113, 1984.

78. Unverferth, D. V., Magiorien, R. D., Altschuld, R., Kolibash, A. J., Lewis, R. P., and Leier, C. V., The hemodynamic and metabolic advantages gained by a 3-day infusion of dobutamine in patients with congestive cardiomyopathy, *Am. Heart J.*, 106, part 1, 29, 1983.

79. Awan, N. A., Evenson, M. K., Needham, K. E., Beattie, J. M., and Mason, D. T., Effect of combined nitroglycerin and dobutamine infusion in left ventricular dysfunction, *Am. Heart J.*, 106, part 1, 35, 1983.

80. Loeb, H. S., Ostrenga, J. P., Gaul, W., Witt, J., Freeman, G., Scanlon, P. and Gunnar, R. M., Beneficial effects of dopamine combined with intravenous nitroglycerin on hemodynamics in patients with severe left ventricular failure, *Circulation*, 68, 813, 1983.

81. MacCannell, K. L., Giraud, G. D., Hamilton, P. L., and Groves, G., Hemodynamic responses to dopamine and dobutamine infusions as a function of duration of infusion, *Pharmacology*, 26, 219, 1983.

82. Bigger, J. T. and Hoffman, B. F., Antiarrhythmic drugs, in *Pharmacological Basis of Therapeutics*, Gilman, A. G., Goodman, L. S., and Gilman, A., Eds., Macmillan, New York, 1980, 761.

83. Stargel, W. W., Shand, D. G., Routledge, P. A., Barchowsky, A., and Wagner, G. S., Clinical comparison of rapid infusion and multiple injection methods for lidocaine loading, *Am. Heart J.*, 102, 872, 1981.

84. Riddell, J. G., McAllister, C. B., Wilkinson, G. R., Wood, A. J. J., and Roden, D. M., A new method for constant plasma drug concentration: application to lidocaine, *Ann. Intem. Med.*, 100, 25, 1984.

85. Salzer, L. B., Weinrib, A. B., Marina, R. J., and Lima, J. J., A comparison of methods of lidocaine administration in patients, *Clin. Pharmacol. Ther.*, 29, 617, 1981.

86. Vaughan, D. P. and Tucker, G. T., General derivation of the ideal intravenous drug input required to achieve and maintain a constant plasma drug concentration: theoretical application to lidocaine therapy, *Eur. J. Clin. Pharmacol.*, 10, 433, 1976.

87. Collins, S. M. and Arzbaecher, R. C., Feedback control in the management of cardiac arrythmias, *ISA Trans.*, 18, 95, 1979.

88. Anderson, J. L., Tucker, E. M., Pasyk, S., Patterson, E., Simon, A. B., Burmeister, W. E., Lucchesi, B. R., Pitt, B., Donahue, R. P. and Conlon, M. E., Long-term intravenous infusion of antiarrhythmic drug using a totally implanted drug delivery system, *Am. J. Cardiol.*, 49, 1954, 1982.

89. Nattel, S. and Bailey, J. C., Time course of the electrophysiological effects of quinidine on canine cardiac Purkinje fibers — concentration dependence and comparison with lidocaine and disopyramide, *J. Pharmacol. Exp. Ther.*, 225, 176, 1983.

90. Margolis, B., Desilva, R. A., and Lown, B., Episodic drug treatment in the management of paroxysmal arrhythmias, *Am. J. Cardiol.*, 45, 621, 1980.

91. Armstrong, P. W., Armstrong, J. A., and Marks, G. S., Pharmacokinetic-hemodynamic studies of intravenous nitroglycerin in congestive heart failure, *Circulation*, 62, 160, 1980.

92. Imhof, P. R., Sieber, A., Hodler, J., Müller, P., Ott, B., Frankhauser, P., Chu, L. C., and Gérrardin, A., Plasma concentrations and hemodynamic effects of nitroglycerin during and after intravenous infusion in healthy volunteers, *Eur. J. Clin. Pharmacol.*, 23, 99, 1982.

93. Dumont, L., Lamoureux, C., Lelorier, J., Stanley, P., and Chartrand, C., Intravenous infusion of nitroglycerin: effects upon cardiovascular dynamics and regional blood flow distribution in conscious dogs, *Can. J. Physiol. Pharmacol.*, 60, 1436, 1982.

94. Armstrong, P. W., Watts, D. G., and Moffat, J. A., Steady state pharmacokinetic hemodynamic studies of intravenous nitroglycerin in congestive cardiac failure, *Br. J. Clin. Pharmacol.*, 16, 385, 1983.

95. Sorkin, E. M., Brogden, R. N., and Romankiewicz, J. A., Intravenous glycerin trinitrate (nitroglycerin): a review of its pharmacological properties and therapeutic efficacy, *Drugs*, 27, 45, 1984.

96. Imhof, P. R., Ott, B., Frankhauser, P., Chu, L. C., and Hodler, J., Difference in nitroglycerin dose-response in venous and arterial beds, *Eur. J. Clin. Pharmacol.*, 18, 455, 1980.

97. Come, P. C. and Pitt, B., Nitroglycerin-induced severe hypotension and bradycardia in patients with acute myocardial infarction, *Circulation*, 54, 624, 1976.

98. Backe, R. J. and Tockman, B. A., Effect of nitroglycerin and nifedipine on subendocardial perfusion in the presence of flow-limiting coronary stenosis in the awake dog, *Circ. Res.*, 50, 678, 1982.

99. Sethna, D. H., Moffitt, E. A., Bussell, J. A., Raymond, M. J., Mathoff, J. M., and Gray, R. J., Intravenous nitroglycerin and myocardial metabolism during anesthesia in patients undergoing myocardial revascularization, *Anesth. Analg.*, 61, 828, 1982.

100. Bussmann, W. D., Bartmann, F., Berghof, E., and Kaltenbach, W. P., Random study on effects of i.v. nitroglycerin on CK and CKMB infarct size, *Circulation*, 56 (Suppl. III) III-65, 1977.

101. Flaherty, J. T., Becker, L. C., Buckley, B. H., Weiss, J. L., Gerstenblith, G., Kallman, C. H., Silverman, K. J., Wei, J. Y., Pitt, B., and Weisfeldt, M. L., A randomized prospective trial of intravenous nitroglycerin in patients with acute myocardial infarction, *Circulation*, 68, 576, 1983.

102. Conti, C. R., Feldman, R. L., Pepine, C. J., Hill, J. A., and Conti, J. B., Effect of glyceryl trinatrate on coronary and systemic hemodynamics in man, *Am. J. Med.*, 74, 28, 1983.

103. Chien, Y. W., Keshary, P. R., Huang, I. C., Sarpotdar, P. P., Comparative controlled skin permeation of nitroglycerin from marketed transdermal delivery systems, *J. Pharm. Sci.*, 72, 968, 1983.

104. Georgopoulos, A. J., Markis, A., and Georgidalis, H., Therapeutic efficacy of a new transdermal system containing nitroglycerin in patients with angina pectoris, *Eur. J. Clin. Pharmacol.*, 22, 481, 1982.

105. Müller, P., Imhof, P. R., Burkart, F., Chu, L. C., and Gerardin, A., Human pharmacological studies of a new transdermal system containing nitroglycerin, *Eur. J. Clin. Pharmacol.*, 22, 473, 1982.

106. Abrams, J., New nitrate delivery systems. Buccal nitroglycerin, *Am. Heart J.*, 105, 848, 1983.

107. Bussmann, W. D., Dries, R. R., and Wagner, W., Controlled release nitroglycerin in buccal and oral form, Karger Verlag, Basel, 1982.

108. Schor, J. M., Davis, S. S., Nigalaye, A., and Bolton, S., Susadrin transmucosal tablets, *Drug Dev. Ind. Pharm.*, 9, 1359, 1983.

109. Buchwald, H., Rohde, T. D., Schneider, P. D., Varco, R. L., and Blackshear, P. J., Long-term continuous intravenous heparin administration by an implantable infusion pump in ambulatory patients with recurrent venous thrombosis, *Surgery*, 88, 507, 1980.

110. Langer, R., Implantable controlled release systems, *Pharmacol. Ther.*, 21, 35, 1983.

111. Chapleau, C. E. and Robertson, J. T., Spontaneously cervical carotid artery dissection: out-patient treatment with continuous heparin infusion using a totally implantable infusion device, *Neurosurgery*, 8, 83, 1981.

112. Brotman, I., Anticoagulation in myocardial infarction, *Am. J. Cardiol.*, 1, 260, 1958.

113. Mosely, P. H., Schatz, I. J., Breneman, G. M., and Keyes, J. W., Long-term anticoagulant therapy, *JAMA*, 186, 914, 1963.

114. Abbrechts, P. H., Oleary, T. J., and Behrendt, D. M., Evaluation of a computer assisted method for individualized anticoagulation — retrospective and prospective studies with a pharmacodynamic model, *Clin. Pharmacol. Ther.*, 32, 129, 1982.

115. Routledge, P. A., Bell, S. M., Davies, D. M., Cavanagh, J. S., and Rawlins, M. D., Predicting patients' warfarin requirements, *Lancet*, 1, 854, 1977.

116. Sheiner, L. B., Computer-aided long-term anticoagulation therapy, *Comp. Biomed. Res.*, 2, 507, 1969.

117. Sawyer, W. T. and Finn, A. L., Digital computer-assisted warfarin therapy: comparison of two models, *Comp. Biomed. Res.*, 12, 221, 1979.

118. O'Leary, T. J. and Abbrecht, P. H., Predicting oral anticoagulant response using a pharmacodynamic model, *Ann. Biomed. Eng.*, 9, 199, 1981.

119. Thijssen, H. H. W. and Hemker, H. C., Orale antistolling, welk anticoagulans?, *Ned. Tijdschr. Geneeskd.*, in press, 1984.

120. Moulopoulos, D. S., Topaz, S., and Kolff, W. J., Diastolic balloon pumping with carbon dioxide in the aorta: a mechanical assistance to the failing circulation, *Am. Heart J.*, 63, 669, 1962.

121. Clark, J. W., Kane, G. R., and Bourland, H. M., On the feasibility of closed-loop control of intraaortic balloon pumping, *IEEE Trans. Biomed. Eng.*, 20, 404, 1973.

122. Sagawa, K., Closed-loop physiological control of the heart, *Ann. Biomed. Eng.*, 8, 415, 1980.

Chapter 8

EFFECTS OF SCHEDULES OF DRUG ADMINISTRATION IN CANCER CHEMOTHERAPY

Branimir Ivan Sikic and Robert W. Carlson

TABLE OF CONTENTS

I. INTRODUCTION

Cancer chemotherapy is significantly limited by the low therapeutic index, or ratio between therapeutic and toxic doses, for most anticancer agents. Continuous intravenous infusion of some of these drugs has been shown to improve their therapeutic index when compared to conventional intravenous bolus injection.[1-8] Recent advances in the technology of implantable catheters and portable infusion pumps have made continuous infusion therapy more practical on an ambulatory basis. However, much of the empirical clinical data supporting continuous infusion therapy is not rigorously controlled. The rationale for such therapy is therefore largely based on theoretical pharmacological considerations and preclinical experiments in animal models.[9,10]

Many variables may contribute to the schedule-dependent effects of anticancer agents. These include the following:

1. *The pharmacokinetics of the drug* — Cytarabine, for example, is rapidly metabolized by deaminases in plasma and tissues. Bleomycin also has a short plasma half-life, with rapid renal excretion and virtually no protein binding. Both of these drugs are most toxic to cells at specific phases of the cell division cycle, during S-phase or DNA synthesis for cytarabine and G_2 and M-phases for bleomycin. Bolus injection of these agents results in a relatively brief exposure of tumor cells to drug, with resulting drug resistance since only a small fraction of cells are in the vulnerable phase of the cell cycle. Continuous infusion may partially overcome such "cytokinetic resistance".

2. *Chemical properties of the drug, namely, stability and solubility* — Many alkylating agents are chemically unstable in solution, and therefore should not be administered by continuous infusion. Etoposide has limited solubility in aqueous solutions, and requires large volumes for safe administration.

3. *The action of the drug relative to the cell cycle* — Most anticancer drugs are proliferation-dependent or selectively toxic to dividing cells. However, the growth fraction of most human cancers is quite low, with the majority of cells in the resting or nonproliferating (G_0) phase of the cell cycle at any given time. Theoretically, prolonged drug infusion will expose a higher fraction of cells during the sensitive phases of the cell cycle, resulting in greater tumor cell kill. Toxicity to normal proliferating tissues, notably the bone marrow and gastrointestinal tract, is also usually increased by such prolonged exposure.

    Bruce et al. have classified cytotoxic drugs by their degree of proliferation dependence and their specificity for a particular phase of the cell cycle.[11] The duration of drug exposure is a major determinant of activity for agents such as cytarabine, bleomycin, and the vinca alkaloids, since cells must enter and progress through the cell cycle for these drugs to be active. The dose-response curves for these drugs exhibit a characteristic plateau, beyond which increasing drug concentrations do not result in increased cell killing, if the duration of exposure is held constant.[9-12]

4. *Threshold effects* — The minimum drug concentration necessary to produce toxicity appears to vary for drugs among various tissues and tumors. In certain cases, administration of a drug by continuous infusion appears to reduce toxicity to a normal tissue without loss of antitumor efficacy. Such avoidance of high peak drug levels appears to reduce the cardiac toxicity of doxorubicin,[5,6,13-18] the pulmonary toxicity of bleomycin,[2-4] and the bone marrow toxicity of 5-fluorouracil.[19-24] The basis for these differences in thresholds of toxicity among various normal tissues and tumors is not well understood.

Table 1
RESPONSE OF L1210 LEUKEMIA IN
MICE (10⁶ CELLS INOCULATED I.P.)
TO VARIOUS SCHEDULES OF
ADMINISTRATION OF CYTARABINE[9]

Dose (mg/kg) i.p.	Schedule	% "Cures" (60-day survivors)
2500	Single dose	0
60	Daily × 6	0
15	Every 3 hr × 8	3
15	Every 3 hr × 16	58

5. *Biochemical drug resistance* — In addition to a low growth fraction resulting in cytokinetic resistance, many human cancers are biochemically resistant to chemotherapeutic agents. In such cases, varying the rate of drug administration does not appreciably increase antitumor effects. The prevalence of such biochemical resistance in human tumors, and the emergence of drug resistant mutations during the course of treatment, are major reasons why the superiority of continuous infusion regimens has been difficult to demonstrate in clinical trials.

Alternative methods of controlled rate delivery for these drugs, such as depot formulations, have not been commercially developed. In part, this is due to the narrow therapeutic index of these drugs, with the requirement for very strict dose and time control, and also the fact that many of these agents are powerful local vesicants and cannot be administered subcutaneously or intramuscularly.

In this chapter, we present the rationale for continuous intravenous infusion therapy of certain anticancer agents, including both preclinical and clinical evidence. We will not discuss the topics of regional arterial perfusion therapy or the effects of the sequencing of drug administration.

II. CYTARABINE

Cytarabine (cytosine arabinoside; Ara-C) is a pyrimidine antimetabolite which inhibits DNA synthesis both by the direct incorporation of the nucleotide ara-CTP into DNA and by inhibition of DNA polymerase. Ara-C kills cells during DNA synthesis, and is thus S-phase specific. It is primarily utilized in the treatment of acute leukemias.

The plasma half-life of Ara-C is only 5 to 15 min, with rapid inactivation due to enzymatic deamination. The short half-life and specificity for killing cells in S-phase suggest that continuous infusion therapy or frequent drug injection might increase Ara-C efficacy. Table 1 indicates that every 3 hr injection of Ara-C in mice bearing L1210 leukemia is superior to single dose or daily injections. Such a schedule-dependent effect is not true for all drugs, as shown for cyclophosphamide in Table 2. In contrast to Ara-C, cyclophosphamide is most effective when given as a single bolus injection. In both Tables 1 and 2, the total drug doses delivered by the various drug schedules were equally toxic to normal tissues, resulting in 10% lethality (LD_{10}). In the case of Ara-C, divided doses increased the therapeutic index, while for cyclophosphamide, dividing the dose decreased the therapeutic index. Table 3 illustrates the LD_{10} doses of Ara-C by various schedules of administration in mice. Myelosuppression is the cause of death in these animals, and it is evident that the bone marrow is also quite sensitive to varying schedules of drug administration.[9] As expected, continuous infusion of Ara-C was also markedly superior to bolus injection in the treatment of L1210 leukemia in mice (Table 4).[12]

Table 2

RESPONSE OF L1210 LEUKEMIA IN MICE
(10^6 CELLS INOCULATED I.P.) TO
SINGLE VS. DIVIDED DOSES OF
CYCLOPHOSPHAMIDE[9]

Dose (mg/kg) i.p.	Schedule	% "Cures" (60-day survivors)
300	Single dose	77
230	Single dose	40
27	Daily × 15	0

Table 3

THE EFFECT OF SCHEDULE OF
ADMINISTRATION ON THE LETHAL
TOXICITY (LD_{10}) OF CYTARABINE IN MICE[9]

Schedule	LD_{10} dose (mg/kg) i.p.	Total dose, LD_{10}
Single injection	2500	2500
Daily × 15	40	600
Every 3 hr × 8	20	160

Table 4

DOSE RESPONSE OF CONTINUOUS INFUSION
VS. BOLUS INJECTION OF CYTARABINE IN
MICE BEARING L1210 LEUKEMIA[12]

	Percent increase in survival	
Schedule	250 gm/kg × 1 (%)	120 mg/kg q4d × 4 (%)
Continuous infusion, s.c. × 24 hr	68	125
Bolus injection, i.p.	17	68

In clinical studies, continuous infusions of Ara-C for 7 days at dosages below 30 mg/m²/day demonstrated no hematologic toxicity.[25] Bolus injections of up to 4.2 g of Ara-C as a single i.v. bolus did not produce myelosuppression.[26] Infusions of 24 hr produced dose-related myelosuppression up to a plateau at 1.5 g. The myelosuppression of infusions of 48 and 96 hr was similar and increased with increasing doses. Nausea and vomiting were noted to be decreased when the drug was given by continuous infusion compared to bolus injection.

A comparison of 5-day infusion vs. daily i.v. bolus injection of Ara-C resulted in greater myelosuppression with infusion therapy at doses of 50 to 100 mg/m².[27] Increasing the dosage of Ara-C by infusion from 100 to 300 mg/m² did not result in a corresponding increase in hematologic toxicity.

The initial studies with continuous infusion Ara-C at 200 mg/m² in acute leukemia produced a remission rate of 39%.[28] The major drug toxicity noted was moderate to severe leukopenia, along with nausea, vomiting, and weight loss. Prolongation of Ara-C continuous infusions from 48 to 120 hr resulted in an increase in complete remission rates from 20 to 38%.[29] The total dose of Ara-C was similar in the two groups, thus confirming the observation from cell culture and animal models that the schedule of administration of this drug was a more important determinant of efficacy than dose.

More recent studies of schedule effects have utilized the drug in combination with other agents, particularly anthracyclines.[1,30,31] The effects of schedules of Ara-C administration in such studies are obscured by other important variables, particularly the high activity of daunorubicin or doxorubicin in leukemias. For example, a prospective randomized study compared 5- or 7-day infusions of Ara-C vs. 5 or 7 days of bolus injections of Ara-C every 12 hr, in combinations with daunorubicin. The complete remission rates were higher in patients who received Ara-C by continuous infusion; however, these differences did not achieve statistical significance.[1]

Continuous infusions of Ara-C result in drug levels in the cerebrospinal fluid which are approximately one half of the plasma values.[32,33] Thus, infusions of Ara-C may play a role in the treatment of leukemias and lymphomas which have a high incidence of meningeal or central nervous system involvement.

Since Ara-C is not a local vesicant, it can be safely administered as a continuous infusion via a standard peripheral venous catheter and even as a continuous subcutaneous infusion. The drug's pharmacokinetics, mechanism of action, and preclinical studies all predict the superiority of continuous infusion regimens, and the available clinical evidence also indicates that continuous infusion appears to have increased efficacy compared with bolus injection in the treatment of acute leukemia.

III. BLEOMYCIN

Bleomycin is a mixture of glycopeptides which are clinically effective in testicular carcinomas, lymphomas, and squamous carcinomas. Bleomycin is of special interest because it lacks bone marrow toxicity, but its dosage is limited by potentially lethal pulmonary toxicity. Pulmonary fibrosis is a serious clinical problem in approximately 10% of patients who have received the drug, and is fatal in 1 to 2%. The mechanism of action of bleomycin involves binding to DNA, activation of molecular oxygen to free radical moieties, and resulting single and double strand cleavage of DNA. It is a highly proliferation-dependent agent, and most effective during the G_2 and M phases of the cell cycle. The half-life of the drug is less than 2 hr in patients with normal renal function. The short half-life and cell cycle phase specificity suggest that bleomycin might be more effective if administered by continuous infusion, compared to bolus injection.

The effect of continuous infusions on the therapeutic index of bleomycin in mice was extensively studied by Sikic et al.[2] The same total doses of bleomycin were delivered either by bolus injection twice weekly (2 doses), bolus injections twice daily (10 doses), or by 7-day continuous infusion (Alzet® minipumps, ALZA Corporation, Palo Alto, Calif.). Antitumor efficacy was assessed in mice bearing Lewis lung carcinoma. Pulmonary toxicity was assessed in mice without tumors by measuring total lung hydroxyproline as an index of lung collagen accumulation. The results are presented in Table 5. Continuous infusion of bleomycin is superior to the bolus injection schedules, both for increased antitumor effects and for decreased pulmonary toxicity. Thus the therapeutic index in this model is dramatically improved by continuous infusion of bleomycin. The mechanism for this schedule-dependent separation of toxic and therapeutic effects is not clear. It is possible that bolus injection results in saturation of pulmonary pathways for drug inactivation or repair. Frequent low-dose injections produced more pulmonary toxicity than less frequent higher-dose injections. Therefore, the threshold for peak plasma levels of bleomycin which produce pulmonary toxicity must be quite low.

Table 5

THE EFFECTS OF SCHEDULE OF
ADMINISTRATION OF BLEOMYCIN ON
PULMONARY TOXICITY AND ANTITUMOR
EFFICACY MICE[2]

Schedule of bleomycin administration, s.c.	Lung toxicity percent increase in lung hydroxyproline (%)	Antitumor efficacy: percent decrease in tumor size (%)
Bolus × 2	20	50
Bolus × 10	31	68
Continuous infusion	10[a]	84[a]

[a]   Continuous infusion resulted in significantly less pulmonary toxicity and greater antitumor efficacy than the two schedules of bolus injections, $p < 0.05$. The total dose administered was the same in the three schedules.[2]

The increased antitumor efficacy of continuous infusion of bleomycin compared to bolus injection was confirmed in mice bearing P388 leukemia.[34] In this study, continuous infusion resulted in a fivefold greater inhibition of leukemia colony forming units compared to bolus injections.

There are no rigorously controlled studies in man comparing the efficacy and toxicity of bleomycin administered by continuous infusion vs. bolus injection. However, several studies have reported either increased antitumor efficacy or decreased pulmonary toxicity with bleomycin infusions, compared to historical controls treated with bolus injections.

In testicular carcinomas, a complete remission rate of 38% was obtained with the combination of bleomycin infusion at 30 U/day for 5 days and vinblastine injection.[35] Prior to the introduction of cisplatin for the treatment of testicular carcinomas, this was the highest complete remission rate reported in patients with advanced pulmonary and abdominal disease. In an earlier study at the same institution, the complete remission rate was only 15% when bleomycin was delivered by i.m. injection rather than infusion. In the infusion study, there was one death from pulmonary toxicity in a patient who had received a total of 600 U of bleomycin. However, the overall incidence of pulmonary toxicity did not appear increased, despite the high total doses of bleomycin which were delivered.

In squamous carcinomas of the cervix, continuous infusion of bleomycin was reported to produce a 30% response rate in 32 patients, including two complete remissions.[4] The response rate for carcinoma of the cervix treated by bolus injections of bleomycin in other studies was only 9%. For several other tumor types which are resistant to bleomycin administered by bolus injection, however, continuous infusion did not significantly increase response rates. Thus optimization of schedule of drug administration may not be sufficient to overcome biochemical drug resistance in human tumors.

In the phase II study of Krakoff et al.,[4] 6 out of 119 patients treated by continuous infusion developed symptomatic pulmonary toxicity, usually 6 to 8 weeks after the completion of the infusions. These cases are not individually analyzed for risk factors such as total drug dose, patient age, prior chest radiotherapy, renal function, and exposure to higher concentrations of oxygen. The incidence of alopecia was higher than with bolus injection (71% vs. 30%), and cutaneous toxicity (hyperkeratosis, hyperpigmentation, and erythema) occurred in almost all patients.

Three schedules of bleomycin administration (weekly, twice weekly, and 4-day infusions) have been compared in combination with vincristine and mitomycin-C in advanced carcinoma of the cervix. The median survival of the patients treated with continuous infusions of bleomycin was slightly but significantly longer than those treated with weekly injections (6 vs. 4 months).[3] Twice-weekly injections produced a somewhat higher response rate than infusion (60% vs. 39%), but the duration of the response was shorter (9 vs. 16 weeks). Severe pulmonary toxicity was significantly more frequent with twice-weekly bleomycin (6 out of 53 patients); whereas no severe pulmonary toxicity was observed among 42 patients treated by continuous infusion.

The effects on pulmonary function of 7-day continuous infusions of bleomycin, 15 $U/m^2/day$, were prospectively studied in a group of 15 patients, 13 of whom had squamous cell carcinomas of the head and neck.[36] Only two patients showed minor decreases in vital capacity and carbon monoxide diffusing capacity, and no patients developed clinically evident pulmonary toxicity.

The rationale favoring continuous infusion bleomycin as the optimal schedule of administration includes the cell cycle phase-specificity of the drug, its pharmacokinetics (short half-life), and preclinical studies which demonstrate increased antitumor efficacy and decreased pulmonary toxicity compared to bolus injection schedules. In addition, several uncontrolled studies in patients suggest that bleomycin may be more effective and/or less toxic when administered by continuous infusion.

IV. DOXORUBICIN

Doxorubicin (Adriamycin®) is an anthracycline antibiotic which is very useful in the treatment of leukemias, lymphomas, and many other types of human cancers. The toxicities of the drug include nausea, myelosuppression, alopecia, and, notably, chronic cardiac toxicity. This cardiac toxicity is cumulative, with a substantially increased risk for congestive heart failure when the total dose of doxorubicin exceeds 450 mg/m^2 by bolus injection.

Several mechanisms of action have been proposed for doxorubicin, including binding to DNA by intercalation, generation of oxygen-derived free radicals, and interactions with the plasma membrane. It is not known whether the mechanisms responsible for the antitumor effects of doxorubicin are identical with the mechanisms responsible for the cardiac toxicity.

The cytotoxicity of doxorubicin to cells in culture is dependent on both drug concentration and duration of exposure.[37,38] The cardiac toxicity of doxorubicin has been shown to be both dose and schedule-dependent in various animal models in vivo, including mice, rats, rabbits, and dogs.[13,14] In some of these models, antitumor efficacy appears to be increased at treatment schedules which exhibit decreased toxicity (Table 6). In this study, administration of the same total dose in 4 divided daily doses was significantly less lethal and resulted in greater antitumor effects when compared to a single bolus injection of doxorubicin.[13] These preclinical data suggest that the cardiotoxic effects of doxorubicin may be separated from its antitumor effects by changes in schedule of administration.

Several clinical studies have suggested that the risk for doxorubicin cardiac toxicity may be decreased by either continuous infusion therapy[5,6] or by administering lower doses of the drug more often (weekly low-dose therapy).[15-18] Unfortunately, none of these studies are prospectively randomized comparisons of these schedules with standard i.v. bolus therapy every 3 weeks. Weekly administration produced less nausea, vomiting, and cardiac toxicity, but more severe stomatitis, than every 3-week therapy. The antitumor efficacy of these two schedules does not appear to be different.

Legha et al.[5,6] have suggested that continuous infusion of doxorubicin decreased the

Table 6
EFFECTS OF SINGLE VS. DIVIDED-DOSE ADMINISTRATION OF DOXORUBICIN IN MICE[13]

Dose schedule (mg/kg)	Peak cardiac doxorubicin level ($\mu g/g$)	Lethal toxicities (%)	Survival, % ILS[a]	
			Lewis lung carcinoma (%)	Mammary carcinoma (%)
15.00 i.v. × 1	24.9	27	3	17
3.75 i.v. × 4	8.0[b]	5	24[b]	64[b]

[a] % ILS = Percent increased life span compared to controls, of mice bearing Lewis lung carcinomas or mammary carcinomas.

[b] $p < 0.05$, single vs. divided doses.

risk for cardiac toxicity in patients with carcinomas of the breast and sarcomas. The nonrandomized control group receiving bolus injections of doxorubicin were mostly patients with carcinoma of the lung who are at higher risk for cardiac disease. Continuous infusion of doxorubicin decreased nausea, vomiting, and cardiac toxicity as assessed by endomyocardial biopsy, while antitumor efficacy and myelosuppression were similar to those expected with bolus injection of doxorubicin. Durations of infusion ranging from 24 to 96 hr were used in these patients and the optimal duration of infusion has not been established.

Doxorubicin is a potent vesicant; therefore, continuous infusion therapy requires placement of a central venous catheter to avoid extravasation of the drug.

V. FLUOROURACIL

Fluorouracil (5-FU) is a pyrimidine antimetabolite which inhibits DNA synthesis by binding to thymidylate synthetase and may also be incorporated into RNA as a fraudulent nucleotide. Its major clinical utility is in the treatment of carcinomas of the breast and gastrointestinal tract. The half-life of fluorouracil in serum is only 10 min in man. This short half-life and a relative specificity for killing cells in S-phase provide a rationale for administering the drug by continuous infusion.

Several clinical studies have demonstrated that fluorouracil can be given safely by continuous infusion at doses of 1.0 to 1.4 g/day, or 22.5 to 30 mg/kg/day, for up to 5 days when the daily infusion was at least 8 hr in duration.[19] Infusion durations of 30 days are well-tolerated at doses up to 300 mg/m²/day.[24] These infusion schedules result in increased gastrointestinal toxicity of fluorouracil, as manifested by stomatitis and diarrhea, but less myelosuppression than with similar doses of intravenous bolus fluorouracil.[20-24,39] Although the spectrum of toxicity of fluorouracil is modified by continuous infusion, there has been no convincing demonstration of increased antitumor efficacy of infusion vs. bolus fluorouracil in clinical trials.[20,22,23,40,41]

The relative lack of myelosuppression of fluorouracil administered by continuous infusion permits combination chemotherapy with other myelosuppressive drugs. Several clinical studies have combined 5-day infusions of fluorouracil with other cytotoxic agents in colorectal and other gastrointestinal cancers.[42-46] Unfortunately, the majority of these cancers are refractory to the agents which were used, so that combination chemotherapy in these studies was not superior to the use of fluorouracil alone. The addition of infusion fluorouracil to cyclophosphamide in ovarian carcinomas yielded superior remission rates and survival than would be expected with cyclophosphamide alone.[47] This study utilized an historical control group, however. It has also been claimed in an uncontrolled study that the addition of infusion fluorouracil improves the results of radiation therapy in patients with esophageal carcinoma.[48]

In summary, administration of fluorouracil by infusion results in less myelosuppression and nausea but greater stomatitis and diarrhea than with bolus injection. There is no major difference in antitumor efficacy by these schedules, however.

VI. VINCA ALKALOIDS

The plant-derived alkaloids vincristine, vinblastine, and vindesine are cell-cycle phase-specific cytotoxic agents which bind to tubulin and inhibit the assembly of microtubules. Despite minor differences in chemical structures, these drugs differ significantly in their spectrum of antitumor efficacy and toxicities. They have conventionally been administered by intravenous bolus injection, but there has been recent interest in infusion therapy because of their phase-specificity. The vinca alkaloids are potent vesicants and require central venous access for safety during prolonged infusions.

The cytotoxic effects of vincristine are markedly dependent on duration of drug exposure in cell culture.[49] The pharmacokinetics and toxicity of continuous infusions of vincristine have been studied in man at doses of 0.5 to 1.0 mg/m²/day for up to 5 days.[50-52] Neurologic toxicities similar to intravenous bolus therapy were found with infusions of 0.5 mg/m²/day. Although a few patients did demonstrate antitumor effects, the overall number of patients studied is quite low, so that the relative antitumor efficacy of infusion vs. bolus administration of vincristine is not known.

Vinblastine has been reported to be effective as a 5-day continuous infusion in patients with refractory breast cancer.[7] Remissions were observed in 40% out of 30 evaluable patients, at dosages ranging from 1.4 to 2.0 mg/m²/day for 5 days. The major toxicity was myelosuppression which was severe at doses greater than 1.8 mg/m²/day. Several patients who responded favorably in this study had failed prior therapy with bolus injections of vinblastine or other vinca alkaloids.

Various infusion schedules of vindesine have been studied clinically.[8,53-55] Five-day infusions every 3 weeks have been compared to bolus injections of the drug in patients with refractory breast cancer.[8,55] Infusions of 1.0 to 1.4 mg/m²/day were more myelosuppressive than bolus administration of 3 to 4 mg/m², while nausea, vomiting, and constipation were more severe with bolus administration. The continuous infusion schedule resulted in a 25% partial remission rate compared to 7% for bolus injection, but the number of patients in this study was too small for this difference to be significant. Four out of eleven patients who failed treatment with bolus injection of vindesine subsequently achieved remissions when the vindesine was administered by continuous infusion.[8]

Although the mechanism of action of the vinca alkaloids and data from tissue culture predict that the vinca alkaloids would be more effective by continuous infusions, clinical studies have not yet shown marked superiority of such schedules. However, there have been several observations of remissions induced by continuous infusion of vinca alkaloids in patients with breast cancer who failed treatment with the same drugs when given by bolus injection.

VII. ETOPOSIDE

Etoposide (VP-16) is an epipodophyllotoxin whose mechanism of action remains unclear. However, the drug appears to be highly phase-specific in the cell cycle, with cells in late S and early G_2 phases being most vulnerable. The drug is especially useful in the treatment of germ cell neoplasms, lymphomas, and small-cell lung cancer.

A major problem in administering etoposide by continuous infusion is its poor solubility in aqueous solutions and instability in dextrose. Thus, at least 1 ℓ of i.v. fluid is required daily to administer the drug by continuous infusion, and since its solubility decreases with time, the infusion solution must be renewed at least every 8 hr. Steady-state plasma levels of etoposide in man are achieved within 3 hr of beginning continuous infusion.[56]

Divided doses of etoposide are superior to single dose therapy in the treatment of L1210 leukemias in mice.[57] Various schedules were also studied in a prospective randomized study of patients with small cell carcinoma of the lung.[58] In this study, weekly bolus injections were compared to oral administration on days 1, 2, and 3 vs. oral administration on days 1 to 5 every 3 weeks. Toxicity, primarily leukopenia, was similar in the 3 regimens. However, the 2 oral schedules of administration were superior to the intravenous bolus injection.

Continuous infusions of etoposide have been administered for 5 days, with myelosuppression being the dose limiting toxicity.[59-61] The large volumes of saline required for etoposide infusion resulted in congestive heart failure in up to 16% of these patients.[60] Two patients in one study developed acute myocardial infarctions during etoposide infusion. Although these patients had a history of prior cardiovascular disease, it is possible that the drug itself may have contributed to these cardiac events, rather than just the fluid loading.

In conclusion, etoposide does appear to demonstrate schedule dependence of antitumor effects. However, repeated intermittent dosing appears to be equivalent to continuous intravenous infusion and may be more safely administered.

VIII. CISPLATIN

Cisplatin (*cis*-diammine-dichloroplatinum) is a coordination complex of the metal platinum whose mechanism of cytotoxicity appears to involve binding and cross-linking of DNA, similar to alkylating agents. The drug has a broad spectrum of activity in human cancers.

Studies in tissue culture suggested that prolonged exposures to low concentrations of cisplatin were as cytotoxic as short exposures to high concentrations.[62,63] In L1210 leukemias in mice, higher total doses of cisplatin were required to achieve equivalent antitumor effects when administered by continuous infusion.[64]

The major toxicities of the drug include severe nausea, kidney damage, and myelosuppression. It has been hypothesized that the nausea and nephrotoxicity of cisplatin were related to high peak levels of the drug given by bolus injection, and that these toxicities might be ameliorated by prolonged continuous infusion. Clinical trials of 24-hr continuous infusion of cisplatin combined with vigorous hydration in patients with head and neck and ovarian cancers has resulted in a low incidence of renal toxicity.[65,66] However, these studies were uncontrolled, and a similar decrease in renal toxicity was observed when cisplatin was given by bolus injection, but with prehydration and mannitol diuresis.[67,68] The antitumor efficacy of 24-hr continuous infusion cisplatin in these studies was similar to that of bolus cisplatin.

Other studies utilizing 5-day infusion of cisplatin have demonstrated less nausea and vomiting than expected with bolus injections, but again these studies were not rigorously controlled.[69-71] The myelosuppression produced by 5-day continuous infusion was dose limiting, with maximal doses of 30 mg/m²/day. Two patients who received 4 courses of cisplatin by continuous infusion developed severe peripheral neuropathy, characterized by generalized muscle weakness, sensory changes, and decreased deep tendon reflexes.[71]

In summary, preclinical data does not support a notable schedule dependence of

Table 7

CHARACTERISTICS OF REPRESENTATIVE AMBULATORY CONTINUOUS
INFUSION PUMPS USED FOR THE ADMINISTRATION OF CYTOSTATICS[a]

Pump	Energy Source	Usable reservoir volume (ml)	Infusion rate (ml/hr)	Weight (g)	Comments
Autosyringe					
AS 2F	Rechargeable battery	5—40	0.02—88.0	482	Mechanical
AS 2FH	Rechargeable battery	5—40	0.01—44.0	482	Mechanical
AS 3B	Nonrechargeable battery	1—5	0.03—1.25	310	Mechanical
Cormed					
M26-4	Rechargeable battery	50	0.16—0.83	530	Peristaltic
M26-6	Rechargeable battery	50	0.4—2.1	530	Peristaltic
M26-8	Rechargeable battery	Up to 2000	25—125	382	Peristaltic
M26-10	Rechargeable battery	Up to 2000	42—208	530	Peristaltic
Travenol					
Infusor®	Elastomer balloon	48	2	~35	Disposable
Infusaid®	Volatile liquid/vapor	22—47	0.04—0.25	165—208	Implantable

[a] Data from the manufacturer's product information.

Reproduced by permission from the *Annals of Internal Medicine* (Vol. 99, 824, 1983).

cisplatin. Vigorous hydration before, during, and after administration appears to be essential to minimize renal toxicity by any schedule. Twenty-four-hour infusions appear to be as efficacious as bolus or short term infusions of the drug. Current controlled clinical trials are ongoing to further study possible schedule effects of cisplatin.

IX. CONCLUSIONS

There is increasing interest in the possible advantages of continuous infusion administration of anticancer agents. Developments in infusion pump technology and intravenous access have made outpatient infusion therapy more practical (cf. Table 7). Special precautions need to be taken when potent vesicants such as doxorubicin and the vinca alkaloids are administered by prolonged infusions. These drugs require the placement of central venous catheters to minimize phlebitis and drug extravasation.

The pulmonary toxicity of bleomycin, the cardiac toxicity of doxorubicin, and the bone-marrow toxicity of fluorouracil all appear to be decreased when the drugs are administered by continuous infusion compared to bolus injection. For bleomycin, in preclinical models, continuous infusion also results in increased antitumor efficacy, so that the therapeutic index is improved both from greater therapeutic effect and decreased lung toxicity. The efficacy of cytarabine and the vinca alkaloids may also be somewhat increased by continuous infusion compared to bolus injection. Etoposide appears to be more efficacious when administered over a 3- to 5-day period compared to a single bolus injection, but continuous infusion does not appear to offer an advantage over frequent intermittent injection.

Despite theoretical considerations and preclinical data which predict schedule-dependent effects of certain anticancer drugs, it has been difficult to demonstrate significant clinical benefit from alterations of drug scheduling. A major problem with many of the clinical studies is the lack of rigorous control groups to compare various schedules for administration. Many studies include too few patients to demonstrate a statistically significant difference between the schedules of drug administration. Finally, biochemical drug resistance to currently available agents appears to be profound in many human cancers, and minimizes the possible advantages of even the optimal schedules of administration. Further controlled clinical trials comparing continuous infusions to conventional intravenous bolus delivery of these drugs are needed to assess the role of infusion therapy in clinical practice.

REFERENCES

1. Rai, K. R., Holland, J. F., Glidewell, O. J., Weinberg, V., Brunner, K., Obrecht, J. P., Preisler, H. D., Nawabi, I. W., Prager, D., Carey, R. W., Cooper, M. R., Haurani, F., Hutchison, J. L., Silver, R. T., Falkson, G., Wiernik, P., Hoagland, H. C., Bloomfield, C. D., James, G. W., Gottlieb, A., Ramanan, S. V., Blom, J., Nissen, N. I., and Bank, A., Treatment of acute myelocytic leukemia: a study by cancer and leukemia group B, *Blood,* 58, 1203, 1981.

2. Sikic, B. I., Collins, J. M., Mimnaugh, E. G., and Gram, T. E., Improved therapeutic index of bleomycin when administered by continuous infusion in mice, *Cancer Treat. Rep.,* 62, 2011, 1978.

3. Baker, L. H., Opipari, M. I., Wilson, H., Bottomley, R., and Coltman, C. A., Jr., Mitomycin C, vincristine, and bleomycin therapy for advanced cervical cancer, *Obstet. Gynecol.,* 52, 146, 1978.

4. Krakoff, I. H., Cvitkovic, E., Currie, V., Yeh, S., and LaMonte, C., Clinical pharmacologic and therapeutic studies of bleomycin given by continuous infusion, *Cancer,* 40, 2027, 1977.

5. Legha, S. S., Benjamin, R. S., MacKay, B., Ewer, M., Wallace, S., Valdivieso, M., Rasmussen, S. L., Blumenschein, G. R., and Freireich, E. J., Reduction of doxorubicin cardiotoxicity by prolonged continuous intravenous infusion., *Ann. Intern. Med.,* 96, 133, 1982.

6. Legha, S. S., Benjamin, R. S., MacKay, B., Yap, H. Y., Wallace, S., Ewer, M., Blumenschein, G. R., and Freireich, E. J., Adriamycin therapy by continuous intravenous infusion in patients with metastatic breast cancer, *Cancer,* 49, 1762, 1982.

7. Yap, Y. H., Blumenschein, G. R., Keating, M. J., Hortobagyi, G. N., Tashima, C. K., and Loo, T. L., Vinblastine given as a continuous 5-day infusion in the treatment of refractory advanced breast cancer, *Cancer Treat. Rep.,* 64, 279, 1980.

8. Yap, H. Y., Blumenschein, G. R., Bodey, G. P., Hortobagyi, G. N., Buzdar, A. U., and DiStefano, A., Vindesine in the treatment of refractory breast cancer: improvement in therapeutic index with continuous 5-day infusion, *Cancer Treat. Rep.,* 65, 775, 1981.

9. Skipper, H. E., *Cancer Chemotherapy,* Vol. 1, University Microfilms International, Ann Arbor, Mich., 1978.

10. Southern Research Institute, *Some Thoughts Regarding the Modes of Action of Drugs on Cells and on Application of Available Pharmacokinetic Data (Anticancer Drugs),* Southern Research Institute, Birmingham, Ala., Booklet 10, 1979.

11. Bruce, W. R., Meeker, B. E., and Valeriote, F. A., Comparison of the sensitivity of normal hematopoietic and transplanted lymphoma colony-forming cells to chemotherapeutic agents administered *in vivo, J. Natl. Cancer Inst.,* 37, 233, 1966.

12. Skipper, H. E., Schabel, F. M., Jr., and Wilcox, W. S., Experimental evaluation of potential anticancer agents. XXI. Scheduling of arabinosylcytosine to take advantage of its S-phase specificity against leukemia cells, *Cancer Chemother. Rep.,* 51, 125, 1967.

13. Pacciarini, M. A., Barbieri, B., Colombo, T., Broggini, M., Grattini, S., and Donelli, M. G., Distribution and antitumor activity of adriamycin given in a high-dose and a repeated low-dose schedule to mice, *Cancer Treat. Rep.,* 62, 791, 1978.

14. Solcia, E., Ballerini, L., Bellini, O., Magrini, U., Bertazzoli, C., Tosana, G., Sala, L., Balconi, F., and Rallo, F., Cardiomyopathy of doxorubicin in experimental animals. Factors affecting the severity, distribution and evolution of myocardial lesions, *Tumori,* 67, 461, 1981.

15. Weiss, A. J., Metter, G. E., Fletcher, W. S., Wilson, W. L., Grage, T. B., and Ramirez, G., Studies on adriamycin using a weekly regimen demonstrating its clinical effectiveness and lack of cardiac toxicity, *Cancer Treat. Rep.,* 60, 813, 1976.

16. Weiss, A. J. and Manthel, R. W., Experience with the use of adriamycin in combination with other anticancer agents using a weekly schedule, with particular reference to lack of cardiac toxicity, *Cancer,* 40, 2046, 1977.

17. Creech, R. H., Catalano, R. B., and Shah, M. K., An effective low-dose adriamycin regimen as secondary chemotherapy for metastatic breast cancer patients, *Cancer,* 46, 433, 1980.

18. Chlebowski, R. T., Paroly, W. S., Pugh, R. P., Hueser, J., Jacobs, E. M., Pajak, T. F., and Bateman, J. R., Adriamycin given as a weekly schedule without a loading course: clinically effective with reduced incidence of cardiotoxicity, *Cancer Treat. Rep.*, 64, 47, 1980.

19. Lemon, H. M., Reduction of 5-fluorouracil toxicity in man with retention of anticancer effects by prolonged intravenous administration in 5% dextrose, *Cancer Chemother. Rep.*, 8, 97, 1960.

20. Reitemeier, R. J. and Moertel, C. G., Comparison of rapid and slow intravenous administration of 5-fluorouracil in treating patients with advanced carcinoma of the large intestine, *Cancer Chemother. Rep.*, 25, 87, 1962.

21. Staley, C. J., Hart, J. T., Van Hagen, F., and Preston, F. W., Various methods of administering 5-fluorouracil, *Cancer Chemother. Rep.*, 20, 107, 1962.

22. Seifert, P., Baker, L. H., Reed, M. L., and Vaitkevicius, V. K., Comparison of continuously infused 5-fluorouracil with bolus injection in treatment of patients with colorectal adenocarcinoma, *Cancer*, 36, 123, 1975.

23. Hum, G. J., and Bateman, J. R., 5-day IV infusion with 5-fluorouracil (5-FU; NSC-19893) for gastroenteric carcinoma after failure on weekly 5-FU therapy, *Cancer Chemother. Rep.*, 59, 1177, 1975.

24. Lokich, J., Bothe, A., Jr., Fine, N., and Perri, J., Phase I study of protracted venous infusion of 5-fluorouracil, *Cancer*, 48, 2565, 1981.

25. Ellison, R. R., Carey, R. W., and Holland, J. R., Continuous infusions of arabinosyl cytosine in patients with neoplastic disease, *Clin. Pharmacol. Ther.*, 8, 800, 1967.

26. Frei, E., III, Bickers, J. N., Hewlett, J. S., Lane, M., Lery, W. V., and Talley, R. W., Dose, schedule and antitumor studies of arabinosyl cytosine (NSC 63878), *Cancer Res.*, 29, 1325, 1969.

27. Burke, P. J., Serpick, A. A., Carbvone, P. P., and Tarr, N., A clinical evaluation of dose and schedule of administration of cytosine arabinoside (NSC 63878), *Cancer Res.*, 28, 274, 1968.

28. Bodey, G. P., Freireich, E. J., Monto, R. W., and Hewlett, J. S., Cytosine arabinoside (NSC 63878) therapy for acute leukemia in adults, *Cancer Chemother. Rep.*, 53, 59, 1969.

29. Southwest Oncology Group, Cytarabine for acute leukemia in adults: effect of schedule on therapeutic response, *Arch. Intern. Med.*, 133, 251, 1974.

30. Bodey, G. P., Coltman, C. A., Hewlett, J. S., and Freireich, E. J., Progress in the treatment of adults with acute leukemia: review of regimens containing cytarabine studied by the Southwest Oncology Group, *Arch. Intern. Med.*, 136, 1383, 1976.

31. Preisler, H., Bjornsson, S., Henderson, E. S., Hrynuik, W., Higby, D., Freeman, A., and Naeher, C., Remission induction in acute nonlymphocytic leukemia: comparison of seven-day and ten-day infusion of cytosine arabinoside in combination with adriamycin, *Med. Pediatr. Oncol.*, 7, 269, 1979.

32. Weinstein, H. J., Griffin, T. W., Feeney, J., Cohen, H. J., Propper, R. D., and Sallan, S. E., Pharmacokinetics of continuous intravenous and subcutaneous infusions of cytosine arabinoside, *Blood*, 59, 1351, 1982.

33. Ho, D. H. W., Potential advances in the clinical use of arabinosyl cytosine, *Cancer Treat. Rep.*, 61, 717, 1977.

34. Peng, Y-M., Alberts, D. S., Chen, H-S. G., Mason, N., and Moon, T. E., Antitumour activity and plasma kinetics of bleomycin by continuous and intermittent administration, *Br. J. Cancer*, 41, 644, 1980.

35. Samuels, M. L., Johnson, D. E., and Holoye, P. Y., Continuous intravenous bleomycin (NSC-125066) therapy with vinblastine (NSC-49842) in stage III testicular neoplasia, *Cancer Treat. Rep.*, 65, 419, 1981.

36. Cooper, K. R. and Hong, W. K., Prospective study of the pulmonary toxicity of continuously infused bleomycin, *Cancer Treat. Rep.*, 65, 419, 1981.

37. Haskell, C. M. and Sullivan, A., Comparative survival in tissue culture of normal and neoplastic human cells exposed to adriamycin, *Cancer Res.*, 34, 2991, 1974.

38. Eichholtz-Wirth, H., Dependence of the cytostatic effect of adriamycin on drug concentration and exposure time *in vitro*, *Br. J. Cancer*, 41, 886, 1980.

39. Sullivan, R. D., Young, C. W., Miller, E., Glatstein, N., Clarkson, B., and Burchenal, J. H., The clinical effects of the continuous administration of fluorinated pyrimidines (5-fluorouracil and 5-fluoro-2'-deoxyuridine), *Cancer Chemother. Rep.*, 8, 77, 1960.

40. Moertel, C. G., Schutt, A. J., Reitemeier, R. J., and Hahn, R. G., A comparison of 5-fluorouracil adminstered by slow infusion and rapid injection, *Cancer Res.*, 32, 2717, 1972.

41. Hartman, H. A., Jr., Kessinger, A., Lemon, H. M., and Foley, J. F., Five-day continuous infusion of 5-fluorouracil for advanced colorectal, gastric, and pancreatic adenocarcinoma, *J. Surg. Oncol.*, 11, 227, 1979.

42. Greco, F. A., Richardson, R. L., Schulman, S. F., and Oldham, R. K., Combination of constant-infusion 5-fluorouracil, methyl-CCNU, mitomycin C, and vincristine in advanced colorectal carcinoma, *Cancer Treat. Rep.*, 62, 1407, 1978.

43. Kane, R. C., Cashdollar, M. R., and Bernath, A. M., Treatment of advanced colorectal cancer with methyl-CCNU plus 5-day fluorouracil infusion, *Cancer Treat. Rep.,* 62, 1521, 1978.

44. Bedikian, A. Y., Stab, R., Livingston, R., Valdivieso, M., Burgess, M. A., and Bodey, G. P., Chemotherapy for colorectal cancer with 5-fluorouracil, cyclophosphamide, and CCNU: comparison of oral and continuous IV administration of 5-fluorouracil, *Cancer Treat. Rep.,* 62, 1603, 1978.

45. Buroker, T., Kim, P. N., Gropp, C., McCracken, J., O'Bryan, R., Panettiere, F., Cottman, C., Bottomley, R., Wilson, H., Bonnet, J., Thigpen, T., Vaitkevicius, V. K., Hoogstraten, B., and Heilbrun, L., 5-FU infusion with mitomycin-C versus 5-FU infusion with methyl-CCNU in the treatment of advanced colon cancer, *Cancer,* 42, 1228, 1978.

46. Buroker, T., Kim, P. N., Groppe, C., McCracken, J., O'Bryan, R., Panettiere, F., Costanzi, J., Bottomley, R., King, G. W., Bonnet, J., Thigpen, T., Whitecar, J., Hass, C., Vaitkevicius, V. K., Hoogstraten, B., and Heilbrun, L., 5-FU Infusion with mitomycin-C versus 5-FU infusion with methyl-CCNU in the treatment of advanced upper gastrointestinal cancer, *Cancer,* 44, 1215, 1979.

47. Isbicki, R. M., Baker, L. H., Samson, M. K., McDonald, B., and Vaitkevicius, V. K., 5-FU Infusion and cyclophosphamide in the treatment of advanced ovarian cancer, *Cancer Treat. Rep.,* 61, 1573, 1977.

48. Byfield, J. E., Barone, R., Mendelsohn, J., Byfield, J. E., Barone, R., Mendelsohn, J., Frankel, S., Quinol, L., Sharp, T., and Seagren, S., Infusional 5-fluorouracil and x-ray therapy for non-resectable esophageal cancer, *Cancer,* 45, 703, 1980.

49. Jackson, D. V., Jr. and Bender, R. A., Cytotoxic thresholds of vincristine in a murine and a human leukemia cell line *in vivo, Cancer Res.,* 39, 4346, 1979.

50. Weber, W., Nagel, G. A., Nagel-Studer, E., and Albrecht, R., Vincristine infusion: a phase I study, *Cancer Chemother. Pharmacol.,* 3, 49, 1979.

51. Jackson, D. V., Jr., Sethi, V. S., Spurr, C. L., Willard, V., White, D. R., Richards, F., 2d, Stuart, J. J., Muss, H. B., Cooper, M. R., Homesley, H. D., Jobson, V. W., and Castle, M. C., Intravenous vincristine infusion: phase I trial, *Cancer,* 48, 2559, 1981.

52. Jackson, D. V., Jr., Sethi, V. S., Spurr, C. L., White, D. R., Richards, F., 2d, Stuart, J. J., Muss, H. B., Cooper, M. R., and Castle, M. C., Pharmacokinetics of vincristine infusion, *Cancer Treat. Rep.,* 65, 1043, 1981.

53. Bayssas, M., Gouveia, J., Ribaud, P., Musset, M., deVassal, F., Pico, J. L., deLuca, L., Misset, J. L., Machover, D., Belpomme, D., Schwarzenberg, L., Jasmin, C., Hayat, M., and Mathe, G., Phase-II trial with vindesine for regression induction in patients with leukemias and hematosarcomas, *Cancer Chemother. Pharmacol.,* 2, 247, 1979.

54. Gilby, E. D., A comparison of vindesine administration by bolus injection and by 24-hour infusion, *Cancer Treat. Rev.,* 7 (Suppl.), 47, 1980.

55. Bodey, G. P., Yap, H-Y., Yap, B-S., and Valdivieso, M., Continuous infusion vindesine in solid tumors, *Cancer Treat. Rev.,* 7(Suppl.), 39, 1980.

56. D'Incalci, M., Farina, P., Sessa, C., Mangioni, C., Conter, V., Masera, G., Rocchetti, M., Pisoni, M. B., Piazza, E., Beer, M., and Cavalli, F., Pharmacokinetics of VP16-213 given by different administration methods, *Cancer Chemother. Pharmacol.,* 7, 141, 1982.

57. Dombernowsky, P. and Nissen, N. L., Schedule dependency of the antileukemic activity of the podophyllotoxin-derivative VP16-213 (NSC-141540) in L1210 leukemia, *Acta Pathol. Microbiol. Scand.,* 81, 715, 1973.

58. Cavalli, F., Sonntag, R. W., Jungi, F., Senn, H. J., and Brunner, K. W., VP-16-213 monotherapy for remission induction of small cell lung cancer: a randomized trial using three dosage schedules, *Cancer Treat. Rep.,* 62, 473, 1978.

59. Lokich, J. and Corkery, J., Phase I study of VP-16-213 (Etoposide) administered as a continuous 5-day infusion, *Cancer Treat. Rep.,* 65, 887, 1981.

60. Aisner, J., Van Echo, D. A., Whitacre, M., and Wiernik, P. H., A phase I trial of continuous infusion VP16-213 (Etoposide), *Cancer Chemother. Pharmacol.,* 7, 157, 1982.

61. Schell, F. C., Yap, H. Y., Hortobagyi, G. N., Issell, B., and Esparza, L., Phase II study of VP16-213 (Etoposide) in refractory metastatic breast carcinoma, *Cancer Chemother. Pharmacol.,* 7, 223, 1982.

62. Drewinko, B., Brown, B. W., and Gottlieb, J. A., The effect of *cis-* diaminedichloroplatinum(II) on cultured human lymphoma cells and its therapeutic implications, *Cancer Res.,* 33, 3091, 1973.

63. Bergerat, J-P., Barlogie, B., and Drewinko, B., Effects of *cis*-dichlorodiaminoplatinum(II) on human colon carcinoma cells, *in vitro, Cancer Res.,* 39, 1334, 1979.

64. Moran, R. E. and Straus, M. J., Effects of pulse and continuous intravenous infusion of *cis*-diamminedichloroplatinum on L1210 leukemia *in vivo, Cancer Res.,* 41, 4993, 1981.

65. Jacobs, C., Bertino, J. R., Goffinet, D. R., Fee, W. E., and Goode, R. L., 24-Hour infusion of *cis*-platinum in head and neck cancers, *Cancer,* 42, 2135, 1978.

66. Bozzino, J. M., Prasad, V., and Koriech, O. M., Avoidance of renal toxicity of 24-hour infusion of cisplatin, *Cancer Treat. Rep.*, 65, 351, 1978.
67. Hayes, D. M., Cvitkovic, E., Golbey, R. B., Scheiner, E., Helson, L., and Krakoff, I. W., High dose *cis*-platinum diamminedichloride: amelioration of renal toxicity by mannitol diuresis, *Cancer*, 39, 1372, 1977.
68. Rainey, R. M., and Alberts, D. S., Safe, rapid administration schedule for *cis*-platinum-mannitol, *Med. Pediatr. Oncol.*, 4, 371, 1978.
69. Yap, H-Y., Salem, P., Hortobagyi, G. N., Bodey, G. P., Sr., Buzdar, A. U., Tashima, C. K., and Blamenschein, G. R., Phase II study of *cis*-dichlorodiammineplatinum(II) in advanced breast cancer, *Cancer Treat. Rep.*, 62, 405, 1978.
70. Salem, P., Hall, S. W., Benjamin, R. S., Murphy, W. K., Warton, J. T., and Bodey, G. P., Clinical phase I-II study of *cis*-dichlorodiammineplatinum(II) given by continuous IV infusion, *Cancer Treat. Rep.*, 62, 1553, 1978.
71. Lokich, J. J., Phase I study of *cis*-diamminedichloroplatinum(II) administered as a constant 5-day infusion, *Cancer Treat. Rep.*, 64, 905, 1980.

Chapter 9

RATE-CONTROLLED DELIVERY OF ANTIBIOTICS

Michel G. Bergeron and Marc LeBel

TABLE OF CONTENTS

I. INTRODUCTION

The question of whether antimicrobial agents should be administered by continuous infusion or by intermittent injections is a matter of controversy.[1-6] Both clinical and experimental investigations dealing with this question have been limited, and convincing proof or evidence of the superiority of either mode of administration has been lacking.[7-12]

To be effective, antibiotics must be active in vitro against the offending agents and must reach sufficient concentrations at the site of infection to control the infection. Early studies have revealed that penicillin was unevenly distributed in accessible body fluids and that the amount of drug detectable in blood was often insufficient to explain therapeutic response.[13] In fact, penicillin could still be detected in infected wound exudates several hours after the antibiotic had disappeared from blood.[13] More so, investigators discovered early on that antibiotics could either diffuse passively into interstitial fluids and tissues, or could be actively transported into body humors or selected sites. These noticeable variations in tissue distribution further encouraged clinicians and researchers to look for new modes of therapy and to investigate whether or not modifications in the modes of administration of antibiotics might influence the outcome of therapy.

Gerber, in 1946, was the first investigator to compare intermittent dosing with continuous infusion of antibiotics.[14] He showed that intermittent administration of penicillin G every 3 hr at daily doses of 25,000 to 50,000 U was more effective than continuous infusion of 100,000 to 500,000 U of penicillin in the treatment of subacute and acute bacterial endocarditis. Early animal studies done by Eagle and Schmidt between 1946 and 1951, and comparing different dosing regimens revealed that by modifying dosage and intervals between dosage, one could affect outcome of therapy.[1-6] In fact, it was found that whatever method of administration one used, in order to be effective, treatment should provide concentration of drug in tissue in excess of the effective levels, i.e., the minimum inhibitory concentration (MIC) of the infecting agent.[1,5,15] In the absence of levels sufficient to prevent growth of surviving bacteria, treatment failure or recurrence of infection may be observed.[16] Continuously maintained bactericidal levels are particularly important in order to achieve cure in cases of severe infection such as bacterial endocarditis or infections in neutropenic patients for whom host defenses may not necessarily operate in conjunction with antimicrobial agents.[4,7-10,17,18] These constant levels of drug, however, may not be indispensable in cases of infection in which both host defenses and drugs are operative.[4,6,11,19-21]

Schmidt has shown that a delay of up to 8 hr with levels below MIC was acceptable in some types of infection; Eagle has also demonstrated that some microorganisms continued to be inhibited even after concentrations of antibiotics had fallen down below MIC while other bacteria would resume multiplication much faster.[1-6]

The objective of this chapter is to review the experimental and clinical evidence on how the use of different dose schedules of antimicrobial agents affects the pharmacological responses. In this chapter, we have reviewed:

- The pharmacokinetic and pharmacodynamic impact of intermittent and continuous administration of antibiotics on:

  A. The tissue distribution of these drugs in humans and animals
  B. The efficacy of these agents in experimental and human infections
  C. The toxicity of antimicrobials in humans and animals

- New antibiotic targeting delivery systems including:

A. Liposomes
B. Other delivery systems

II. INTERMITTENT VS. CONTINUOUS ADMINISTRATION OF ANTIBIOTICS

Although a wealth of literature has been published on the issue of whether or not antibiotics should be administered by intermittent administration or by continuous infusion, it is extremely hard to draw any conclusion. The difficulty resides in the fact that most investigators have limited their animal or clinical investigations to the pharmacokinetic aspects of antimicrobial agents, or else have evaluated the clinical outcome of antibiotic therapy without specifically analyzing simultaneously the distribution of drugs at the site of infection. Both issues rarely have been dealt with concurrently. This is of critical importance. In fact, besides the commonly known factors including the physicochemical properties of antibiotics, blood supply to the site of infection, binding of drugs to proteins in serum, interstitial fluid or tissue, membrane permeability and active transport which might influence tissue distribution, the inflammatory process and the presence of enzymes from bacteria which may locally destroy antibiotics should always be remembered as factors which may influence positively or negatively the concentration of drugs in tissues and modify the outcome of therapy.

Beside the above factors which may influence à la fois tissue distribution and the outcome of therapy, several other variables render the critical interpretation of published data extremely difficult. The experimental model used, the animal species, the type of microorganisms, the status of the host, the dosage regimen, and even the metabolic transformation of antibiotics are all factors which may affect tissue distribution and outcome. For example, rabbits will desacetylate antibiotics to a greater degree than humans so that the metabolized antibiotic, which is not as active as the nontransformed antibiotic, might be less effective in rabbits than in humans.[22]

All of the above factors must thus be taken into consideration before drawing any conclusion on the role of modes of administration of antibiotics on success of therapy. For the purpose of the discussion, we will present several comparative studies on intermittent vs. continuous administration of antibiotics.

A. Tissue Distribution of Antibiotics Following Intermittent or Continuous Administration

1. Animal Studies

Several animal models have been used to investigate whether or not tissue distribution of antimicrobials would be affected by different modes of administration. Tissue fluid pharmacokinetic models including interstitial fluid, tissue cages, and the fibrin clot model have been most commonly used to study the passive diffusion of antibiotics from serum to tissue fluid. The interstitial fluid models are rapidly equilibrating models where tissue fluid antibiotic levels will equilibrate rapidly with serum while the latter two are slowly equilibrating models.

Table 1 summarizes some of the available data on the peripheral distribution of antibiotics following intermittent injection (very rapid bolus or short infusion) or continuous administration of antimicrobials. Essential components of the investigations including the experimental models, sample size, antibiotics studied, modes of administration, dose, infusion time, interval between doses, and the number of doses are presented so that these factors, which may all influence tissue penetration, can be compared. When available, we have used the ratio (%) of the area under the curve (AUC) in tissue over serum ($AUC_{t/s}$) as a better indicator of tissue penetration than the ratio peak tissue over peak serum which may vary considerably from one protocol to the

Table 1

TISSUE PENETRATION OF ANTIBIOTICS FOLLOWING INTERMITTENT OR CONTINUOUS ADMINISTRATION IN "TISSUE FLUID PHARMACOKINETIC MODELS"

Interstitial Fluid

Experimental models	Sample size	Antibiotic	Mode of administration	Dose	Infusion time (hr)	Interval (hr)	Number of dose(s)	$\frac{Peak_t}{Peak_s}$	$\frac{AUC_t}{AUC_s}$	Results, conclusions	Ref.
Experimental wound infection in rabbits	6 rabbits (4 wounds each)	Cephaloridine	Intermittent i.v.	200 mg	Bolus	6	1 and 2	27.2 and 136.4	N.A.	Higher concentration in the wound in a shorter period of time	23
			Continuous i.v.	L.D. 50 mg then 30 mg	6	—	1	29.6			
Paper disc s.c. in rabbits	15 rabbits (5—6 discs each)	Penicillin G	Intermittent i.v.	22.5 mg/kg	0.25	3	2	56	N.A.	Bolus yielded higher concentration in "interstitial fluid" but percentage of penetration is fairly similar	24
			Continuous i.v.	45 mg/kg	6	—	1	40			
		Gentamicin	Intermittent i.v.	6 mg/kg	Bolus	—	1	99		Bolus produced faster peak but smaller percentage of penetration	25
			Continuous i.v.	6 mg/kg	6	—	1	164			
Paper disc s.c. in rabbits	4 rabbits (8—12 discs each)	Aztreonam	Intermittent i.v.	25 mg/kg	0.5	6	4	58	171	Both regimens achieved similar peak levels; bolus produced faster peak and better tissue penetration according to AUC	26
			Continuous i.v.	100 mg/kg	24	—	1	60	94		
Paper disc s.c. in rabbits	8 rabbits (8—12 discs each)	Cefuroxime	Intermittent i.v.	25 mg/kg	0.5	6	4	46	45	Opposite results of tissue penetration, whether they are expressed according to peak or AUC	
			Continuous i.v.	100 mg/kg	24	—	1	65	35		
		Ampicillin	Intermittent i.v.	25 mg/kg	0.5	6	4	43	59	Same	
			Continuous i.v.	100 mg/kg	24	—	1	61	38		

Tissue Cage

Experimental models	Sample size	Antibiotic	Mode of administration	Dose	Infusion time (hr)	Interval (hr)	Number of dose(s)	$\frac{Peak_t}{Peak_s}$	$\frac{AUC_t}{AUC_s}$	Results, conclusions	Ref.
S.C. stainless steel cylinders in dogs	3 dogs (4 cylinders each)	Ampicillin Gentamicin Clindamycin Tetracycline Cephalothin	Intermittent i.v.	25 mg/kg	Bolus	6	4	41.7, 81.8, 70	N.A.	I.V. intermittent "push" showed comparable levels in wound fluid 4—12 times faster than continuous method after 12 hr; highest levels in wound fluid achieved with intermittent	27
			Intermittent i.m.	2 mg/kg		6	4	N.D.			
			Continuous i.v.	4 mg/kg	24	—	1	58.3, 40.8, 14.3			
				7 mg/kg				?, 25.0, 30.0			
								109, 71.5, 69.2			
I.P. chambers in rabbits	6 rabbits (4 chambers each)	Gentamicin	Intermittent i.v.	1.7 mg/kg	Bolus	—	1	10.3	N.A.	Bolus administration gave higher capsula fluid levels over first 2 hr, then no difference was seen	28
			Continuous i.v.	1.7 mg/kg	0.5	—	1	46.8			
S.C. tissue cage in rabbits	20 rabbits (1 cage each)	Cephalothin	Intermittent i.v.	30 mg/kg	Bolus	3	3	3.4	N.A.	The 0.25 hr infusion yielded higher interstitial level ($p < 0.001$); cumulative effect after multiple dose	29
			Intermittent i.v.	30 mg/kg	0.25	3	3	9.5			
			Continuous i.v.	30 mg/kg	1	3	3	12.6			
			Intermittent i.m.	30 mg/kg	—	3	3	10			

Model	Animals	Drug	Administration	Dose				Concentration		Comments	Ref.
S.C. tissue fluid chambers in rabbits	5 rabbits studied twice (4 chambers each)	Cefazolin	Intermittent i.m.	30 mg/kg	—	4	3	Saline: 2.8 Serum: 17.5 Saline: 10 Serum: ~100	N.A.	In situation close to equilibrium, continuous infusion is more efficient at delivering drug to extravascular space; apparent stable levels are reached earlier with intermittent injection	30
S.C. tissue fluid chambers in rabbits	14 rabbits studied twice (4 chambers each)	Ampicillin	Intermittent i.m.	30 mg/kg	—	4	6	20.5	N.A.	At steady-state conditions, only for ampicillin, constant infusion achieved greater tissue fluid levels; with the three others no difference could be detected	31
			Continuous i.v.	195 mg/kg	26	—	1	~80			
		Oxacillin	Intermittent i.m.	30 mg/kg	—	4	6	22.4			
			Continuous i.v.	195 mg/kg	26	—	1	~66			
		Gentamicin	Intermittent i.v.	4 mg/kg	—	4	7	25.7			
			Continuous i.v.	24 mg/kg	24	—	1	~100			
		Amikacin	Intermittent i.m.	8 mg/kg	—	4	3	44.0			
			Continuous i.v.	24 mg/kg	12	—	1	~80			

Fibrin Clots

Model	Animals	Drug	Administration	Dose				Concentration		Comments	Ref.
Infected s.c. fibrin clots in rabbits	15 rabbits (5—6 clots each)	Penicillin G	Intermittent i.v.	22.5 mg/kg	0.25	3	2	4	N.A.	Bolus yielded higher peak clot levels but lower percentage of penetration	24
		Gentamicin	Continuous i.v.	44 mg/kg	6	—	1	27		Same	
			Intermittent i.v.	6 mg/kg	Bolus	—	1	20			
			Continuous i.v.	6 mg/kg	6	—	1	65			
Infected s.c. fibrin clots in rabbits	8 rabbits (8—12 clots each)	Aztreonam	Intermittent i.v.	25 mg/kg	0.5	6	4	10.1	49	Both regimens produced similar peak levels but intermittent administration achieved high levels more rapidly	25
			Continuous i.v.	100 mg/kg	24	—	1	60.2	60.5		
		Cefotaxime	Intermittent i.v.	25 mg/kg	0.5	6	4	5	20	Both regimens achieved similar tissue penetration	
			Continuous i.v.	100 mg/kg	24	—	1	22	20		
Infected s.c. fibrin clots in rabbits	8 rabbits (8—12 clots each)	Ampicillin	Intermittent i.v.	25 mg/kg	0.5	6	4	2	6	Intermittent administration produced peak levels alsome MIC and trough levels below MIC	26
			Continuous i.v.	100 mg/kg	24	—	1	2	20		
		Cefuroxime	Intermittent i.v.	25 mg/kg	0.5	6	4	4	15	Intermittent administration achieved higher peak clot levels	
			Continuous i.v.	100 mg/kg	24	—	1	10	17		

Note: N.A. = not available; N.D. = no data.

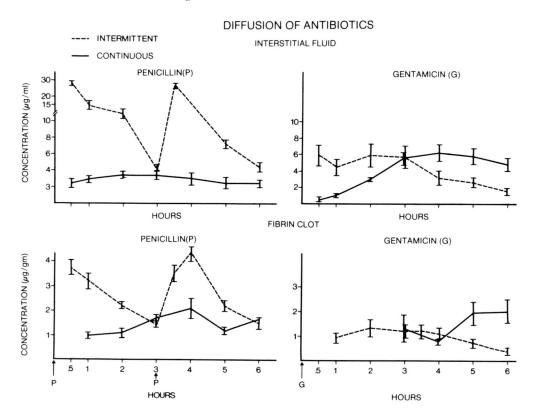

FIGURE 1.   Mean concentrations of antimicrobial agents in interstitial fluid and fibrin clots of rabbits after two bolus injections of 37,500 U of penicillin G/kg given at 0 and 3 hr, or after one bolus injection of gentamicin/kg given at 0 hr (pulse), or during a continuous infusion of either 75,000 U of penicillin G/kg, or 6 mg of gentamicin/kg over a period of 6 hr. Each point gives the mean value for five animals: vertical bars indicate ± SE. (From Bergeron, M. G. et al., *Rev. Infect. Dis.*, 3, 84, 1981. With permission from University of Chicago.)

other.[32] This former ratio was not always available, so that both ratios were presented in this study. Whether one is dealing with interstitial fluid models, tissue cages, or fibrin clots, intermittent rapid injections induced, in general, much higher levels of drugs than continuous infusions.[23-31]

In fact, peak concentrations were usually higher with bolus (or rapid) injection, especially during the first few hours after a single administration. Most of the time, tissue levels were higher after intermittent administration than after continuous infusion. In some instances, the AUC was similar with the two modes of delivery; however, in others, the AUC in peripheral sites was substantially greater with rapid intermittent injections.

Figure 1 further stresses the importance of modes of administration of drugs on the penetration of antibiotics in interstitial fluid and fibrin clots. Following a bolus injection, the levels of penicillin G in interstitial fluid reached values up to eight times those observed during the continuous infusion. In fibrin clots, delays in reaching maximum levels after continuous infusion were even more striking.

Minimal change in the time of infusion was also shown to greatly affect tissue distribution. This is well illustrated in Table 2 where we have compared the influence of time of infusion on the ratio AUC_t/AUC_s of several antibiotics in different animal models. The similitude between the results is quite striking. A constant finding is that

Table 2

INFLUENCE OF TIME OF INFUSION ON THE RATIO AUC$_t$/AUC$_s$
FOLLOWING THE INJECTION OF SEVERAL ANTIBIOTICS

Antibiotic	Dose (mg/kg)	Time of infusion	$\dfrac{\text{AUC}_t}{\text{AUC}_s}$	Models	Ref.
Gentamicin	1.7	2.5 min	0.84	Cage	28
		30 min	1.50		
Gentamicin	6	15 min	0.56	Clots	33
		6 hr	0.28		
Cephalothin	30	1 min	0.94	Cage	
		15 min	1.41		
		60 min	0.67		
Erythromycin	44	60 min	0.86	Clots	Simard and Bergeron
		4 hr	0.62		(unpublished)
Chloramphenicol	50	60 min	0.91	Clots	Simard and Bergeron
		4 hr	0.35		(unpublished)
Cefotaxime	100	30 min	0.67	Clots	25
		24 hr	0.23		

the ratio (AUC$_t$/AUC$_s$) is much lower following a long infusion than after a bolus, suggesting again that the penetrability of antibiotics is favored by short courses of antibiotics and that to reach high tissue levels rapidly, the drug should be given as a bolus.[34]

Other animal models, besides tissue fluid models, have been used to investigate the influence of modes of administration on drug penetration. These include models of meningitis and of eye penetration where the active transport of antibiotics into specialized sites including CSF and vitreous humor can be evaluated.

In contrast with tissue fluid pharmacokinetic models where levels of antibiotics were in general higher following intermittent injections, rate penetrations were quite variable, and both CSF and intraocular penetrations were in general not greatly influenced by modes of administrations (Table 3).

2. Human Studies (Clinical Trials)

Human experimentation trying to answer the above questions is very limited, but as shown in Table 4, tissue levels in bile and bronchial secretions were in general higher following bolus or intermittent administration of antibiotics.

3. Conclusion on Tissue Levels

Although there was a general trend in favor of intermittent administrations of antibiotics, it is clear from the data presented that there are few discrepancies which are hard to fully explain, especially when one deals with data from the same animal models. Van Etta et al. have pointed out that some of the inconsistencies noted previously may have been due to a failure to achieve steady state, which may take up to 24 hr in some experimental models.[31] For example, Peterson et al. using the visking chambers have shown that cefazolin required 10 hr to reach stable tissue fluid concentrations by intermittent injections, and 26 hr by constant infusion.[30] Also of importance is the fact that these authors did not find that intermittent pulse dosing resulted in higher mean extravascular levels than did constant infusion of the drug.

These studies further stress the need for better standardization of animal models and protocols aimed at studying the influence of modes of administration on tissue distribution of antibiotics.

Table 3
TISSUE PENETRATION OF ANTIBIOTICS FOLLOWING INTERMITTENT OR CONTINUOUS ADMINISTRATION IN SPECIALIZED SITES WHERE ANTIMICROBIALS ARE ACTIVELY TRANSPORTED

Experimental models	Sample size	Antibiotic	Mode of administration	Dose	Infusion time (hr)	Interval (hr)	Number of dose(s)	Percentage of tissue penetration		Results, conclusions	Ref.
								$\dfrac{Peak_1}{Peak_2}$	$\dfrac{AUC_1}{AUC_2}$		
CSF in normal dogs and aseptic meningitis in dogs	76 dogs	Penicillin G	Intermittent i.m.	30,000 U/kg	Bolus	—	1	Serum levels exceed upper limit of assay	N.A.	Highest immediate CSF levels with intermittent schedule; highest concentrations at 4 and 6 hr after administration	12
			Intermittent i.v.	6 mg/kg	4 and 6	0 and 2	1 and 3				
			Continuous i.v.	60,000 and 90,000 U/kg		—	1				
CSF of normal dogs	20 dogs	Amoxicillin	Intermittent i.v.	1 g	Bolus	—	1		N.A.	Higher CSF levels with "slow intravenous infusion" (continuous) No significant difference between two regimens	35
			"Continuous" i.v.	1 g	1	—	1				
		Penicillin G	Intermittent i.v.	1,200 mg	Bolus	—	1				
			"Continuous" i.v.	1,200 mg	1	—	1				
CSF in pneumococcal meningitis in rabbits		Penicillin G	Intermittent i.v.		8	4	2		N.A.	Bolus highest peak at 5 hr, killing identical	36
			Continuous i.v.		—	—	1				
Infected vitreous humor of rabbits	55 rabbits (110 eyes)	Gentamicin	Intermittent i.m.	4.16 mg/kg	—	3	4	24.5%	N.A.	Intraocular penetration not influenced by mode of administration	37
			Continuous i.v.	L.D. = 1.6 mg/kg then 19.2 mg/kg	12	—	1	42%			

Table 4

PENETRATION OF ANTIBIOTICS FOLLOWING INTERMITTENT OR CONTINUOUS ADMINISTRATION IN BILE AND BRONCHIAL SECRETIONS

Diseases in human	Sample size (patients)	Antibiotic	Mode of administration	Dose	Infusion time (hr)	Interval (hr)	Number of dose(s)	Peak,/Peak,	AUC,/AUC,	Results, conclusions	Ref.
Bronchial secretions from bronchopulmonary infections or tracheobronchitis	10	Netilmicin	Intermittent i.v.	2.5 mg/kg	0.033	8	3	8.8%	19.2%	Similar percentage of tissue penetration but higher bronchial secretions level after intermittent schedule	38
			Continuous i.v.	7.5 mg/kg	24	—	1	18.2%	19.3%		
Bronchial secretions from bronchopulmonary infections or tracheobronchitis	12	Amoxicillin	Intermittent i.v.	16.7 mg/kg	0.033	8	3	8.3%	N.A.	Higher tissue penetration and higher bronchial secretions level after short-injection	39
			Continuous i.v.	16.7 mg/kg	1.0	8	3	4.2%			
Cholecystectomized patients	6	Cefazolin	Intermittent i.v.	1.5 g	Bolus	6	4	N.A.	N.A.	Authors report higher levels in bile with intermittent schedule for first 3 hr and lowest from 3-6 hr. Note that one patient is mainly responsible for higher values in first 3 hr	40
			Continuous i.v.	6 g	24	—	1	N.A.	N.A.		

B. Efficacy of Antibiotics Following Intermittent or Continuous Administration
1. Animal Studies

Eagle et al. and Schmidt et al. were the first ones to try to determine optimal dosage of penicillin for the treatment of treponemal and streptococcal infections induced in animals.[1-6] These studies generally involved a very large sample size and a wide range of dosing. Since these early studies were also designed to establish the optimum formulation of penicillin, they often compare repository forms of penicillin (penicillin G procaine, penicillin G procaine in oil) to immediate release forms (penicillin G aqueous).

As shown in Table 5, these early studies have demonstrated that massive doses of penicillin G were no more effective than lower dosages, providing concentrations were in excess of the minimum inhibitory concentrations. For example, for the treatment of intraperitoneal infections due to Group B and Group A β-hemolytic streptococci or *Streptococcus pneumoniae,* larger doses of antibiotics were needed when longer intervals were used. Administration of a large single dose or repeated administration of relatively low doses would yield similar results.

These investigators can be considered as "pioneers" that stimulated other researchers to better define new approaches for the treatment of infectious diseases.[1-6] It took more than 25 years before these concepts were addressed again.[24] In fact, Bergeron and co-workers in 1978 (cf. Tables 1 and 5) compared continuous and intermittent administrations of antibiotics in an attempt to correlate distribution in tissue with efficacy in vivo. They were the first to extensively analyze the influence of administration of these drugs on the dynamic interaction that exists between the penetration of the drugs into tissues and their efficacy in vivo. In these experiments, they used the fibrin clot model in rabbits infected with *Streptococcus faecalis.* In fact, this model seems to be one of the most appropriate models to study both tissue penetration and in vivo efficacy.[34] In contrast to tissue cage models in which the protein content of the so-called interstitial fluid is high and where inflammatory cells are observed, leukocytes and immunoglobulins are absent in fibrin clots. Therefore, the bacteria and antimicrobial drugs can interact without the help of host defenses, a situation that is prevalent in neutropenic patients or the vegetation of bacterial endocarditis.[34] As shown in Figure 2, these experiments demonstrated that bolus injections resulted in a more rapid achievement and greater degree of bactericidal activity in serum and efficacy in vivo than did continuous infusion. These data also suggest that the area under the curve for serum was not a good indicator of the efficacy of the drugs in vivo. With this model, there was a good correlation between the bactericidal activity in serum and the elimination of *Streptococcus faecalis* from the clots. Synergism in vivo, as determined by counts of live bacteria in the clots, was demonstrated after intermittent injections of penicillin G and gentamicin, but constant infusion of the combination was not synergistic.[24]

In the continuous infusion experiments, both penicillin G and gentamicin diffused slowly; at 4 and 5 hr after administration was begun, the levels of drug in serum had barely reached the MICs against the enterococcus (Figure 2). A bolus injection followed by a continuous infusion might have improved the efficacy of the drugs in vivo in our model, but these methods would have necessitated an increase in the total amount of drug given over the same period of time.[24] The use of the lowest effective dose possible is critical when one deals with potentially toxic antimicrobial agents such as aminoglycosides for which there might be a very small margin of security between bactericidal activity and toxicity.

Intermittent injections of antibiotics are thus crucial for the rapid killing of bacteria. Recent studies from our laboratory suggest that bolus injections allow a rapid penetration of antibiotics into the core of the fibrin clots, thus inhibiting the microorganisms which otherwise would have been protected if drugs would have only penetrated the

Table 5

COMPARATIVE EFFICACY OF INTERMITTENT AND CONTINUOUS ADMINISTRATION IN EXPERIMENTAL MODELS OF INFECTIONS

Experimental models	Sample size	Microorganism	Antibiotic	Dosing regimen	Age of infection at time of treatment	Results, conclusions	Ref.
Syphilis in rabbits	355	Treponema pallidum	Penicillin G i.m. (aqueous)	1.2 to 38.4 mg/kg q 0.25,1,2, 4,12,24, 96 hr for 4 doses	6 weeks	Q 12 hr administration gives optimum results; larger doses needed if shorter or longer interval used	1
"I.P. infection" in rabbits	66	Group B streptococcus	Penicillin G i.m.	0.6 to 512 mg/kg q 3,6,9,24 hr for 4 doses and q 1,3 hr for 10 doses	6 hr	Larger doses needed when given in single injection than divided doses	2
		Group A β-hemolytic streptococcus			0		
		Streptococcus pneumoniae			0		
"I.M. infection" in mice	105	Group A β-hemolytic streptococcus	Penicillin G i.m. (aqueous)	200 mg/kg q 24 hr for 1 day	0 and 24 hr	Massive doses no more effective than procaine penicillin in oil	3
			Penicillin G i.m. (procaine, in oil)	45 mg/kg for 1 dose	0 and 24 hr		
"I.M. infection" in mice	320	Group A β-hemolytic streptococcus	Penicillin G i.m. (aqueous)	0.05 to 200 mg/kg q 0.75 to 24 hr for 1 to 16 doses	2 hr	"Continuous" (i.e., q 0.75 hr) most effective	4
Meningitis in rabbits	30	Streptococcus pneumoniae	Penicillin G	240 mg over 2 min q 4 hr for 2 doses L.D. 60 mg then 60 mg/hr for 8 hr	16—18 hr	Initial acceleration in bactericidal rate with bolus between time 1 and 2 hr; after 2 hr same bactericidal killing	36

Table 5 (continued)
COMPARATIVE EFFICACY OF INTERMITTENT AND CONTINUOUS ADMINISTRATION IN
EXPERIMENTAL MODELS OF INFECTIONS

Experimental models	Sample size	Microorganism	Antibiotic	Dosing regimen	Age of infection at time of treatment	Results, conclusions	Ref.
Acute pneumonia in guinea pigs	60	*Pseudomonas aeruginosa*	Tobramycin i.p.	20 and 40 mg/kg over 24 hr[a] or 1 bolus for 3 doses	5 hr	Better decrease in colony count with intermittent dosing	41
Chronic pneumonia in rats	72	*Pseudomonas aeruginosa*	Tobramycin i.p.	10,20,40 mg/kg over 24 hr[b] or 1 bolus for 7 doses	120 hr	No statistical difference between mode of administration	41
Endocarditis in rabbits	47	*Pseudomonas aeruginosa*	Tobramycin i.p.	22.5 mg/kg over 24 hr or 1 bolus for 7 doses	24 hr	No statistical difference between mode of administration	41
Peritonitis in rats with neutropenia	270	*Pseudomonas aeruginosa*	Amikacin and/or ticarcillin i.m.	Doses adjusted to give same AUC for both schedule	4 hr	Constant infusion significantly better than intermittent bolus	42
"I.P. infection" in rats	684	*Streptococcus pneumoniae*	Penicillin G i.m. (aqueous)	4,8,16 mg/kg q 2,4,8,12,24 hr for 2 and 4 doses	4 hr	Q 2,4,8 hr administration more effective than 12,24 hr	5
			Penicillin G i.m. (procaine, aqueous)	4,8,16 mg/kg q 24 hr for 2 and 4 doses	4 hr		
Lobar pneumonia in rats	260	*Streptococcus pneumoniae*	Penicillin G i.m. (aqueous)	2,4,8 mg/kg q 2,4,8,12,24 hr for 4 doses	24 hr	Q 8 hr administration is the best regimen	6
			Penicillin G i.m. (procaine, aqueous)	2,4,8,16 mg/kg q 24 hr for 4 doses	24 hr		
S.C. fibrin clots in rabbits	(5—6 clots each)	*Streptococcus faecalis*	Penicillin G i.v.	45 mg/kg over 6 hr or ÷ 2 bolus	<0.5 hr	Bolus injection of both drugs yielded better killing power	17

Model	No. of clots	Organism	Antibiotic	Dosage regimen	$t_{1/2}$	Results	Ref.
			Gentamicin	6 and 9 mg/kg over 6 hr or 1 bolus	<0.5 hr	Intermittent bolus were significantly more effective	25
S.C. fibrin clots in rabbits	8—12 clots each	Haemophilus influenzae (β-lactamase +)	Aztreonam i.v.	100 mg/kg over 24 hr or ÷ 4 bolus every 6 hr	0.5 hr	Intermittent bolus were significantly more effective only for the first 3 hr	25
		Haemophilus influenzae (β-lactamase +)	Cefotaxime i.v.	100 mg/kg over 24 hr or ÷ 4 bolus every 6 hr	0.5 hr		
Fibrin clots in rabbits	(8—12 clots each)	Haemophilus influenzae (β-lactamase −)	Ampicillin i.v.	100 mg/kg over 24 hr or ÷ 4 bolus every 6 hr	0.5 hr	Both regimen showed similar efficacy	26
		Haemophilus influenzae (β-lactamase +)	Cefuroxime i.v.	100 mg/kg over 24 hr or ÷ 4 bolus every 6 hr	0.5 hr	Same	26

[a] Osmotic pumps, Alzet®

[b] S.C. pump, Infusaid®

IN VIVO EFFICACY

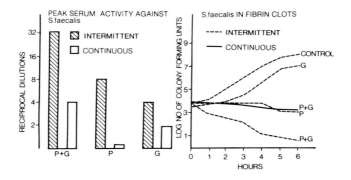

FIGURE 2.   Peak bactericidal activity of serum and log number of
cfu or *Streptococcus faecalis* in fibrin clots in rabbits after i.v. bolus
injections (pulse) or continuous infusion of penicillin G (P) and gentamicin (G) given alone or in combination. (From Bergeron, M. G. et
al., *Rev. Infect. Dis.,* 3, 84, 1981. With permission.)

fibrin superficially. A large gradient between serum and tissue is probably necessary to
allow antibiotics to penetrate into all the layers of infected tissues. Continuous infusion
may allow drugs to penetrate deeply into the fibrin, but it takes a long time. This long
time may allow bacteria to multiply and produce more enzymes which may destroy the
antibiotics at the site of infection. This is especially true when drug penetrates the tissue
very slowly and in very small amounts, as we have observed in continuous infusion
experiments. In fact, we have recently shown the in vivo enzymatic destruction of
cefoperazone by a β-lactamase-producing strain of *Hemophilus influenzae* inserted
into the clots.[25] These data further stress the importance of taking into consideration
the concentrations of active (nondestroyed) drug at the site of infection.

As shown in Table 5, aztreonam and cefotaxime administered intermittently were
more effective against β-lactamase positive *H. influenzae.* Such difference could not
be demonstrated with ampicillin and cefuroxime. We have also demonstrated that a
single large bolus which allows good levels in tissues is often more effective than intermittent injections with lower doses.

Using their experimental meningitis model in rabbits, Sande et al. (cf. Table 5) observed an enhanced bactericidal effect with intermittent infusion of penicillin early in
the treatment period (only between the first and second hours of therapy), a reflection
of higher CSF levels.[36] Over the remaining 6 hr of treatment, the magnitude of bacterial killing (change in log titer) was identical in groups of animals receiving either intermittent or continuous dosages.

Powell et al.[41] have recently reported on the effects of antibiotic concentration oscillation on in vivo efficacy and toxicity of tobramycin. One daily dose rapidly injected
was as efficacious or even more effective than continuous infusion using osmotic
pumps (Alzet®) or Infusaid® pumps. These results are in accordance with our data
in fibrin clots, but one must be careful before suggesting that a single large daily dose
should be given instead of standard intermittent or continuous therapy. On the other
hand, innovative approaches to therapy should be considered seriously, since it may at
the same time improve efficacy and quality of care. As long as antibiotics are maintained at levels above MIC in tissues, we strongly believe that breakthrough bacteremia
or recurrence of infection should be prevented.[16,43] Large doses of antibiotics at long
intervals should be investigated further in clinical trials. In addition to tissue levels of
antibiotics which are crucial to the outcome of therapy, in vivo postantibiotic effects

(PAE) observed recently by Sande et al. should also be discussed here.[36] PAE, an in vitro phenomenon, refers to a period of several hours after complete removal of the antibiotic, during which there is no growth of the target organism. PAE varies depending on the antibiotic used and the bacteria studied.[44] The duration of PAE is dependent on both the concentration of drug and duration of exposure. For *Staphylococcus aureus,* most antimicrobial agents produce a postantibiotic effect lasting 1.5 to 3 hr; streptococci exhibit even longer-lasting effects. For β-lactam antibiotics, this effect on Gram-positive microorganisms is observed at concentrations approximately five times the MIC. In contrast, Gram-negative bacteria show a more variable pattern; β-lactam antibiotics cause a negligible PAE against strains of *Escherichia coli, Enterobacter* and *Pseudomonas aeruginosa.*[44-45] In Craig's experimental model, regrowth of *E. coli, Klebsiella pneumoniae,* and *P. aeruginosa* occurred almost immediately after serum levels feel below MIC.[46]

However, drugs which inhibit protein synthesis, such as chloramphenicol or tetracycline, or interfere with RNA synthesis, such as rifampin, generally produce a substantial PAE lasting some 0.5 to 2.5 hr with Gram-positive and Gram-negative organisms.[44]

For aminoglycosides, the time course of antibacterial effects on Gram-negative bacilli is much different than with β-lactam antibiotics. Intermittent exposure of these organisms to aminoglycosides results in a marked reduction in the number of viable organisms that is rapid and dose dependent. When levels fall below the MIC, the organisms do not immediately recover, but are maintained in a suppressed phase for several hours prior to regrowth. Using an in vivo model, Gerber et al. have observed that the activity of aminoglycosides lasted up to 10 hr even though levels exceeded the MIC for only 2 hr.[47]

It is hard to draw any conclusion on PAE from the data presented, but if one combines both tissue levels and postantibiotic effect, it may be suggested that with antibiotics which have a long postantibiotic effect, intermittent dosing at long intervals may be effective, while shorter intervals between doses or even bolus injection followed by continuous injection may be preferable if antibiotics with no PAE are used.

It is too early to make any recommendations, but, as we will see in the next sections dealing with clinical trials, only two studies have shown some advantages with intermittent dosing over continuous infusion for the treatment of Gram-negative bacteria with aminoglycosides.[41,48] Others have shown no difference.[41]

2. Human Studies (Clinical Trials)

Most of the data on the role of intermittent vs. continuous administration of antimicrobials have been generated in one center. As shown in Table 6, Bodey and co-workers have gathered a vast experience on the use of aminoglycosides in cancer and/or neutropenic patients.[50] They have argued for years that in these patients with limited host defenses, subinhibitory aminoglycosides serum concentrations, which may result from intermittent dosing, may favor the multiplication and dissemination of infection. They thus have used continuous infusion of the aminoglycosides to ensure that serum concentrations exceeded the MIC and MBC at all times. None of their studies clearly demonstrated any advantage to be gained from continuous infusion of aminoglycosides. However, in one trial where they have used a combination of tobramycin and cefamandole, this latter drug was given as a continuous infusion, and it has resulted in improved efficacy.[10]

Feld suggested that aminoglycosides alone may be preferably given by continuous infusion, but that this benefit was probably lost when they were given in combination with β-lactam antibiotics.[51] He also made the point that an excess of 600 patients would be needed to show any statistical difference between these two regimens.[8,51] This comment probably applies to all these reports presented in Table 6.

Table 6

COMPARATIVE EFFICACY OF ANTIBIOTICS FOLLOWING INTERMITTENT AND CONTINUOUS ADMINISTRATION IN CLINICAL TRIALS

Diseases or conditions	Sample size	Antibiotic	Mode of administration	Loading dose	Regular daily dose	Infusion time (hr)	Interval (hr)	Concomitant therapy	Results, conclusions	Ref.
Endocarditis (Subacute and acute)	25 patients and historical experience	Penicillin G / Penicillin G (aqueous)	Intermittent i.m. / Continuous i.v.	50—100,000 U / —	25—50,000 U / 100—500,000 U	— / 24	3 / —	None	Intermittent injection more effective	14
Cancer patients with fever ≥ 38.3°C	160 patients 195 febrile episodes	Amikacin	Intermittent i.v. / Continuous i.v.	— / 50 mg/m²	150 mg/m²[a] / 800 mg/m²[b]	0.5 / 24	6 / —	None	Continuous infusion in patients with neutrophil counts of <100/mm³ as good as intermittent therapy in patients with adequate neutrophil counts	7
Cancer patients with fever ≥ 38.3°C and neutropenia (<1000/mm³)	120 patients 133 febrile episodes	Sisomicin	Intermittent i.v. / Continuous i.v.	30 mg/m²	30 mg/m² / 120 mg/m²	0.5 / 24	6 / —	None	Response rate of 61% by continuous infusion and 41% by intermittent dosing (p > 0.05)	8
Cancer patients with fever ≥ 38.3°C and neutropenia (<1000/mm³)	92 patients 100 febrile episodes	Netilmicin	Intermittent i.v. / Continuous i.v.	— / 60 mg/m²	60 mg/m² / 240 mg/m²	0.5 / 24	6 / —	None	Continuous infusion as effective as intermittent administration	9
Cancer patients with fever ≥ 38.3°C	460 febrile episodes	Cefamandole / Cefamandole / Tobramycin	Intermittent i.v. / Continuous i.v. / Continuous i.v.	— / 3 g / 90 mg/m²	3 g / 12 g / 360 mg/m²	0.5 / 24 / 24	6 / — / —	Carbenicillin 5 g q 4 hr over 2 hr	Cefamandole continuous infusion regimen was superior to	10

Pneumococcal	123 patients	Penicillin G procaine	Intermittent i.m.	—	360 mg	—	—	None	intermittent schedule with cefamandole or continuous infusion with tobramycin (p < 0.05)	
		Penicillin G	Continuous i.v.	—	12 g	24	—		Continuous infusion of large doses did not lower the mortality compared to low doses (p < 0.75)	49
Exacerbations of pulmonary infections in cystic fibrosis patients	52 patients	Tobramycin	Intermittent i.v.	—	11 mg/kg	0.33	24	None	Inconclusive results for efficacy	41
			Continuous i.v.	—	11 mg/kg	24	—			
			Intermittent i.v.	—	10 mg/kg	0.33	24			
			Intermittent i.v.	—	12 mg/kg	0.33	24			

a   Approximately 1.5 mg/kg

b   Dose adjusted to try to maintain a serum concentration of 12—16 μg/mℓ

Technical problems, such as necessity to maintain two i.v. sites in these very ill patients, have also been considered as obstacles to this method. Recent studies from Bodey and co-workers seem to suggest that they have decided to abandon the use of continuous infusion of aminoglycosides, but still favored discontinuous infusion (ceftazidime or cefoperazone have been given over 2 hr every 4 hr) of β-lactam antibiotics.[52-53]

Other recent studies have failed to support the contention that one mode of administration of either β-lactam or aminoglycoside may be advantageous over the other, but these latter studies were not performed in neutropenic or cancer patients.[41,49]

The use of newer antibiotics like ceftriaxone, which have a very long half-life ($t_{1/2}$ = 6 to 8 hr) and which "mimics" continuous infusion, may well have in the future an important therapeutic impact. Clearly, further investigations are needed in order to establish the clinical importance of mode of administration (or dosing intervals) in immunodepressed and nonimmunodepressed patients.

C. Toxicity of Antibiotics Following Intermittent and Continuous Administration in Experimental Models and Clinical Studies

As shown in Table 7, animal and clinical antibiotic studies on toxicity have been limited to aminoglycosides.

Continuous intravenous infusion of aminoglycosides in seriously ill cancer patients has been thought to be less nephrotoxic than when comparable doses were given as intravenous injections every 6 hr. The results shown in Table 7 are conflicting. Nephrotoxicity defined as a serum creatinine above 1.4 mg/dℓ and a BUN above 20 mg/dℓ was more frequently observed following intermittent infusion in one study, while two other investigators have demonstrated the opposite situation, and no difference was found in another study.[7-10]

In animal studies where the experiments can be controlled much more easily than in clinical trials, intermittent administrations of aminoglycosides were less toxic than continuous infusion. These data were confirmed in cystic fibrosis patients where auditory, cochlear, and nephrotoxicity was very low in the group receiving a single daily dose of aminoglycosides.[41]

Further investigations comparing single large doses, multiple daily doses, or continuous infusions of aminoglycosides with variable doses are thus needed to further delineate the role of intermittent vs. continuous infusion of antibiotics on the toxicity of these agents. Animal data done in normal *noninfected* animals are of interest, but they may not reflect what happens in an infected patient with all of his underlying pathology.

III. ANTIBIOTIC TARGETING DELIVERY SYSTEMS

Antibiotic delivery systems are in their early phase of investigation and experimentation with these systems has been limited.

A. Liposomes

From new developments in drug formulation, liposomes are one of a number of macromolecular drug carriers presently under investigation. They are phospholipid vesicles with a bilayered lipid membrane which completely encloses an aqueous compartment.[55] They are easily prepared, biodegradable and nontoxic. Furthermore, their distribution and pharmacokinetics can be modified by altering their lipid composition, size, charge, and membrane fluidity.[56] The liposomes have also the potential to reduce toxicity and favorably alter the pharmacokinetics of entrapped drugs. Finally, their structure impacts a certain degree of tissue specificity upon the trapped drug for the reticulo-endothelial system (passive targeting).[57]

Table 7

COMPARATIVE TOXICITY OF ANTIBIOTICS FOLLOWING INTERMITTENT AND CONTINUOUS
ADMINISTRATION IN EXPERIMENTAL MODELS AND CLINICAL STUDIES

Experimental model or diseases in human	Sample size	Antibiotic	Mode of administration	Dosing regimen	Results, conclusions	Ref.
Female mongrel dog	40 dogs	Gentamicin	Intermittent i.v. Continuous i.v.	45 mg/kg once a day over 10 min	Continuous infusion of gentamicin or tobramycin leads to a greater decrease in renal function than in- termittent administration	54
		Tobramycin	Intermittent i.v. Continuous i.v.	L.D. = 4.05 mg/kg then 45 mg/kg/day		
Female mongrel dog	93 dogs	Gentamicin	Intermittent i.v. Intermittent i.v.	45 mg/kg once a day 45 mg/kg/day divided q 4 hr	Same; previous results con- firmed	41
		Tobramycin Netilmicin	Continuous i.v.	L.D. = 45 mg/kg/day		
Exacerbations of pulmonary infections in cystic fibrosis patients	52 patients	Tobramycin	Intermittent i.v. Continuous i.v. Intermittent i.v. Intermittent i.v.	11 mg/kg/day over 10 min 11 mg/kg/day over 24 hr 10 mg/kg/day over 10 min 12 mg/kg/day over 10 min	Possible low toxicity (ne- phro, cochlear, or audi- tory) with single intermit- tent daily schedule	7
Cancer patients with fever >38.3°C	160 patients 195 febrile episodes	Amikacin	Intermittent i.v. Continuous i.v.	150 mg/m² q 6 hr L.D. = 800 mg/m²/day[b]	Nephrotoxicity more com- mon with intermittent in- fusion: 21 and 6%, re- spectively	8
Cancer patients with fever >38.3°C and neutropenia (<1000/mm³)	120 patients 133 febrile episodes	Sisomicin	Intermittent i.v. Continuous i.v.	30 mg/m² q 6 hr L.D. = 120 mg/m²/day	Nephrotoxicity in 13 and 21%, respectively	8
Cancer patients with fever >38.3°C and <1000/mm³)	92 patients 100 febrile episodes	Netilmicin	Intermittent i.v. Continuous i.v.	60 mg/m² q 6 hr L.D. = 240 mg/m²/day	Nephrotoxicity in 12 and 12%, respectively	9
Cancer patients with fever >38.3°C	460 febrile episodes	Cefamandole Cefamandole Tobramycin	Intermittent i.v. Continuous i.v. Continuous i.v.	3 g q 6 hr L.D. = 12 g /day L.D. = 360 mg/m²	Nephrotoxicity in 13, 12 and 12%, respectively	10

ᵃ Approximately 1.5 mg/kg

ᵇ Dose adjusted to try to maintain a serum concentration of 12—16 μg/mℓ.

Applications of lipsomes targeting delivery system to antimicrobial chemotherapy have been recently reviewed.[58] The vast variety of microorganisms, which can survive intracellularly and cause infections, gives some idea of the area in which liposomally-entrapped antimicrobials may be used. Nonbacterial infections including leishmaniasis, malaria, Q fever, and Rocky Mountain spotted fever are probably the prime candidates for this new approach. Bacterial diseases should include brucellosis, leprosy, tuberculosis, and listeria infections. Viral diseases, especially those limited to the liver, spleen, or the lymphatics such as hepatitis, yellow fever, and cytomegalovirus infections may also be ideal targets for liposomal antimicrobial therapy.[58]

In the experimental treatment of leishmaniasis, liposomes reduce toxicity of antimonial drugs and are also much more effective than the nonentrapped drugs.[59-61] One hopes that leishmaniasis will be the first application of liposomally-entrapped drugs in the treatment of an infectious disease in man. Liposomes also offer interesting possibilities for the future of malaria treatment. Two studies reported positive results with antimalarial agents.[62-63]

Few studies have been conducted in the area of liposomes as drug carriers for treating diseases caused by bacteria. Their use in the treatment of experimental tuberculosis have been reported; liposome-associated dihydrostreptomycin has also been investigated in vitro on the killing of phagocytosed *Staphylococcus aureus*.[64-65]

Recent studies have shown that topically applied liposomes may prove to be very effective for the ocular delivery of drugs including antiherpetic drugs and certain antibiotics.[66-67] Interferon has also been successfully used with this method in the treatment of murine hepatitis, and also amphotericin B in experimental histoplasmosis, murine cryptococcosis, and candidosis.[68-71] The latter three infections are not caused by intracellular organisms, but exemplify the potential of liposome targeting delivery system to decrease toxicity and modify pharmacokinetics of encapsulated drugs.

In the area of antimicrobial chemotherapy, the future of liposome systems lies in the ability of the lipid membrane to protect entrapped materials from degradation and to alter the tissue penetration, pharmacokinetics, and toxicity of the new drugs formulation.[58]

B. Other Antibiotic Targeting Delivery Systems

Among other antibiotic targeting delivery systems, the best-established method is the gentamicin-polymethylmethacrylate (PMMA) beads used in the treatment of chronic osteomyelitis. These beads consist of a macromolecular carrier, the PMMA, and 4.5 mg of gentamicin base, an antibiotic which is especially suitable for mixing with PMMA because of its bacteriological and physicochemical properties.[72] Chains with 30 beads are used singly or threaded on a stainless multistranded steel wire. These provide high antibiotic concentrations at the site of implantation which persist for many weeks and greatly exceed the levels required to kill infecting bacteria. The results obtained by 16 different groups of investigators in 1045 patients treated with gentamicin-PMMA beads have been published.[73] Preliminary results with the use of this formulation as prophylaxis against infection in major head and neck surgery has also been reported.[66] It should be kept in mind that such an antibiotic delivery system is an "ancillary treatment" of chronic osteomyelitis which can only be effective if there is appropriate surgical intervention: this remains the most important element of treatment.[74]

Other attempts to bind antibiotics to cement and dacron grafts have also been reported.[75,76] These studies are always aimed at obtaining slow release of antibiotics at therapeutic levels in the adjacent tissue. The above methods, and probably others presently in their early investigational stages, are very appealing systems which should be further evaluated.

IV. CONCLUSION

In this chapter we have summarized the available data on the importance of antibiotic dosage on tissue distribution and clinical efficacy. Based on our own experience combined with those of others, we can conclude that further studies should be done to better delineate the role of variable modes of administration of antibiotics in both humans and animal experimentations.

On the basis of animal experimentation dealing with the comparative distribution of antimicrobial agents in tissues, intermittent therapy may result in greater levels of drugs in tissues than does continuous infusion. In fact, such observation probably holds true for interstitial fluid and fibrin clots but continuous infusion may result in better diffusion of drugs into specific body humors, including cerebrospinal fluid (CSF), the aqueous humor of the anterior chamber of the eye, and bile, fluids into which penetration of both penicillins and cephalosporins is influenced by active transport mechanisms.[12,36-37,40] From available data, we can state that the frequent administration of drugs at short intervals may possibly be an alternative approach to constant infusion. In fact, this method has resulted in a significant accumulation of antibacterial agents in interstitial fluid, ascites, and tissues. The use of probenecid in conjunction with antibiotics has not been discussed in this chapter. In fact, this agent, which blocks tubular secretion of most β-lactams and other drugs, can induce higher levels of antibiotics in serum and tissues but does not influence the percentage of penetration of these drugs in tissues.[77-80]

For humans suffering from severe infections, including bacterial endocarditis and severe neutropenia, some investigators have suggested that continuous infusion of antibacterial agents is the safest and most effective therapy.[1,7-10] From a practical point of view, continuous i.v. infusion may expose the patients to in vitro and in vivo drug incompatibility and possible drug toxicity and allergic reaction, whereas high concentrations of drugs given as bolus injections may induce phlebitis.[54,81-87]

Finally, we believe that intermittent administration of drug is probably the safest and more practical way to administer antibiotics. Large bolus at long intervals is a very appealing new approach to the therapy of infectious diseases, but its role should be confirmed clinically before further suggestions are made.

New methods of drug delivery system, although appealing, need much improvement before they can be recommended as future modes of therapy. Finally, for a treatment to be effective, tissue levels of free (nonprotein bound or tissue bound), antibiotic may not need to be at all times above the MIC. The importance of postantibiotic effects on the in vivo efficacy and antimicrobial agents need to be evaluated further. Finally, it is clear from the literature that much needs to be done to better elucidate the question of whether antimicrobials should be administered by continuous infusions or by intermittent injections.

ACKNOWLEDGMENTS

The authors wish to acknowledge Gaétan Lavoie for his useful comments and Mrs. Lise Villeneuve for the preparation of the manuscript. This work was supported by grant MA5527 and DG 132 from the Medical Research Council of Canada.

REFERENCES

1. Eagle, H., Magnuson, H. J., and Fleischman, R., The effect of the method of administration on the therapeutic efficacy of sodium penicillin in experimental syphilis, *Bull. Johns Hopkins Hosp.*, 77, 168, 1946.
2. Eagle, H., Fleischman, R., and Musselman, A. D., Effect of schedule of administration on the therapeutic efficacy of penicillin, *Am. J. Med.*, 9, 280, 1950.
3. Eagle, H., Experimental approach to the problem of treatment failure with penicillin, *Am. J. Med.*, 13, 389, 1952.
4. Eagle, H., Fleischman, R., and Levy, M., "Continuous" vs. "discontinuous" therapy with penicillin: the effect of the interval between injections on therapeutic efficacy, *N. Engl. J. Med.*, 248, 481, 1953.
5. Schmidt, L. H., Walley, A., and Larson, R. D., The influence of the dosage regimen on the therapeutic activity of penicillin G., *J. Pharmacol. Exp. Ther.*, 96, 258, 1949.
6. Schmidt, L. H. and Walley, A., The influence of the dosage regimen on the therapeutic effectiveness of penicillin G in experimental lobar pneumonia, *J. Pharmacol. Exp. Ther.*, 103, 479, 1951.
7. Barza, M., Principles of tissue penetrations of antibiotics, *J. Antimicrob. Chemother.*, 8 (Suppl C), 7, 1981.
8. Feld, R., Valdivieso, M., Bodey, G. P., and Rodriguez, V., A comparative trial of sisomicin therapy by intermittent versus continuous infusion, *Am. J. Med. Sci.*, 274, 179, 1977.
9. Yap, B. and Bodey, G. P., Netilmicin in the treatment of infections in patients with cancer, *Arch. Intern. Med.*, 139, 1259, 1979.
10. Bodey, G. P., Ketchel, S. J., and Rodriguez, V., A randomized study of carbenicillin plus cefamandole or tobramycin in the treatment of febrile episodes in cancer patients, *Am. J. Med.*, 67, 608, 1979.
11. Barza, M., Brusch, J., Bergeron, M. G., and Weinstein, L., Penetration of antibiotics into fibrin loci in vivo. III. Intermittent vs. continuous infusion and the effect of probenecid, *J. Infect. Dis.*, 129, 73, 1974.
12. Plorde, J. J., Garcia, M., and Petersdorf, R. G., Studies on the pathogenesis of meningitis. IV. Penicillin levels in the cerebrospinal fluid in experimental meningitis, *J. Lab. Clin. Med.*, 64, 960, 1964.
13. Florey, M. E., Turton, E. C., and Duthie, E. S., Penicillin in wound exudates, *Lancet*, 2, 405, 1946.
14. Gerber, I. E. and Schwartzman, G., Penetration of penicillin into foci of infection, *JAMA*, 130, 761, 1946.
15. Hall, W. H., Gerding, D. N., and Schierl, E. A., Penetration of tobramycin into infected extravascular fluids and its therapeutic effectiveness, *J. Infect. Dis.*, 135, 957, 1977.
16. Anderson, E. T., Young, L. S., and Hewitt, W. L., Simultaneous antibiotic levels in "breakthrough" gram-negative rod bacteremia, *Am. J. Med.*, 61, 493, 1976.
17. Merrikin, D. and Rolinson, G. N., Antibiotic levels in experimentally infected mice in relation to therapeutic effect and antibacterial activity in vitro, *J. Antimicrob. Chemother.*, 5, 423, 1979.
18. Geraci, J. E. and Martin, W. J., Antibiotic therapy of bacterial endocarditis. VI. Subacute enterococcal endocarditis: clinical, pathologic and therapeutic consideration of 33 cases, *Circulation*, 10, 173, 1954.
19. Chan, R. A., Benner, E. J., and Hoeprich, P. D., Gentamicin therapy in renal failure: a nomogram for dosage, *Ann. Intern. Med.*, 76, 773, 1972.
20. Weinstein, L. and Dalton, A. C., Host determinants of response to antimicrobial agents, *N. Engl. J. Med.*, 279, 467, 524, 580, 1968.
21. Bigger, J. W., Treatment of staphylococcal infections with penicillin by intermittent sterilization, *Lancet*, 2, 497, 1944.
22. Bergeron, M. G., Nguyen, B. M., Trottier, S., and Gauvreau, L., Penetration of cefamandole, cephalothin and desacetylcephalothin into fibrin clots, *Antimicrob. Agents Chemother.*, 12, 682, 1977.
23. Ehrlich, H. P., Licko, V., and Hunt, T. K., Kinetics of cephaloridine in experimental wounds, *Am. J. Med. Sci.*, 265, 33, 1973.
24. Bergeron, M. G., Nguyen, B. M., and Gauvreau, L., Influence of constant infusion versus bolus injections of antibiotics, *Infection*, 6 (Suppl. 1), 3, 1978.
25. Brousseau, L., Lavoie, G., Simard, P., and Bergeron, M. G., Comparative in vivo efficacy of azthreonam, cefotaxime, moxalactan and cefoperazone: inoculum size effect and enzymuria destruction of cefoperazone, 22nd Interscience Conference of Antimicrobial Agents and Chemotherapy, Miami Beach, October 1982.
26. Lavoie, G. and Bergeron, M. G., Relation between efficacy and β-lactamase stability of antibiotics in an in vivo model, 23rd Interscience Conference of Antimicrobial Agents and Chemotherapy, Las Vegas, October 1983.

27. Alexander, J. W. and Alexander, N. S., The influence of route of administration on wound fluid concentration of prophylactic antibiotics, *J. Trauma,* 16, 488, 1976.

28. Kozak, A. J., Gerding, D. N., Peterson, L. R., and Hall, W. H., Gentamicin intravenous infusion rate: effect on interstitial fluid concentration, *Antimicrob. Agents Chemother.,* 12, 606, 1977.

29. Carbon, C., Chau, V. P., Contrepois, A., and Lamothe-Bisailon, S., Tissue cage experiments with β-lactam antibiotics in rabbits, *Scand. J. Infect. Dis.,* 14, (Suppl.), 127, 1978.

30. Peterson, L. R., Gerding, D. N., and Fasching, C. E., Effects of method of antibiotic administration on extravascular penetration: cross-over study of cefazolin given by intermittent injection or constant infusion, *J. Antimicrob. Chemother.,* 7, 71, 1981.

31. Van Etta, L. L., Kravitz, G. R., Russ, T. E., Fasching, C. E., Gerding, D. N., and Peterson, L. R., Effect of method of administration on extravascular penetration of four antibiotics, *Antimicrob. Agents Chemother.,* 21, 873, 1982.

32. Bergan, T., Pharmacokinetics of tissue penetration of antibiotics, *Rev. Infect. Dis.,* 3, 45, 1981.

33. Bergeron, M. G., Beauchamp, D., Poirier, A., and Bastille, A., Continuous vs. intermittent administration of antimicrobial agents: tissue penetration and efficacy in vivo, *Rev. Infect. Dis.,* 3, 84, 1981.

34. Bergeron, M. G. and Brousseau, L., Tissue fluid pharmacokinetic models in humans and animals, in *Animal Models in the Evaluation of Chemotherapy of Infectious Diseases,* Sande, M., Zak, O., Eds., Academic Press, New York, 1985, in press.

35. Auvergnat, J. C., A comparative experimental study of the circulation of amoxycilin and penicillin G in the cerebrospinal fluid of dogs as a function of the type of intravenous administration, *J. Int. Med. Res.,* 2, 189, 1974.

36. Sande, M. E., Korzeniowski, O. M., Allegro, G. M., Brennan, R. O., Zak, O., and Scheld, W. M., Intermittent or continuous therapy of experimental meningitis due to *Streptococcus pneumoniae* in rabbits: preliminary observations on the postantibiotic effect in vivo, *Rev. Infect. Dis.,* 3, 98, 1981.

37. Barza, M., Kane, A., and Baum, J., Comparison of the effects of continuous and intermittent systemic administration on the penetration of gentamicin into infected rabbit eyes, *J. Infect. Dis.,* 147, 144, 1983.

38. Klastersky, J., Thys, J. P., and Mombelli, G., Comparative studies of intermittent and continuous administration of aminoglycosides in the treatment of bronchopulmonary infections due to Gram-negative bacteria, *Rev. Infect. Dis.,* 3, 74, 1981.

39. Granthil, C., Blanc, M., Charrel, C. T., Jamet, M., and Dumont, J. C., Diffusion intrabronchique de l'amoxicilline administrée selon deux modalités d'injection différentes, *Pathol. Biol.,* 30, 337, 1982.

40. Thys, J. P., Vanderkelen, B., and Klastersky, J., Pharmacological study of cefazolin during intermittent and continuous infusion: a cross-over investigation in humans, *Antimicrob. Agents Chemother.,* 10, 395, 1976.

41. Powell, S. H., Thompson, W. L., Luthe, M. A., Stern, R. C., Grossniklaus, D. A., Bloxham, D. D., Groder, D. L., Jacobs, M. R., DiScenna, A. O., Cash, H. A., and Klinger, J. D., Once-daily vs. continuous aminoglycoside dosing: efficacy and toxicity in animal and clinical studies of gentamicin, netilmicin, and tobramycin, *J. Infect. Dis.,* 47, 918, 1983.

42. Mordenti, J. J., Nightingale, C. H., and Quintiliani, R., Combination antibiotic therapy: comparison of constant infusion and intermittent bolus dosing in an experimental animal model, 23rd Interscience Conference of Antimicrobial Agents and Chemotherapy, Las Vegas, October 1983.

43. Weinstein, M. P. and Reller, L. B., Clinical importance of "breakthrough bacteremia", *Am. J. Med.,* 76, 175, 1984.

44. Bundtzen, R. W., Gerber, A. U., Cohn, D. L., and Craig, W. A., Postantibiotic suppression of bacterial growth, *Rev. Infect. Dis.,* 3, 28, 1981.

45. Kagan, J. P., Zunner, S. H., Keating, M. H., Moon-McDermott, L., and Peter, G., In vitro continuous and bolus infusions of new-β-lactams and gentamicin against *Klebsiella pneumoniae* using a capillary model, 22nd Interscience Conference of Antimicrobial Agents and Chemotherapy, Miami Beach, October 1982.

46. Craig, W. A., The time course of antibacterial effects of aminoglycosides, 13th International Congress of Chemotherapy, Vienna, August-September, 1983.

47. Gerber, A. U., Craig, W. A., Brugger, H. P., Feller, C., Vastola, A. P., and Brandel, J., Impact of dosing intervals on the activity of gentamicin and ticarcillin against *Pseudomonas aeruginosa* in granulocytopenic mice, *J. Infect. Dis.,* 147, 910, 1983.

48. Gerber, A. U., Wiprachtiger, P., Stettler-Spichiger, V., and Lebek, G., Constant infusions vs. intermittent doses of gentamicin against *Pseudomonas aeruginosa* in vitro, *J. Infect. Dis.,* 145, 554, 1982.

49. Brewin, A., Arango, L., Hadley, W. K., and Murray, J. F., High-dose penicillin therapy and pneumococcal pneumonia, *JAMA,* 230, 409, 1974.

50. Bodey, G. P., Valdivieso, M., and Yap, B. S., The role of schedule in antibiotic therapy of the neutropenic patient, *Infection,* 8 (Suppl. 1), S75, 1980.

51. Feld, R., Optimal dosage of beta-lactam antibiotics in neutropenic patients. 13th International Congress of Chemotherapy, Vienna, August-September 1983.
52. Garcia, I., Fainstein, V., Smith, R. G., and Bodey, G. P., Multiple dose pharmacokinetics of ceftazidime in cancer patients, *Antimicrob. Agents Chemother.*, 24, 141, 1983.
53. Bolivar, R., Fainstein, V., Elting, L., and Bodey, G. P., Cefoperazone for the treatment of infections in patients with cancer, *Rev. Infect. Dis.*, 5 (Suppl. 1), S181, 1983.
54. Reiner, N. E., Bloxham, D. D., and Thompson, W. L., Nephrotoxicity of gentamicin and tobramycin given once daily or continuously in dogs, *J. Antimicrob. Chemother.*, 4 (Suppl. A), 85, 1978.
55. Bangham, A. D., Standish, M. M., and Watkins, J. C., Diffusion of univalent ions across the lamellae of swollen phospholipids, *J. Mol. Biol.*, 13, 238, 1965.
56. Juliano, R. L., Interactions of liposomes with the reticulo-endothelial system: implications for the controlled delivery drugs, in *Optimization of Drug Delivery,* Bungard, H., Hansen, A. B., and Kofud, H., Eds., Monskgaard, Copenhagen, 1982, 405.
57. Scherphof, G., Roerdink, F., Hoekstra, D., Zbrowski, J., and Wisse, E., Stability of liposomes in presence of blood constituents: consequences for uptake of liposomal lipid and entrapped compounds by rat liver cells, in *Liposomes in Biological Systems,* Gregoriadis, G., Allison, A. C., Eds., John Wiley & Sons, New York, 1980, 179.
58. Richardson, V. J., Liposomes in antimicrobial chemotherapy, *J. Antimicrob. Chemother.*, 12, 532, 1983.
59. Black, C. D., Watson, G. J., and Ward, R. J., The use of pentostam liposomes in chemotherapy of experimental leishmaniasis, *Trans. R. Soc. Trop. Med. Hyg.*, 71, 550, 1977.
60. Alving, C. R., Steck, E. A., Chapman, W. L., Waits, V. B., Hendricks, L. D., Swartz, G. M., and Hanson, W. L., Liposomes in leishmaniasis: therapeutic effects of antimonial drugs 8-aminoquinolins and tetracycline, *Life Sci.*, 26, 223i, 1980.
61. Trouet, A. V., Pirson, P., Steiger, R., Masquelier, M., Baurain, R., and Gillet, J., Development of new derivatives of primaquine by association with lysomotropic carriers, *Bull. WHO,* 59, 449, 1981.
62. Pirson, P., Steiger, R. F., Trouet, A., Gillet, J., Herman, F., Primaquin-6-methoxy-8-(4'-amino-1'-methylbutyl-amino)quinoline, *Ann. Trop. Med. Parasitol.*, 74, 383, 1980.
63. Alving, C. R., Schneider, I., Swartz, G. M., Jr., and Steck, E. A., Sporozoite-induced malaria: therapeutic effects of glycolipids in liposomes, *Science,* 205, 1142, 1979.
64. Vladimirskii, M. A., Liposomes as vehicles for antitubercular drugs, a new approach to experimental chemotherapy of tuberculosis, *Probl. Tuberk.*, 7, 53, 1980.
65. Bonventre, P. and Gregoriadis, G., Killing of intraphagocytic *Staphylococcus aureus* by dihydro-streptomycin entrapped within liposomes, *Antimicrob. Agents Chemother.*, 113, 1049, 1978.
66. Smolin, G., Okumoto, M., Feiler, S., and London, D., Ioduridine-liposome therapy for herpes simplex keratitis, *Am. J. Ophthalmol.*, 91, 220, 1981.
67. Schaeffer, H. E. and Krohn, D. L., Liposomes in topical drug delivery, *Invest. Ophthalmol.*, 22, 220, 1982.
68. La Bonnadière, C., Preliminary data on protective effect of interferon coupled with liposomes in the mouse-virus model for murine hepatitis, *Ann. Microbiol. (Paris),* 129, 397, 1978.
69. Taylor, R. L., Williams, D. M., Craven, P. C., Graybill, J. R., and Drutz, D. J., Amphotericin B in liposomes: a novel therapy for histoplasmosis, *Am. Rev. Respir. Dis.*, 125, 610, 1982.
70. Graybill, J. R., Craven, P. C., Taylor, R. L., Williams, D. M., and Magee, W. E., Treatment of murine cryptococcosis with liposome associated amphotericin B, *J. Infect. Dis.*, 45, 748, 1982.
71. Lopez-Berestein, G. et al., Treatment and prophylaxis of disseminated infection due to *Candida albicans* in mice with liposome-encapsulated amphotericin B, *J. Infect. Dis.*, 147, 939, 1983.
72. Wahlig, H., Gentamicin-PMMA beads: a drug delivery system in the treatment of chronic bone and soft tissue infections, *J. Antimicrob. Chemother.*, 10, 463, 1982.
73. Grieben, A., Clinical results of septopal R in bone and soft tissue infections. A survey of clinical trials. Local antibiotic treatment in osteomyelitis and soft-tissue infections, in *International Congress Series,* No. 556, Van Rens, T. J. G. and Kayser, F. J., Eds., Excerpta Medica, Amsterdam, 144, 1981.
74. Barton, R. P. E. and Moir, A. A., Use of local gentamicin preparation ("garamycin" chains) as prophylaxis against infection in major head or neck surgery: a pilot study, *Pharmacotherapeutica,* 3, 327, 1983.
75. Josefsson, G., Lindberg, L., and Wiklander, B., Systemic antibiotics and gentamicin-containing bone cement in the prophylaxis of post-operative infections in total hip arthroplasty, *Clin. Orthop. Relat. Res.*, 159, 194, 1981.
76. Harvey, R. A., Tesoriero, J. V., and Greco, R. S., Noncovalent bonding of penicillin and cefazolin to dacron, *Am. J. Surg.*, 47, 205, 1984.

77. Lee, R. D., Brusch, J. L., Barza, M. J., and Weinstein, L., Effect of probenecid on penetration of oxacilin into fibrin clots in vitro, *Antimicrob. Agents Chemother.,* 8, 105, 1975.

78. Gibaldi, M. and Schwartz, M. A., Apparent effect of probenecid on the distribution of penicillins in man, *Clin. Pharmacol. Ther.,* 9, 345, 1968.

79. Gibaldi, M., Davidson, D., Plant, M. E., and Schwartz, M. A., Modification of penicillin distribution and elimination by probenecid, *Int. J. Clin. Pharmacol.,* 3, 182, 1970.

80. Barza, M., Brusch, J., Bergeron, M. G., Kemmotsu, O., and Weinstein, L., Extraction of antibiotics from the circulation by liver and kidney: effect of probenecid, *J. Infect. Dis.,* 131 (Suppl.), S86, 1975.

81. Simkerkoff, M. S., Thomas, L., McGregor, D., Shenkein, I., and Levine, B. B., Inactivations of penicillins by carbohydrate solutions at alkaline pH, *N. Engl. J. Med.,* 283, 116, 1970.

82. Fowler, T. J., Some incompatibilities of intravenous admixtures, *Am. J. Hosp. Pharm.,* 24, 450, 1967.

83. Rapp, R. P., Wermeling, D. P., and Piecoro, J. J., Jr., Guidelines for the administration of commonly used drugs, *Drug Intell. Clin. Pharm.,* 18, 217, 1984.

84. Henderson, J. L., Polk, R. E., and Kline, B. J., In vitro inactivation of gentamicin, tobramycin, and netilmicin by carbenicillin, azlocillin, or mezlocillin, *Am. J. Hosp. Pharm.,* 38, 1167, 1981.

85. Pickering, L. K. and Rutherford, I., Effect of concentration and time upon inactivation of tobramycin, gentamicin, and netilmicin and amikacin by azlocillin, carbenicillin, mecillinam, mezlocillin, and piperacillin, *J. Pharmacol. Exp. Ther.,* 217, 345, 1981.

86. Neftel, K. A., Walti, M., Spengler, H., and deWeck, A. L., Effect of storage of penicillin-G solutions on sensitivation to penicillin G after intravenous administration, *Lancet,* 1, 986, 1982.

87. Bergeron, M. G., Brusch, J. L., Barza, M., and Weinstein, L., Significant reduction in the incidence of phlebitis with buffered versus unbuffered cephalothin, *Antimicrob. Agents Chemother.,* 9, 646, 1976.

Chapter 10

RATE-CONTROLLED DELIVERY OF ENDOCRINE AGENTS: SOME PARADOXICAL CONSEQUENCES OF CONTROLLING THE INPUTS

F. Eugene Yates and Timothy Poston

TABLE OF CONTENTS

I. INTRODUCTION

When a physician prescribes a hormone or a metabolite that is normally present in the human body, he is trying to couple into a complex system that evolved its own internal command-control and communication systems. In using hormones or metabolites as agents of his purpose (to get the patient "well"), the physician depends upon his understanding of the informational and dynamical aspects of endocrine systems. Conventional endocrinology, however, is largely a morphological and biochemical science; our understanding of endocrine "messages" is primitive. In this chapter, we examine the limitations of current knowledge and suggest some extensions. Our aim is to rationalize the design of therapeutic systems for the delivery of endocrine agents.

At the outset, there is a difficulty: the power of dynamical approaches to informational and intentional systems is being lost or ignored by biologists. In its place, an information theoretic has arisen that treats natural systems without meeting the requirements of physical dynamics. As an example of the permeation of an "information" metaphor into science, consider that biologists often speak about their systems in casual anthropomorphisms such as:

- DNA "codes" "information"
- Hormones are or provoke "messengers"
- The "fidelity" of protein synthesis is assured by kinetic "proofreading"
- Aging and death are the result of "error" catastrophes
- Animal (or plant) development follows a "program"

Use of such linguistic metaphors in science and especially in biology usually represents failure to solve a fundamental dynamical problem and the sneaking of unjustified "smart" elements into the account. Dennett[1] has written clearly about this deception:

Any time a theory builder proposes to call any event, state, structure, etc., in any system (say the brain of an organism) a *signal* or *message* or *command* or otherwise endows it with content, he takes out a *loan of intelligence.* He implicitly posits along with his signals, messages, or commands, something that can serve as a signal-*reader,* message-*understander,* or *commander,* else his "signals" will be for nought, will decay unreceived, uncomprehended. This loan must be repaid eventually by finding and analyzing away these readers or comprehenders; for, failing this, the theory will have among its elements unanalyzed manalogues endowed with enough intelligence to read the signals, etc., and thus the theory will *postpone* answering the major question: what makes for intelligence? The intentionality of all such talk of signals and commands reminds us that rationality is being taken for granted, and in this way shows us where a theory is incomplete.

If endocrinologists have any common mission that they all endorse, it should be to account for the richness of behavior of organisms, at all their levels of organization, by a theory of chemical signaling and dynamical stability that does not require a loan of intelligence.

Science is unitary at its foundation; it is a mistake to suppose that information has an independent nondynamical representation in natural systems. The changing of the dynamic contingencies of a system by any kind of chemical flux capable of altering its states requires matching of the amplitudes or the configurations of the flux to the configurations and energies of the system. This is a physical problem. Command-control-communication theories and models that ignore this coupling problem usually lead to contrived feedback networks that are dynamical fictions and pseudomathematizations. In this chapter, we shall try to identify within quotation marks terms that come from metaphors of information science and explain or replace these with ideas that come from dynamics.

The normal performance of endocrine systems deploys chemical agents to convey "messages" according to "designs" arrived at by evolutionary processes not requiring the aid of physicians or the intervention of man. In 1974, Sebeok[2,3] proposed the term *endosemiotics* to describe studies of regulatory systems within the body. He noted that within a human being, for example, an array of mechanisms exists that may be thought to be involved in "signaling". The array includes the molecular "code" at the "lower" end of the scale and the verbal "code" at the "upper". Semiotics is devoted to the scientific study of signs and signaling behavior within and between living systems of the same species, as well as across species. Endocrinology is thus encompassed by endosemiotics. We shall later examine the "representation" of "information" and "meaning" in endocrine systems and try to give these a dynamical account. Again, our aim is to set forth some theoretical principles that can underlie the rational design of therapeutic systems delivering endocrine agents.

II. ENDOCRINE "SIGNALS" IN BLOOD

A. Are Plasma Concentrations the Relevant Variables?

Endocrinologists no longer insist that an endocrine "signal" be carried only by a classical hormone of the thyroid, gastrointestinal tract, adrenals, gonads, parathyroids, pancreas, or pituitary. Some neurotransmitters, neuropeptide modulators, paracrines, growth factors, substrates, oxygen or hydrogen ions may be chemical vehicles for "commands", "messages", or other kinds of influences that can partially determine or change the operating point of the metabolic system or of behavior. Furthermore, because endocrinology is so comprehensive, it seems overly restrictive to focus just on endocrine signals in systemic blood plasma — as we shall do. The justification for this narrowness is both methodological and theoretical: chemicals in plasma can be collected and assayed more easily than can those in most other fluids or regions, and thus we have more data to examine from plasma. More importantly, however, we note that plasma interfaces physiologically with all other body fluids in one way or another; concentrations of chemical agents in plasma therefore either directly or indirectly influence or reflect the "signaling" activity of endocrine systems. Theoretically, intracellular or interstitial fluid concentrations would be perhaps more relevant, but we shall have to confine our attention to concentrations of chemical agents in plasma.

All the chemical agents we have in mind have endogenous sources; they are hormones or metabolites.

B. Waveforms (Patterns) of Plasma Concentrations

A logically exhaustive classification of patterns of time histories of the plasma concentration of hormones or metabolites would be: (1) steady-state or (2) fluctuating. Steady-state concentrations may be near-constant or near-periodic. Fluctuating concentrations may have any shape of time history (waveforms), except for the two forms of steady states. It should be noted, though, that the steady states may be intermittent — a hormonal level may be constant for a while, then oscillate, and perhaps later fluctuate. Time histories of endocrine variables are likely to be nonstationary in a statistical sense. This characteristic poses difficulties for theoretical analysis, and such nonstationarities apply to physiological variables other than endocrine ones as well. For example, Figure 1 shows a spontaneous transition from one waveform to another in a regional blood flow. The occurrence and disappearance of alpha rhythms in the human extracranial EEG is a well-known example of such nonstationarity. Steady states of either kind may sometimes be appropriate "signaling" and at other times be pathological — a particular waveform or pattern may have some interval over which it is effective or appropriate, but it may be pathological if extended beyond that interval. The effective intervals may themselves be recurrent in a near-periodic fashion.

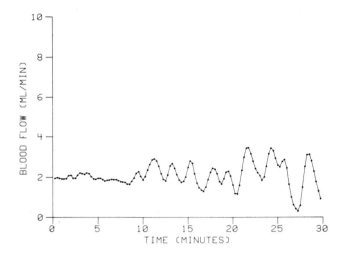

FIGURE 1.   Spontaneous transition from steady to oscillatory blood flow in adrenal gland of conscious, normal, resting dog. (Data from unpublished experiment of L. A. Benton, L. L. Loring, and F. E. Yates.)

C. What Aspects of Concentration Waveforms Possess "Information"?

Information in its narrowest, simplest technological sense is measured by the bit — the selection of either one of two alternatives that are equally likely. More generally, selective information consists of making choices from a finite set of alternatives of known but not necessarily equal probabilities. The larger the set, the greater the amount of selective information in a particular choice. (For further description of the limited, but precise technological information theory — a coding theory — see Cherry,[4] Pierce,[5] and Shannon and Weaver.[6] Yates[7] has discussed technological information as it may apply to endocrine communication systems.)

A *sign* is a physical entity that can be observed or measured. An *event* is a change in time. A *signal* is a *sign event* and is the physical manifestation of a message. A *message* consists of a sign event (signal) or a sequence of sign events (signals). These terms emphasize that a signal must have an element of surprise or change in it. (Constancy is not a signal but a static bias, if there could be no other value.) Messages are made up of signals that can be generated, transmitted, received, "decoded", and "interpreted" according to a "context". A physical event is a signal only in a context established by the rules of transmission of a sender or the rules of detection and "interpretation" of a receiver. Messages require *rules* at both transmission and receiving ends, and the rules must in some way be matched appropriately for communication or command to occur.

Rules are commonly syntactical and are not physical laws, although in operation they obey physical laws. Note that there is no information in a physical law, because the law *must* be obeyed, without surprise. Novelty and variety (and therefore signals and messages) arise from the boundary conditions or constraints on the field of action of physical laws. These issues are discussed in Section IV.A below.

Selective information is too narrow a concept to account for endocrine communications. If we fully understood the "information" content of endocrine signals, perhaps we could reduce that information to selective information representations. Because we cannot now do that, we shall instead discuss (in natural language) five aspects of waveforms that might convey endocrine "information". These are level, frequency, phase, threshold, and rate-of-change.

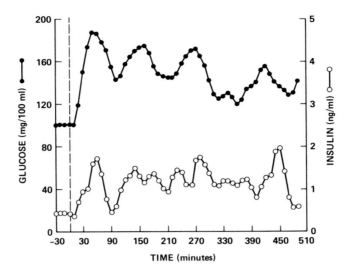

FIGURE 2. Approximately 90-min periodicity in arterial plasma concentrations of glucose and insulin. Data were obtained from un-restrained, conscious, normal dog receiving an intravenous infusion of glucose at 10 mg/kg/min started at zero time (vertical dashed line).

1. Level (Static Dose-Response)

The simplest idea about endocrine "information" is that it is conveyed by the level of a hormone in plasma. Static dose-response curves (with or without semilogarithmic transformations of the data) are the typical example — the higher the level, the more the effect (such as activation or inhibition). The dose-response relationship shows the nonlinearities of at least minimum effective doses (thresholds) and maximum effects (saturation). The biologist's intuition that some endocrine systems may be amplitude modulated (that is, level-sensitive) is natural and causes no confusion. It is patently true for some agents.

2. Frequency of an Oscillation

Many endocrine variables have near-periodic waveforms, at least over some inter-vals. Periods range from minutes to months. Figure 2 shows spontaneous oscillations of glucose and insulin with an ultradian period of 90 min in the blood of a conscious, unrestrained dog. Many circadian rhythms within biological systems are, of course, now extremely well known, and they have dominated the study of biological rhythms. The monthly menstrual cycle is equally prominent. We now know that near-periodic behavior characterizes many of the processes of living systems at all their levels of organization (for detailed discussion, see Yates[8]), but we have very little evidence yet that any endocrine signals are frequency modulated. The famous and perhaps only example is that of GnRH flux to the pituitary, which can modulate the ratio of LH and FSH release rates or concentrations in plasma by changes in its frequency.[9]

3. Phase of an Oscillation

The phase of an oscillation can be profoundly important to the handling of either signals or noise that may impinge on the oscillatory process. To illustrate, we consider here a simple, classical model of a thermodynamically valid kinematic oscillator origi-nally described by Van der Pol. The energy dissipative requirements of the second law of thermodynamics assure that in systems above the level of atoms there are no linear, harmonic, ideal oscillators. All real oscillators are nonlinear, and the archetype is the

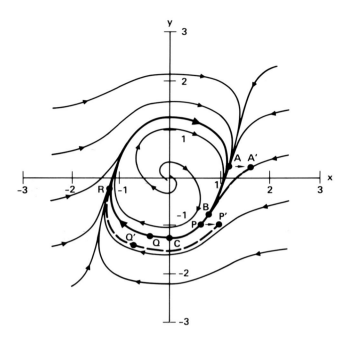

FIGURE 3.   Van der Pol limit cycle (nonlinear) oscillator shown as
the phase portrait corresponding to Equations 1 and 2, showing tracks
along which (x,y) evolves; time is not explicit. Points A and P are on
the cycle (heavy curve) to which all tracks (except unstable constancy
at (0,0)) tend, and they are regularly revisited. Perturbations to A', P'
originate tracks which return to the cycle, although with different relaxation times (Figures 4 to 6).

limit cycle, such as that produced by the Van der Pol oscillator. This oscillator model
can be described (after a Lienard transformation) by the equations:

$$\dot{x} = y - x^3 + x \tag{1}$$

$$\dot{y} = -x \tag{2}$$

The evolution of this system is shown in the phase portrait in Figure 3. Starting at
any point (x,y) in the plane, the system evolves along whatever curve of the figure
passes through that point in the direction of the arrows. From *any* initial conditions
(except (0,0) exactly) the system heads toward the rounded-parallelogram limit cycle
visible in the figure and follows it round and round. For example, starting when time
t = 0 at (x,y) = (1.2,0.2), i.e., at point A, the time histories of x and y are as shown in
Figure 4. Points B and C are reached at times t = 1 and t = 2, respectively (as may be
seen by converting the number pairs (x(1),y(1)) = (0.8,−0.8) and (x(2),y(2)) =
(0.0,−1.3), read from Figure 4 into coordinates in Figure 3). The cyclic movement has
replaced a static value of (x,y) as the normal, ''equilibrium'' behavior of the system.
Now we examine the importance of phase. Suppose x is suddenly increased by 0.4 as
the system passes A, moving it to A'. Because for simplicity we have chosen an oscillator with no external forcing term (just as the circadian body rhythm of temperature
continues to run in the absence of a light/dark cycle, although shifted in phase), there
is a small phase shift that we discount by moving the time histories beginning at A' a
little to the left in Figure 5, where they superimpose well on those from A by the time

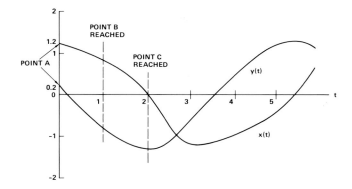

FIGURE 4. The time histories of x and y in the Van der Pol model as they obey Equations 1 and 2, with initial data x = 1.2, y = 0.2, corresponding to point A in Figure 3. The evolving coordinates of a point following the cycle are shown.

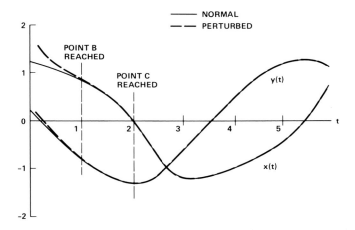

FIGURE 5. The time histories of the Van der Pol model of conditions of Figure 4 (light curves), superimposed with those from the off-cycle initial conditions x = 1.6, y = 0.2 (broken heavy curves). When x is perturbed to increase abruptly by 0.4, the return to the normal cyclic behavior is essentially complete by time t = 1.

t = 1. (In a forced nonlinear oscillation, this move would not be necessary; but the picture analogous to Figure 3 would be more complicated.)

In contrast, consider the same increase in x by 0.4 at a different phase as the system passes point P in Figure 6, where (x,y) = (0.6,−1). By again adjusting the phase so that the time histories from P and the disturbed point P′ eventually settle to running together, we see that they disagree (in both x and y) until nearly t = 2, when they both (approximately) pass through the point R. At t = 1 they are still separated as they pass through the points Q and Q′, respectively.

No term in Equations 1 and 2 corresponds to a greater "responsiveness" of x to perturbation when (x,y) = (1.2,0.2) than when (x,y) = (0.6,−1). Indeed, $\dot{x} = -0.328$ at A′, while $\dot{x} = -0.616$ at P′; and x is "responding" — at least, changing in response to the state of the system — nearly twice as fast. But it still takes twice as long to return to the normal cycle of values. This is an emergent property of the whole system described by Equations 1 and 2 (which are, by definition, a *complete* description of the dynamics producing the time histories shown); this is not a result of a "signal" called

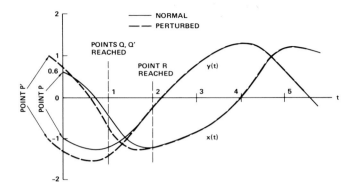

FIGURE 6.   Time histories of the Van der Pol model from initial data (x,y) = (0.6,−1) = P, on the normal cycle (light curves) and from (1,−1) = P′, following a perturbation that increases x by 0.4 (broken heavy curves). The return to approximately normal takes twice as long as in Figure 5, which shows the same perturbations occurring at a different phase.

"increase x by 0.4" being differently "interpreted" by some localizable "sensor" whose output and/or states would contribute identifiable terms to the dynamics.

Because the emergent, phase-dependent response just described is common in nonlinear oscillators, it is misleading for endocrinologists to interpret some of their experiments in the way they do. For example, suppose an endocrinologist wants to answer the question: is the adrenocortical response to ACTH a function of a circadian rhythm in the adrenal gland? To answer, he may then inject boluses of ACTH into normal animals at different times of the day and measure the adrenal secretory response or changes in the plasma levels of adrenocortical hormones such as cortisol or corticosterone. If the response to a given fixed dose of ACTH is different at different times of day, it is then sometimes argued that there is a circadian rhythm in adrenal "responsiveness" to ACTH. This conclusion may be defective because the circadian rhythm in the overall glucocorticoid system is itself a nonlinear oscillator. The ACTH bolus may merely act as one kind of perturbation, and according to the dynamics intrinsic to nonlinear oscillators of the limit cycle type, it should be *expected* that the glucocorticoid response to the perturbation would be a function of phase of the circadian rhythm. There is no justification for postulating a separate, local circadian rhythm in adrenal "responsiveness" to ACTH.

Recognition that the phase of a biological oscillation may be a very important consideration in designing therapeutic interventions has been strengthened by the work of Halberg et al.[10] Nevertheless, we still have little clear evidence on whether and how physicians should take advantage of the phase of an endogenous rhythm to optimize hormonal therapy.

4. Threshold (for Switching)

A simple concept of endocrine information is that the level of a hormone in blood must cross some threshold in order to have an effect, but that above that threshold variations in the level are not important. This is the "permissive action" view of hormone effects (some is needed, but more is irrelevant) that was popularized by Dwight Ingle in the 1950s. Both the preparation of estrogen for the surge in LH and the surge itself may have such characteristics. The idea of a threshold can be elaborated into strength-duration products such that the product itself has a threshold rather than the strength (level). The old ideas of "chronaxy" and "rheobase" in neurophysiology were of this character.

5. Rate-of-Change of Level (or Frequency)

Engineers use derivative control (rate-of-change sensitivity) as a means to anticipate necessary adjustments of system behavior. Some endocrine and metabolic systems appear to derive "information" from the slope (roughly, from the first time derivative) of the level (plasma concentration) of an agent.[11] It seems likely to us that many instances of such rate-of-change sensitivity of levels may be discovered in biochemical systems, but most experimental protocols are designed for other purposes and do not address this question. Rate-of-change of *frequency* could, in principle, be a higher-order signal, but as far as we know there is no example in endocrinology. (Indeed, a "changing frequency" is not even well-defined except when the change is slow on the time scale set by the period.)

III. SHAPING THE WAVEFORMS

The time history of the plasma concentration of a hormone or metabolite (its waveform) may be shaped naturally by the internal arrangements of the system, or it may be shaped by technological interventions. We examine each of these means briefly below.

A. Natural Means

Waveforms may be shaped internally either by regulation or by control. Regulation is accomplished by the intrinsic dynamics of a system and does not require an extrinsic controller or even feedback. In contrast, classical engineering control requires the presence of some element outside the system to be controlled that can accomplish measurement, amplification, comparison with reference "ideal" values, and feedback. Controllers require the presence of "information" outside the system that specifies the "desired" operation of the system. Control is not intrinsic to the dynamics of the system itself. The shortcomings of the control theory metaphor to describe most biological regulations have been pointed out by Yates.[8]

Below we discuss four means by which endocrine wave forms are shaped naturally.

1. Self-Regulation by Protein Binding

The multiple mass action theory that establishes the "buffering" effects of protein binding of hormones can be found in Yates and Urquhart[12] or Keller et al.[13] These effects have also been discussed by Yates.[7] Just as hydrogen ion is stabilized in plasma by multiple mass actions that involve proton donors and acceptors, so can the concentration of a free hormone in blood by stabilized by adsorption and release reactions that are either specific (involving carrier proteins) or nonspecific (e.g., with albumin). A computer simulation of the binding of thyroid hormones has demonstrated the stabilizing effect.[14] A waveform of the plasma concentration of a hormone that undergoes protein binding tends toward constancy because of the damping effect of the mass action reactions.

2. Self-Regulation by First-Order Elimination

Elimination of a hormone can occur either by chemical transformation into an inactive substance or by excretion from the body. In each case, if the elimination process follows first-order kinetics:

$$\text{rate of removal of x} = -Kx \tag{3}$$

as is usually at least approximately true, fluctuational increases or decreases in the concentration of x are then automatically compensated for by increases or decreases in reaction rates or transports eliminating x. (Any order of process higher than zero will provide some compensatory action. First-order reactions are usually postulated, although not necessarily in linear form.) The coefficient of Equation 3 may itself be dependent on substance x, giving a nonlinear relationship:

$$\text{rate of removal of x} = -K(x)x \qquad (4)$$

In this case, the nonlinearity can enhance the compensatory effectiveness of the self-regulatory process.

Protein binding and first-order elimination together do not provide very precise bounding of plasma concentrations. There are "load errors", and these can be large. However, for substances in which the regulation band (the range of the variable in which variation makes no physiological difference) is wide, the two self-regulatory processes described above may provide adequate compensation for disturbances. Such dynamic regulations are much more common in biology than are controls.[15] When the time history of a physiological variable is carefully monitored, it is usually found that the regulation band (or the peak-trough amplitude in the case of near-periodic variations) covers a range of at least 2 to 1, and sometimes 4 to 1. But there are variables such as core temperature that are bounded more closely, and controls may have been added to self-regulatory processes in the course of evolution.

3. Control of Inputs (Secretion Rates)

Control may be of two types: open-loop or closed-loop.

Open-loop control — In open-loop control the output obeys a time-varying input because of tight couplings in the causal chain between input and output. This is the manner in which the secretion of somatotropin and adrenal medullary hormones seems to be adjusted.

Closed-loop control — As is well known, the secretion rates of thyroid hormones, adrenocorticoid hormones, parathyroid hormones, testosterone, and estradiol (as examples) seem to be adjusted by a closed-loop control. However, in the so-called "stress" response of the adrenal cortex and in the LH surge, open-loop control may take over and dominate. The details of conversions from one type of control to another within one endocrine system have been difficult to work out and are still not clear.

4. Control of Effects

The time history of a plasma concentration of a hormone can be altered indirectly by changing the effects of the hormone, either through variations in receptor recognition or in the subsequent activation stages. By changing the effects, the physiological state is changed; other systems adjust their operating points accordingly, the changes of which may then influence the secretion rate, and, finally, the plasma concentration of the hormone. The cause-and-effect relationships in such a case may be very obscure, but "up and down regulation" of receptor number in cellular targets for hormones is one of the possiblities for adjusting the flow of "messages" in endocrine systems.

B. Technological Means

1. Comment on Current Methods

Current technology has almost no means to vary hormonal waveforms by adjusting the extent of protein binding. (Displacements of an active substance by an inactive substance through competitive protein binding can shape the waveform of the active substance, but this well-known principle has not yet been used in therapy.) Similarly, little can be done by adjusting elimination rates, except in those extreme cases when renal dialysis is used to alter the chemical composition of plasma or, less extremely, when acid-base balance is deliberately perturbed to change excretion of a weakly acidic or basic substance. Most of the technology used in medicine to shape waveforms of hormones in blood focuses on exogenous inputs (infusions, injections, pills, implantations, suppositories, etc.). Recently this approach has taken on a new sophistication in the creation of "therapeutic systems".[16] These systems, such as those designed and developed by the ALZA Corporation, have been described by Heilmann,[17] Urquhart,[18] and Urquhart et al.[19]

Almost all of the current therapeutic systems control the input mass fluxes of the endocrine agents and, in so doing, accomplish "rate-controlled" delivery (that is, control of the input mass flux, which must be distinguished from control of or by rate-of-change of plasma concentrations). Because of the lack of stable, reliable and small chemical sensors, almost all rate-controlled delivery systems operate open-loop. Furthermore, for obvious reasons of simplicity, these systems mainly attempt to guarantee *constancy* of input. Only feebly can they imitate or impose circadian rhythms.[20]

2. Constancy and "Clamping"

Administration of hormonal agents by rate-controlling delivery systems operating under open-loop control with constant fluxes will lead to "clamping" of the input rates either if the endogenous source is missing or if it is shut off by closed-loop internal controls. A consequence of clamping the input is near-constancy of the plasma concentration of the hormone — and that is usually the intended result. In many cases, that intention is proper, justified, and effective. There are surprising hazards, however, as described below.

IV. COUNTERINTUITIVE CONSEQUENCES OF CLAMPING INPUTS OR LEVELS OF HORMONAL AGENTS

A. The Problem

It is intuitively obvious that if one clamps a hormonal level or input rate at some average value when the normal pattern is (for example) a near-periodic function, then the average may not convey the same "message" that the periodic waveform did. But what is *not* obvious is that when one clamps an endogenous variable that (most of the time) appears to be spontaneously constant, so as seemingly to replace constancy with constancy, dramatic changes in system dynamics may occur.

B. Illustration by Mathematical Models

It is often experimentally observed that some variable in a given natural system is approximately constant and that perturbations of that variable die away exponentially. (Indeed, the time constant can be an important practical test for pathology, as in the glucose tolerance test for diabetes.) It is almost as often deduced that if such a naturally constant level is experimentally or medically *held* constant, as when a hormone concentration is maintained by constant-input replacement therapy, the result will be an essentially equivalent system. But this may not be so.

In the stability of its equilibrium with other variables with which it interacts, the dynamic response of a variable is in general as crucial as its value. As a simple illustration of this idea, consider a continuously stirred tank reactor containing two chemicals, X and Y, undergoing the reaction

$$X + 2Y \underset{18/65}{\overset{9/5}{\rightleftarrows}} 3Y \tag{5}$$

with the rate constants shown. An inflow with concentration 3/2 of x and 1/6 of y occurs at the rate 1, and fluid with the instantaneous, stirred concentrations x and y is withdrawn at the same rate.

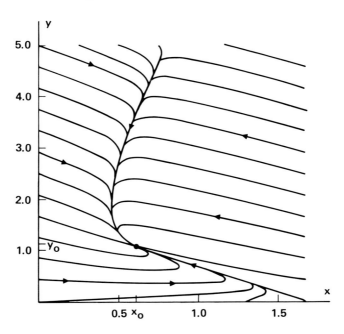

FIGURE 7.   Phase portrait of Model 1 (Equations 6 and 7). All trajectories relax to (x_o, y_o).

By ordinary mass action arguments we obtain the equations

$$\dot{x} = \left[\frac{3}{2} \right] - \left[x \right] + \left[\frac{18}{65} y^3 - \frac{9}{5} xy^2 \right] \tag{6}$$

$$\dot{y} = \left[\frac{1}{6} \right] - \left[y \right] + \left[\frac{9}{5} xy^2 - \frac{18}{65} y^3 \right] \tag{7}$$

inflow   efflux   reaction

whose phase portrait is shown in Figure 7. ($\dot{x}$ and $\dot{y}$ are rates of change of the respective concentrations.)

As is clear from the figure, there is a unique equilibrium point $(x_o, y_o) = (0.606, 1.062)$ at which $\dot{x}$ and $\dot{y}$ vanish, and to which all trajectories flow. A simple perturbation of the system, such as an increase in the concentration y, is followed by a smooth return to the value (x_o, y_o).

Notice, however, that the return of y is not monotonic. The immediate response to an increase in y (in the zone $x > x_o$) is that y increases further, while x decreases. (Reaction 5 goes to the right.) The decrease in x is due to the contribution of X to the rate of synthesis of Y, until the synthesis and influx of Y together are less than the combination of efflux with the back reaction in Reaction 5. For a short while, x and y then decrease together; finally x increases as y decreases, and the point of equilibrium is reached again.

Suppose, however, that the value of x is *constrained* at its normal equilibrium value, x_o, by a "therapeutic system". In the tank, this could be approximated by suitably*

---

*   The usual forms of buffering do not reproduce the effects described here; X must be held in approximate equilibrium with some Z at saturation, and thus attached to the specific concentration x_o.

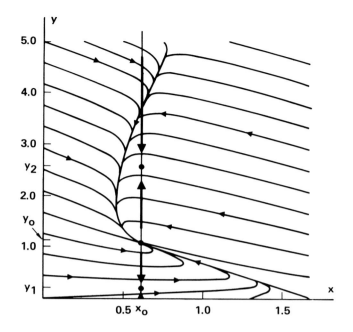

FIGURE 8. Model 1 when (x,y) is on (or close to) the line $x = x_o$ (see Equation 8). Now y increases when between y_0 and y_2, because if x is not allowed to change, (x,y) cannot follow the flow to the left, where it can move downward; it can only move upward to (x_0,y_2). Similarly, between y_0 and y_1, (x,y) moves down to (x_0, y_1). New dynamical equilibria have emerged from clamping x at its previous equilibrium value.

buffering X; in a hormonal system, a gland might be replaced by a steady exogenous infusion at some "representative" secretion rate. If there is a perturbation in the system now, the preliminary decrease in x that is essential to a decrease in y no longer occurs, and the initial increase in y is not turned off. Thus y continues to increase (Figure 8) as long as it is below the newly created equilibrium value $y_2 = 2.652$.

Similarly, a small decrease from y_o with fixed $x = x_o$ continues (unchecked by a briefly increasing excursion in x as previously allowed) as long as $y > y_1 = 0.2136$.

Algebraically, we have replaced Equations 6 and 7 by

$$\dot{y} = \frac{1}{6} - y + \frac{9}{5} x_0 y^2 - \frac{18}{65} y^3 \tag{8}$$

which is approximately

$$\dot{y} = 0.1667 - y + 1.088\, y^2 - 0.277\, y^3$$

whose right hand side is graphed in Figure 9. The zeros y_1 and y_2 (Figure 8) are the new equilibria, because the nonvanishing of x is made irrelevant by the constraint on x.

The destabilization of the system by clamping x is not a result of its nonlinear character. (Clamped at $x = 0$, the linear system $x = 8y - 19x$, $y = y - 8x$ will destabilize along the y-axis in just this manner.) The nonlinear terms merely allow other equilibria for y to exist (a linear or affine equation having at most one isolated zero), so that in the clamped model, y does not depart exponentially for $\pm\infty$.

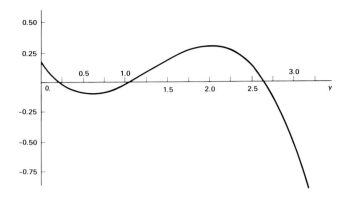

FIGURE 9.   Graph of $\dot{y}$ vs. y in Model 1 (Equation 8), where x is held fixed at the equilibrium value x_o. The original equilibrium value for y (y_o in Figure 7) and the two new possible values after clamping (y_1 and y_2, Figure 8) are shown as zeroes for $\dot{y}$.

This is a more subtle phenomenon than the well-known (and unsubtle) loss of stability against *large* perturbations that can result from fixing a normally variable level. For example, the return of the body to it normal state after certain "stresses" requires a temporary increase in cortisol. While steady replacement therapy for cortisol in Addison's disease produces an equilibrium stable against small perturbations, it is not adequate against large ones. Extreme stress such as surgery requires temporary administration of cortisol at levels that would be very damaging on a regular basis.

The contrast between these two phenomena — (1) an equilibrium ceasing to be attractive at all or (2) the equilibrium being only *globally* attractive — can be illustrated by the equations

$$\dot{x} = x + 4y - x^3 \tag{9}$$

$$\dot{y} = 3(-x - 2y + 3y^2 - y^3) \tag{10}$$

whose phase portrait is shown in Figure 10. Clamping x = 0 appears analogous to fixing cortisol level; small perturbations of the remaining system variable y die out, but after perturbations above the level $q_1 = 1$ the level of y heads for the distant point $q_2 = 2$. Perturbation to the level m in Figure 10 also would die away in the unclamped system, although its effect would be the large excursion shown by the dotted trajectory involving a temporary surge in x. (Compare to this the cortisol surge required for recovery from surgery or the temperature excursion — fever — during illness and return to health.) The clamped system goes from m to q_2.

By contrast, clamping y = 0 reproduces the subtle effect discussed above. The system becomes unstable against even *small* perturbations, and ordinary noise will send it off to one of the new equilibria p_1 or p_2.

Equations 9 and 10 are, of course, offered not as a specific model for a biochemical interaction, but as simple illustrations of unexpected phenomena that can in principle occur equally easily in the multivariable systems that provide the dynamics of hormonal interaction. It is important to realize that these phenomena do not depend on highly special choices of equations; their occurrence is *structurally stable*. Loosely, this means that a small perturbation of Equations 6 and 7, or of Equations 9 and 10, and/ or of the clamping values chosen (they need not be exactly the equilibrium values for the corresponding variables) will not qualitatively change the results. They are robust phenomena.

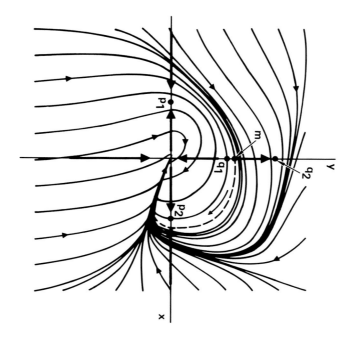

FIGURE 10.   Phase portrait of Model 2. Behaviors of Equations 9 and 10 are shown together (curves) and separately (arrows on axes) with x or y clamped at the equilibrium value 0. For the unclamped model, (0,0) is universally attractive. If x is clamped at 0, (0,0) remains attractive, although some initial conditions lead to (0,2); if y is clamped at 0, (0,0) is destabilized.

Much research has gone into avoiding "overdose-underdose" fluctuations by developing steady-release pills, soluble implants, and therapeutic systems. *But a steady clamped variable may be inadequate to replace a normally steady, but dynamically responsive one.*

More elaborate behavior can easily occur in a clamped system containing a larger number of variables. For example, consider

$$\dot{a} = b - 1 \tag{11}$$

$$\dot{b} = 7 - a - 11b + 6b^2 - b^3 \tag{12}$$

$$\dot{c} = 3d - 2b \tag{13}$$

$$\dot{d} = 9 - c - 11d + 6d^2 - d^3 \tag{14}$$

Because Equations 11 and 12 involve only a and b, the behavior of these two variables is wholly accounted for by the phase portrait in Figure 11. There is a unique equilibrium at $a = b = 1$, to which all trajectories tend. Thus after transient variations in (a,b) die away, we may assume $b = 1$ in Equation 13 to achieve an equilibrium value $d = 2/3$, $c = 2.037$. That this unique equilibrium is globally attractive is clear by inspection of the phase portrait (Figure 12) of Equations 13 and 14 with b at its asymptotic value of 1.

If, however, a is clamped at its equilibrium value, b is given two stable equilibria

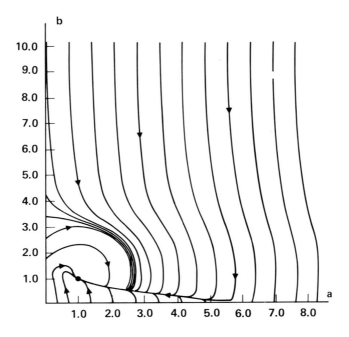

FIGURE 11. Phase portrait of Equations 11 and 12 (in Model 3). All trajectories flow to equilibrium point (a,b) = (1,1). In Model 3, the variable a is equal or proportional to the influx of cortisol (endogenous secretion plus exogenous infusion) received by a conscious, resting dog, studied experimentally under the conditions discussed with respect to Figures 16, 17, and 18.

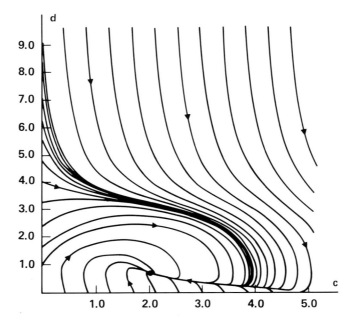

FIGURE 12. Phase portrait of Equations 13 and 14 (in Model 3) under conditions such that Equations 11 and 12 are at equilibrium, as shown in Figure 11. In Model 3 the variable d represents the secretion rate of cortisol from the adrenal glands.

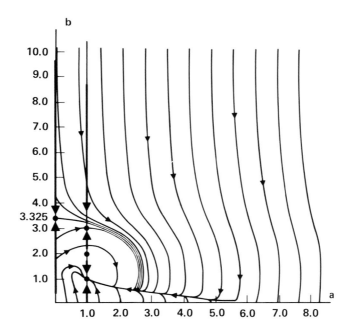

FIGURE 13. The effect of clamping influx variable a in Model 3 (Equations 11 and 12) at its equilibrium value a = 1. The behavior of variable b now becomes very dependent on initial conditions, and two new equilibrium points appear for b.

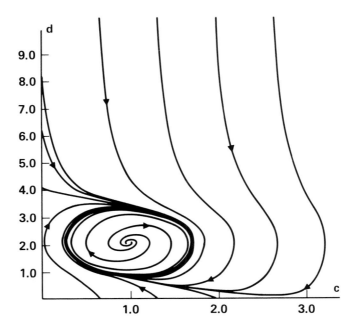

FIGURE 14. Effect of clamping a = 1 in Model 3 when the initial conditions for b are b > 2. If b < 2, the result is the same as that shown in Figure 12. When b = 2, the system is unstable and is responsive to small fluctuations that drive it either to b = 1 or to b = 3. When b > 2 the behavior of d becomes oscillatory.

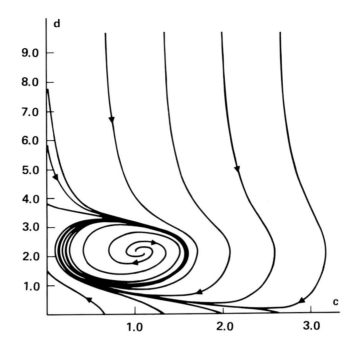

FIGURE 15.   Effect of clamping a = 0 in Model 3. The behavior of
d is now oscillatory regardless of initial conditions.

(Figure 13) at 1 and 3. Initial conditions with b < 2 lead asymptotically to b = 1, and
the previous analysis of c and d applies. The original stable behavior continues.

However, with initial b > 2, asymptotically b→3. This gives via Equation 13 unique
equilibrium values d = 2, c = 1; but these values are *unstable* (Figure 14), and the
asymptotic behavior of c and d is oscillatory: they follow a limit cycle.

Depending upon the initial conditions, then, the clamped system *either* stabilizes at
the usual unclamped equilibrium *or* it oscillates — with the range of oscillation of d
not even including the unclamped steady value, let alone having it as mean.

By contrast, if a is clamped to the nonequilibrium value 0, the system *must* oscillate.
Equation 12 has then the unique equilibrium b = 3.325, and instead of a choice between
the behaviors shown in Figure 12 and Figure 14, the asymptotic behavior of c and d is
now invariably dominated by the limit cycle shown in Figure 15.

C. Example of a Replacement Infusion

A real example of the potential problems that may arise when an endogenous variable such as a hormonal concentration or secretion rate is clamped is illustrated in Figures 16 to 18. The data show total spontaneous cortisol secretion rates from both
adrenal glands of a conscious, unrestrained dog under conditions in which none of the
cortisol secreted was returned to the dog, although his blood volume was maintained.
(This preparation is diagrammed in Yates et al.[21]) Under the experimental conditions,
cortisol was secreted by the animal in an open-loop manner, because the physiological
negative feedback was disrupted by on-line removal of all the secreted cortisol.

Figure 16A shows the normal, closed-loop operating conditions and 16B the consequences of opening the control loop by removing cortisol. When the loop inhibiting
secretion of cortisol was broken by *clamping* the cortisol input at zero, cortisol secretion rate rose and oscillated (but, of course, did not enter the dog in this open-loop
condition).

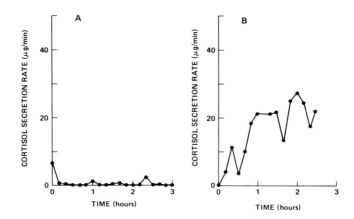

FIGURE 16. Cortisol secretion rate (both adrenals) in quiet, normal unrestrained dog when adrenal glucocorticoid system is operating either (A) closed-loop (normal mode) or (B) open-loop (experimental mode). (See Reference 21 for details.) Loop opened at "zero" time. Opening the loop, panel B, clamped cortisol secretion rate (from the point of view of the dog's adrenocortical system) at zero. (The maximum possible secretion rate in the experimental mode B was 34 μg/min.) The conditions illustrated in panel 4 are simulated in Figures 11 and 12; those of panel B are simulated in Figure 15.

Figures 17 and 18 show two different results obtained when a replacement infusion of cortisol *clamped* at a constant rate approximately equal to that secreted spontaneously by the dog) was started at the time the loop was opened. The intuitive result was that endogenous secretion of hormone would now remain unaffected by opening the loop, because the exogenous infusion exactly replaced the hormone being removed and there were no changes within the system. Indeed, Figure 17 shows such a result in which the system remained relatively quiet and the endogenous secretion rate did not rise after the loop was opened and the replacement infusion was administered.

In other similar experiments, however, clamping the level of cortisol by means of exogenous rate-controlled delivery destabilized the system, as shown in Figure 18. Here the replacement infusion, although again approximately matched to the initial secretion rate before the cortisol loop was opened, seemed to lead to erratic behavior of the system, unlike that shown in either Figure 16 or 17. In some experiments, this behavior was oscillatory. This unexpected result occurred so often that we thought there was some important, missing feedback signal in the adrenal effluent that we had left out of our cortisol-only replacement infusion (as still might be true). But later analysis, as shown above, raised the possibility that the erratic results were instead a direct consequence of clamping the cortisol input. We now believe that this latter interpretation is one that must be considered whenever rate-controlled delivery of an endocrine agent is used in such a way as to clamp an endogenous variable.

In the experiments described above, opening the loop constituted clamping cortisol production (normally a variable intricately responsive to others) at zero. Opening the loop and simultaneously infusing cortisol clamped cortisol input at its normal, resting value but did *not reconstitute the original system,* because the replacement infusion did not replace the *responsiveness* of cortisol to fluctuations in other physiological variables. There is in this physiological case at least a topological resemblance to the mathematical behavior of Equations 11 to 14 above. Of course, Equations 11 to 14 are not offered as a quantitative model for the canine cortisol system. However, the topological pattern of existences of attractive points and cycles *is* a model, of a qualitative kind; the equations serve as an existence proof that such a pattern is possible.

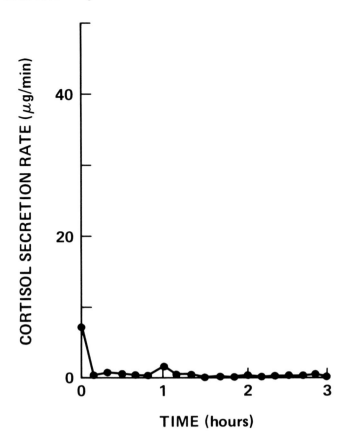

FIGURE 17. Cortisol secretion rate (both adrenals) under same open-loop conditions as shown in Figure 16B, except that an exogenous i.v. infusion of cortisol at 3 μg/min was given throughout the experiment. The results look very much like those shown in Figure 16A (closed-loop), as expected. Here the "secretion rate" (exogenous) provided a clamp at a typical endogenous rate. These conditions are simulated in Figures 12 and 13; the variable b in the model is at low initial value.

Above all, the ideas and data discussed above illustrate that the equilibrium or oscillatory asymptotic behavior of a free-running system can be a very poor predictor of the behavior of the same system clamped to those same patterns. Nevertheless, ours is not a general argument against clamped experiments, such as the Hodgkin and Huxley "voltage clamp". Their data were quite properly compared with computations from the model equations, correspondingly clamped; the false assumption, that clamping an equilibrium level produces a system equivalent to the unclamped one at equilibrium, was not made. In the context of the dynamics of major excursions from equilibrium — such as nerve impulses — this false assumption is not usually made. However, in the study of steady systems (whether constant or oscillatory) it can easily slip in unrecognized. Thus, it should always be considered that forcing a variable to confine its trajectory to the trajectory it was previously showing can lead to a changed dynamic regime! Moreover, the clamping of *any* waveform of an endogenous variable can lead to the changed dynamical regime — it does not have to be clamped only at constancy. The implications of this feature of dynamics for rate-controlled delivery of endocrine agents is obvious: if we imitate exactly what we consider to be normal rates and patterns of delivery, we may be unpleasantly surprised.

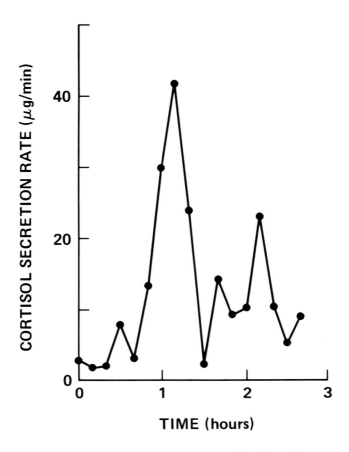

FIGURE 18. Cortisol secretion rate (both adrenals) under same open-loop conditions with cortisol replacement (clamping) infusion as shown in Figure 17. Surprisingly, the fixed replacement infusion failed to prove equivalent to the spontaneous, steady, endogenous secretion at the same rate. The system dynamics became unstable and oscillatory. A possible explanation was later found by mathematical study (see text). The conditions of this experiment are simulated in Figure 14.

We emphasize that *the analysis we have given of some of the surprises and dangers of clamping through rate-controlled delivery applies only to agents that are endogenous.* Drugs and foreign substances that have no endogenous sources and no cooperative arrangements concerning those molecules are not subject to the problems described above, as long as they are not surrogates for (derivatives of) endogenous variables.

V. ENDOSEMIOTICS — A DIFFERENT VIEW OF ENDOCRINE INFORMATION

Up to this point, we have tried to show that traditional ideas about selective information are too limited to account for endocrine signals. As shapely patterns, endocrine waveforms have at least five attributes in their variations that might convey messages. We have shown that the dynamics of endocrine systems are sufficiently subtle that even if a therapeutic system for rate-controlled delivery *exactly* reproduced an endocrine waveform, it might destablize the system by that seemingly desirable act. We need a richer view of endocrine information and its relation to dynamics if we are to rationalize the designs of rate-controlling delivery devices. Pattee[22] and Rosen[23] have separately tried to sharpen discussions of biological information and dynamics, and their different approaches may help us clarify the issues. We outline some of their work below.

A. Dynamic and "Linguistic" Modes of Complex Systems

Pattee[22] has taken the view that complex, living systems differ from other kinds of dynamical systems in that they contain a self-description. That description is written in the sense of the genetic code, and in that form, it is static or rate-independent. But the information is connected to the dynamical system, because it influences the formation of structures that constrain the subsequent dynamics. By careful reasoning, which we shall not attempt to reproduce here, Pattee concludes that living systems must be viewed both from an informational perspective and from a dynamic perspective. These two separate perspectives are related in the sense that they have the same referent — the living system — although epistemologically they are complementary accounts (in the Bohr sense). Neither description is complete; no experiments conducted in the framework of one account can produce contradictions in the framework of the other; and neither can be subsumed by the other. (Most biologists, to judge by our personal experiences, seem to behave according to Pattee's philosophy — they move easily and without apology from linguistic to dynamic metaphors in talking about living systems.) In this view, questions about endocrine messages or signals do not need to be cast in dynamical terms, and it is not likely to be helpful to do so. Instead, we should seek functional terms (as discussed later) to specify chemical "commands".

B. Dynamic Nature of Information

Recent work by Robert Rosen[23] attempts to avoid the complementarity proposed by Pattee and to subsume at least certain kinds of information within the scope of dynamics. Rosen's approach is sketched briefly below.

1. Activation and Inhibition as Primitives

Rosen notes that the work of Higgins (see Rosen) demonstrated that in complex, chemically coupled networks, activation and inhibition (which can be defined mathematically) are themselves primitives of an informational system. Rosen expands on that idea by offering a generalized dynamical equation of motion under conditions of a system containing many-to-few mappings (as will be explained below). The equation of motion has implicit in it three different kinds of information in the framework of dynamics.

2. Three Kinds of Information in Equations of Motion

Rosen's generalized equation of motion is:

$$Z(t) = \int_0^t \Phi g(Z, u(\tau)) d\tau + Z(0) \tag{15}$$

where Z is the state vector of the system (made up of its configurational state variables), U is a vector of external input variables, Z (0) represents the initial conditions, ϕ is representative of the dynamics of the system under constraints, and g represents the "genetic" variables that determine the structural aspects of the constraints and give the system its "identity".

Rosen then notes that changes in the g variables can be considered to be (in the Aristotelian sense) formal causes; variations in the initial conditions, Z(0), can be thought of as material causes, and changes in the operation ϕ, in concert with the input variable U, can be thought of as efficient causes. The effect of the causes is Z(t), or a change in the set of configurational variables making up the state vector Z. Rosen then defines what we shall here call "dynamical information" by the following partials:

$$\frac{\partial}{\partial(\text{cause})} \left(\frac{d}{dt} (\text{effect}) \right) \tag{16}$$

For each cause there is a connection to effect according to the terms in Equation 16. Thus there are three different kinds of dynamical information, one obtained when the cause is formal, one when it is material, and one when it is efficient. For convenience, Rosen refers to these three kinds of information as "genetic", "somatic", and "external" or "environmental", respectively. He emphasizes that these three different kinds of information have the following important features: (1) they are dynamical in that they are parts of an equation of motion; and (2) they are distinctly different from each other. They are not complementary to dynamics, but are aspects of the dynamics. This is the view that we believe should be further explored (in contrast to earlier agreement[7,8] with Pattee's view that information and dynamics were complementary). As we invoke Rosen's work, we imagine that endocrine information is usually the somatic kind, although it is sometimes the external kind (with respect to a subsystem, such as the liver for example). But then we have a problem: endocrine messages often cause structural changes (such as smooth-rough transitions in endoplasmic reticulum). These structures, according to Pattee's work, are information converted to or manifested as nonholonomic constraints on dynamics, and they might affect Rosen's genetic information by changing the function ϕ_g. Thus a description of endocrine information seems to need the ideas of both Rosen and Pattee. Is there a synthesis or another approach? We shall suggest a partial answer; it requires consideration of semiotics.

C. Implications of Endosemiotics for Research and Therapy

It is the province of semiotics to deal with messages — any messages whatsoever. As Sebeok[24] has remarked: "Since every message is composed of signs according to some ordered selection, semiotics has been variously identified as the doctrine ... or science, or the theory... of signs. Correspondingly, the study designated semiotics comprises the set of general principles that underlie the structure of all signs, constituting a code, which was defined by Cherry[4]... as an agreed transformation, or set of unambiguous rules, whereby messages are converted from one representation to another ... Semiotics is concerned, successively, with the generation and encoding of messages, their propogation in any ... appropriate form of physical energy, their decoding and interpretation." We agree with Sebeok and urge the consideration of pharmacosemiotics (Yates previously referred to this inexactly as "pharmacolinguistics")[25] or, better, endosemiotics, as the approach to the design of therapeutic systems to command changes in or repair of human physiological dynamic contingencies by means of administering endocrine agents.

Before proceeding further, we must clarify that communication, which is under discussion here, differs from "language", which in turn differs from "speech". There is a regrettable tendency to confound these terms. Endosemiotics, as we employ it, refers to chemical communications within living systems. ("Language" and "speech" are reserved for the anthroposemiotic aspects of zoosemiotics, which is the general study of signaling behavior among and across animal species. We are not here interested in language or speech.)

We turn now to the matter of Cherry's "agreed transformations" or "unambiguous rules". We have noted that a physical event is not a sign event except in the "context" of the rules of transmission of a sender or the rules of detection and interpretation of a receiver. A sender may generate a message for which there is no effective receiver, or a receiver may be ready to detect a message that is never sent. Either way, there is no communication. But these two extreme cases cannot apply to endocrine signaling, because metabolic, reproductive, and other biological systems have evolved with senders and receivers matched to each other. The agreement about transformations and the unambiguous rules is the residue of evolutionary selective processes and must be accounted for by an evolutionary theory. With respect to the design of therapeutic systems, we can assume that such transformations and rules exist. The job then is to work with those rules in order to command physiological state changes in a patient.

Messages require rules at both the transmission end (in this case, in the therapeutic system) and at the receiving end, and the rules must be matched appropriately for communication or command to occur. Rules are commonly syntactical and are not physical laws, as we have previously noted. The "meaning of a message" does not reside in the transmitted signal, which is a purely physical manifestation without semantic content. Meaning is found in the receipt of a message in the context of the receiver. The context of the receiver is established both by the states of its memory and the current dynamical state of the system, as well as by its recent past dynamical states as they influence the current dynamical state. Thus the arrival of a message can *provoke* responses or *evoke* responses (if memory is triggered); or it can merely change the probabilities — the dynamic contingencies — instead of the ongoing processes. Thus, we can never be certain that a cell did *not* receive a meaningful message just because we failed to see it do anything different after the message was transmitted. Unless we know the cellular "context," we cannot be sure about "interpretations" of endocrine messages. Because of this limitation (as Yates has written elsewhere):[7]

It is likely that we shall discover only the obvious messages, those that cause an immediate change in observable behavior. But we must never forget that *meaningful messages change contingencies as well as processes*, and the former, though perhaps unobservable, may be more important in the life of a cell ...To get at meanings, we shall have to decide how many different modes of behavior and how many internal states a receiving cell can have. My guess is that the number in each case will be relatively small (< 10), but different for different specialized cells ... We may find in endocrine signals ... the use of very *functional commands* ... patterns of concentrations in plasma may ultimately be interpreted as a broad command for a cell to divide. Or the message may be : 'Grow!' or 'Secrete!'. We need to find out what aspect of concentration level was the essential part of the functional command. What we learn from such studies, if they are undertaken systematically, would have a potentially profound effect on the design of pharmacist's dosage forms and delivery systems.

D. Endosemiotics and Physics

The broad scope of semiotics needs some physical specification or restricting if it is to sharpen our images of communications by means of chemically conveyed messages in plants and animals. One of our colleagues, A. Iberall, has been attempting a physical account of what he calls "languages". (We would rather use the term "communications" or "messages" — only some which are properly linguistic.) Messages, in this generalized notion, arise in complex systems (those with a large number of internal degrees of freedom and delays in energy equipartitioning) as a means to switch behavior from one (nonlinear) action mode to another. Messages are catalytic in the sense of being of low energy or low amplitude (or mass) compared to the processes they influence. Nonlinear couplings and dissipations assure that messages are received, swept into the ongoing dynamics or memories of the complex system, and are effectively matched to those processes so that they change dynamic contingencies.

Out of the endosemiotics of chemical messages come dynamic cooperatives such as "families", "neighborhoods" and "cultures" — in a technical, physical sense. These physical ideas and metaphors differ from those of Pattee and Rosen, but do not, we think, conflict with them. Neither, unfortunately, do they synthesize them. All notions of endosemiotics and the modulations of biological dynamics seem merely partial glimpses of a better, larger theory, not yet invented. Meanwhile, Yates has tried to apply Iberall's view to the problems of metabolic regulations[8] and biological adaptations.[27]

VI. SUMMARY

We suggest the following approach to the design of research models of therapeutic systems for rate-controlled delivery of endocrine agents. First, the therapeutic systems (which for the foreseeable future will operate open-loop because we do not yet have adequate chemical or physical sensors to support closed-loop designs) should be switchable by action of the patient. Second, the switching should occur at onset of each of four physiological states: (1) sleep, (2) wakefulness, (3) exercise, and (4) meal eating and digestion (allowing 2 to 3 hr to complete the postabsorptive state). Other states, such as sexual activity, would not be addressed until the next round of designs. Third, the therapeutic system should deliver fixed amplitude pulses of the endocrine agent. Whatever the power supply that delivers the pulses (osmotic, electrical, mechanical), the programming of the pulses will have to be electronic and will require participation of the patient. Because the phase of physiological systems and their internal clockworks may differ substantially from external clock time and even drift (as in jet lag), it would not be effective, in general, to schedule the pulses by use of an external clock in the therapeutic system. Through electronic programming, however, the *scheduling* of the pulses could be arranged so that the pulse train could be variable — pulses close together, or widely spaced, or with adjustable spacing. The low-pass filtering characteristics of all pharmacokinetic systems would allow the pulse trains to be smoothed and shaped into time-varying waveforms that might be near-periodic (e.g., a circadian rhythm) or fluctuating. The pulse trains could be arranged to approximate ramps, sinusoids, steps, exponentials, or other deterministic waveforms in plasma. Pseudorandom binary signals could also be imitated. In this way, the pharmacodynamic aspects of the system could be probed to determine what pattern of signaling would be most effective for a desired result.

In many cases, it may be optimal simply to imitate the waveforms observed in the plasma of normal subjects in the four physiological states mentioned above. That is exactly what is being attempted with insulin pumps. But because this approach involves clamping, with imitation of values but not of responsiveness, it could in some cases be destabilizing, as we have shown here. In the absence of a technology for reproducing responsiveness, only experiments can determine what is a safe waveform. Constancy will sometimes be a safe waveform in cases in which using the original fluctuating waveform as the clamping pattern would destabilize the system. There are strange dynamical paradoxes encountered when one tries to control inputs of endogenous agents.

Endocrinology must be viewed ultimately as a science of communication, dynamic regulation, and control. It is only incidentally the science of morphology, biochemistry, molecular biology, cell biology and physiology. Each of these specialties has much to offer endocrinology, but it seems to us that only by considering the communicational and dynamical issues raised here can we ultimately rationalize the design of rate-controlled delivery systems for endocrine agents.

ACKNOWLEDGMENTS

This work was supported by USPHS Grant GM 23732, and by the Crump Institute for Medical Engineering, UCLA.

We thank Laurel Benton for her criticism of and help with this manuscript.

REFERENCES

1. Dennett, D. C., *Brainstorms: Philosophical Essays on Mind and Psychology,* Bradford Books, Montgomery, Vt., 1978, 12.
2. Sebeok, T. A., *Current Trends in Linguistics,* Vol. 12, Sebeok, T. A., Ed., Mouton, The Hague, 1974, 213.
3. Sebeok, T. A., *Contributions to the Doctrine of Signs,* Research Center for Language and Semiotics Studies, Bloomington, 1976, 3.
4. Cherry, C., *On Human Communication,* 3rd ed., MIT Press, Cambridge, Mass., 1978.
5. Pierce, J. R., *Symbols, Signals and Noise. The Nature and Process of Communication,* Harper Torch, New York, 1965.
6. Shannon, C. E. and Weaver, W., *The Mathematical Theory of Communication,* University of Illinois Press, Urbana, 1964.
7. Yates, F. E., Analysis of endocrine signals: the engineering and physics of biochemical communication systems, *Biol. Reproduct.,* 24, 73, 1981.
8. Yates, F. E., Systems analysis of hormone action: principles and strategies, in *Biological Regulation and Development,* Vol. IIIA, Goldberger, R. F. and Yamamoto, K., Eds., Plenum, New York, 1982, chap. 2.
9. Knobil, E., The neuroendocrine control of the menstrual cycle, *Recent Prog. Horm. Res.,* 36, 55, 1980.
10. Halberg, F., Hans, E., Cardoso, S. S., Scheving, L. E., Kühl, J. F. W., Shiotsuka, R., Rosene, G., Pauly, J. E., Runge, W., Spalding, J. F., Lee, J. K., and Good, R. A., Toward a chronotherapy of neoplasia: tolerance of treatment depends upon host rhythms, *Experientia,* 29, 909, 1973.
11. Dallman, M. F. and Yates, F. E., Dynamic asymmetries in the corticosteroid negative feedback paths and distribution-binding-metabolism elements of the adrenocortical system, *Ann. N. Y. Acad. Sci.,* 156, 696, 1969.
12. Yates, F. E. and Urquhart, J., Control of the plasma concentrations of adrenal cortical hormones, *Physiol. Rev.,* 42, 359, 1962.
13. Keller, N., Sendelbeck, L. R., Richardson, U. I., Moore, C., and Yates, F. E., Protein-binding of corticosteroids in undiluted rat plasma, *Endocrinology,* 79, 884, 1966.
14. Brown-Grant, K., Brennan, R. D., and Yates, F. E., Simulation of the thyroid hormone-binding protein interactions in human plasma, *J. Clin. Endocrinol. Metab.,* 30, 281, 1970.
15. Yates, F. E., Outline of a physical theory of physiological systems, *Can. J. Physiol. Pharm.,* 60, 217, 1982.
16. Yates, F. E., Benson, H., Buckles, R., Urquhart, J., and Zaffaroni, A., Engineering designs for improved therapy through controlled delivery of drugs, *Adv. Biomed. Eng.,* 5, 1, 1975.
17. Heilmann, K., *Therapeutic Systems: Pattern-Specific Drug Delivery — Concept and Development,* G. Thieme, Stuttgart, 1978.
18. Urquhart, J., *Controlled-Release Pharmaceuticals,* Urquhart, J., Ed., Academy of Pharmaceutical Sciences, Washington, D.C., 1981.
19. Urquhart, J., Fara, J. W., and Willis, K. L., Rate-controlled delivery systems in drug and hormone research, *Annu. Rev. Pharmacol. Toxicol.,* 24, 199, 1984.
20. Lynch, H. J., Rivest, R. W., and Wortman, R. J., Artificial induction of melatonin rhythms by programmed microinfusion, *Neuroendocrinology,* 31, 106, 1980.
21. Yates, F. E., Maran, J. W., and Marsh, D., The adrenal cortex, in *Medical Physiology,* 14th ed., Mountcastle, V. B., Ed., C. V. Mosby, St. Louis, 1980, 1577.
22. Pattee, H. H., Dynamic and linguistic modes of complex systems, *Int. J. Gen. Syst.,* 3, 259, 1977.
23. Rosen, R., Information and cause, in *Proc. Orbis. Scient.,* Dirac 80th Festschrift, Coral Gables, Fla., 1983.
24. Sebeok, T. A., Zoosemiotic components of human communication, in *How Animals Communicate,* Sebeok, T. A., Ed., Indiana University Press, Bloomington, 1977, chap. 38.
25. Yates, F. E., Integrative pharmacology — beyond structure-activity relationships into pharmacolinguistics, *Am. J. Physiol./Reg., Integ. Comp. Physiol.,* 6, R251, 1979.
26. Iberall, A. S., What is "language" that can facilitate the flow of information? A contribution to a fundamental theory of language and communication, *J. Theor. Biol.,* 102, 347, 1983.
27. Yates, F. E., The dynamics of adaptation in living systems, in *Adaptive Control of Ill-Defined Systems,* Selfridge, O. G., Rissland, E. L., and Arbib, M. A., Eds., Plenum, New York, 1984, 89.

INDEX

A

H

I

saturation, 88, 91
Klebsiella pneumoniae, 235

L

β-Lactam antibiotics, 235, 238
β-Lactamase-producing strain of *Hemophilus influenzae*, 234
Lactic acid, 25
Laplace s-domain, 55
Laplace transforms, 56
Large single dose of antibiotics, 230
Leishmaniasis, 27, 240
Leprosy, 37, 39, 40, 240
Leucine, 25
Leukemia, 207—211, 214
Levels
   nonlinearity of, 110
   rate-of-change of, 255
   steady-state, 4
LH, see Luteinizing hormone
Lidocaine, 19, 36, 193, 194
Limitations of controlled drug delivery, 43—44
Linearity, in phamacokinetics, 88, 90
Linguistic modes of complex systems, 268—269
Lipid exchange, 27
Liposomes, 27, 163, 238—240
   insulin in, 163
Listeria, 240
Lithium, 19
Lithium sulfate, 18
Local delivery, 84
   systemic delivery vs., 85—95
Long-lasting insulin, 146
Long-term vascular control, 177
Lormetazepan, 72
Low doses
   of antibiotics, 230
   of insulin, 154
   of prodrugs, 102—103
Lung cancer, 213, 214
Luteinizing hormone (LH), 119, 127, 255, 256
Luteinizing hormone releasing factor (LHRH), 119
Lymphomas, 209, 211, 213
Lysine, 148

M

Macromolecules, 24
MADDS, see Monoacetyl-metabolite
Magnetic controlled release, 28
Magnetic particles within matrix, 27—28
Magnetic systems, 27—28
Malaria, 26, 240
Mass balance, 85, 88, 92, 97
MAT, see Mean absorption time
Maternal-fetal relationships, 122
Matrix, 4, 23—27

acrylate polymeric, 26
bioerodible, 25
hemispheric, 24
magnetic particles within, 27—28
polymeric, 24
porous, 24
state transition, 52
MBC, 235
MDD, see Microsealed drug delivery
Mean absorption time (MAT), 73
Mean residence time, 70
Mean retention time (MRT), 70—72
Mean times, 56, 70—72
Mean transit time (MTT), 52, 55, 59, 72, 73
Mechanical pumps, see also specific types, 44
   for insulin delivery, 147—153
Median transit time, 52, 55
Medical devices, see also specific types, 2, 116
Medroxyprogesterone acetate (MPA), 35, 37
α-Melanin stimulating hormone (MSH), 119
Melatonin, 134
Membranes
   biophysics of, 11
   hydrogel, 24, 26
   polymer, 24
Meningitis, 227, 234
Meperidine, 72
Metabolic control, 160—161
Metabolic input functions, 77—78
Metabolic profiles in insulin-infused diabetic animals, 158—161
Metabolites
   concentration profile of, 78
   intermediary, 148, 151, 154
   osmotic pump delivery of, 119
Metals, see also specific metals; specific types, 119
Methadone, 72
Methenamine, 95
Methoxyesterone, 119
Methoxyflurane, 20
Mexiletine, 193
MIC, see Minimum inhibitory concentration
Michaelis-Menten equations, 97
Microalbuminuria, 151
Microcapsules, 37
Microorganisms, see also Bacteria, 230
Microperfusion, 123
Microsealed drug delivery system (MDD), 4, 43
Microspheres, 37, 40
Minerals, see also specific minerals, 119
Miniaturization of pumps, 7, 9
Minimization of stress, 117—121
Minimum inhibitory concentration (MIC), 222, 235
   of antibiotics, 230, 234, 235
Minocycline, 20
Mitomycin-C, 211
Modal transit time, 52, 55
Models, see also specific types
   animal, see Animal studies